Haematology and Immunology

For the MLA and Medical Exams

First edition author

Saimah Arif

Arjmand Mufti

Second edition author

James Griffin

Third edition authors

Gareth Kitchen

Fourth edition authors

Yousef Gargani

Fifth edition authors

Gus Redhouse White

Olivia Vanbergen

6th Edition
CRASH COURSE

SERIES EDITOR
Philip Xiu
MA (Cantab), MB BChir, MRCP, MRCGP, MScClinEd, FHEA, MAcadMEd, RCPathME
Honorary Senior Lecturer
Leeds University School of Medicine
PCN Educational Lead
Medical Examiner
Leeds Teaching Hospital Trust
Leeds, UK

FACULTY ADVISOR
Varun Mehra
MBBS, MRCP (UK), FRCPath (Haematology)
Consultant Haematologist in Stem Cell Transplantation and Cellular therapies
King's College Hospital
London, UK

Haematology and Immunology
For the MLA and Medical Exams

Priya Sriskandarajah
MBBS, BSc, MRCP, PhD, FRCPath
Consultant Haematologist
Guy's Hospital
London, UK

Maheen Ahsan
MBBS, BSc, MRCP
Internal Medicine Trainee
King's College Hospital
London, UK

Ioanna Lazana
MD, PhD, MRCP, FRCPath
Consultant Haematologist
King's College Hospital
London, UK

Michael Lim
MBBS, MRCP, PhD
Haematology Registrar
Guy's Hospital
London, UK

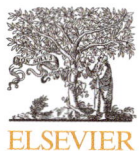

ELSEVIER

First edition 1998

Second edition 2003

Third edition 2007

Reprinted, 2008, 2010 (twice)

Fourth edition 2012

Updated Fourth edition 2015

Fifth edition 2019

Sixth edition 2025

ISBN: 978-0-4432-4996-9

Content Strategist: Trinity Hutton; Jennifer Dooley

Content Project Manager: Ayan Dhar

Design: Miles Hitchen

Marketing Manager: Deborah Watkins

Printed in India

Last digit is the print number: 9 8 7 6 5 4 3 2 1

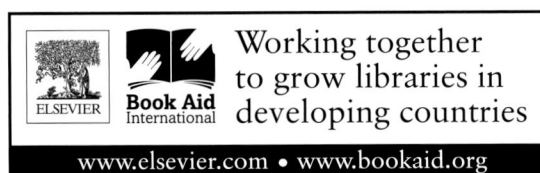

Working together to grow libraries in developing countries

www.elsevier.com • www.bookaid.org

Series editor's foreword

With great honour and pride, we present the latest edition of the *Crash Course* series. This series has traversed a journey of nearly a quarter-century, stemming from the vision of Dr. Dan Horton-Szar, and his legacy continues to walk with us on this pathway of knowledge.

The series has been popular with students worldwide, selling over **1 million copies** and being translated into more than **8 languages**, reinforcing our commitment to global learning.

We remain extremely grateful for your unwavering trust. The series has once again been refreshed and fully upgraded in accordance with the rapidly changing medical guidelines, ensuring the content is comprehensive, accurate and fully up-to-date.

This latest series continues our tradition of integrating clinical practice with basic medical sciences, tailored meticulously for today's medical undergraduate curriculum. A central highlight of this instalment is our emphasis on high-yield exam content designed specifically for the MLA curriculum.

The addition of the **Rapid MLA Index** at the beginning of the book enhances this offering, serving as a valuable aid to students to track their exam preparation efficiently. We have also revised all self-assessment questions to align with the single best answer format in line with the latest MLA examination style. We have also added ***High-Yield Association Tables***. These are essential tools designed to aid students in recognizing clinical patterns and acing vignette-style exam questions. By condensing complex medical scenarios into digestible, manageable insights, these tables ensure efficient learning. They connect symptoms, diagnosis and treatment, bolstering understanding and confidence in tackling the rigorous MLA exams. This comprehensive approach makes these tables an indispensable asset in your exam preparations.

Utilizing student feedback, we have strived to maintain the core principles of this series: delivering precise and readable text that brings together depth and clarity. The authors are experienced junior doctors who successfully navigated these exams recently, ensuring practical and tested guidance. A team of expert faculty advisors from across the United Kingdom ensures the content's accuracy, making it resilient and reliable.

As we turn a new chapter with the latest edition, we honour the past, cherish the present and embrace the promise of the future. We wish you every success in your journey of learning and growth and hope that this series adds value to your life, both as students and as future medical professionals.

Philip Xiu

Preface

Authors

Being able to work in a field such as haematology and immunology allows us to combine laboratory diagnostics with the clinical picture. In everyday medicine, we encounter patients impacted by conditions within these disease areas almost on a daily basis. Regretfully, in medical schools, limited time is spent in either of these specialties, and speaking from experience, it can be daunting managing a patient with a newly diagnosed haematological cancer.

What we hope to achieve with this volume of *Crash Course: Haematology and Immunology* is to relieve some of these fears and present common haematological and immunological conditions in a systematic manner. As with any specialty within pathology, we integrate the pathophysiology of the condition with the key laboratory findings and clinical management. Importantly, we highlight common clinical emergencies in order to support the transition from student to doctor, including a quick reference guide relevant to key clinical signs and symptoms.

In keeping with the latest MLA examination style, we have removed the extended matching questions and expanded the single best answer question bank, as well as included clinical scenarios with blood film interpretation.

We hope this volume will be a valuable resource and potentially support others hoping to pursue a career in either haematology or immunology.

Priya Sriskandarajah, Maheen Ahsan, Ioanna Lazana and Michael Lim

Faculty advisor

Haematology is at the forefront of some very exciting developments and changing the understanding of how we can utilise the best of immunology and cancer therapeutics in improving our patient outcomes for both non-malignant and malignant disorders. These are helping drive wider research in non-haematological conditions including autoimmune diseases, using re-engineered immune therapies. The 6th Crash Course series in Haematology and Immunology provides important updates in the basics of these specialist disease areas, while keeping the core strength of self-learning through concise text, comprehension check boxes and hints and tips boxes. The key salient points are presented in a user-friendly and easy-to-read manner that enables the rapid assimilation of core knowledge and provides an invaluable foundation for application to clinical practice.

I would like to thank our series editor Dr Xiu and our Authors, colleagues and friends, Dr Sriskandarajah, Dr Ahsan, Dr Lazana and Dr Lim, who worked very hard to help revise this edition and produce a fantastic overview of common haematological and immunological conditions and help enhance subject understanding. My hope is that this will be a 'must have' valuable resource for current and prospective medical professionals like you and help in your careers and most importantly improving care for our patients.

Varun Mehra

Acknowledgements

I would like to thank my sister Ramya Sriskandarajah, who, as a medical student, was an invaluable resource in the development of this latest edition. I am grateful for your feedback and for being a sounding board for the questions! In addition, I would like to thank my husband Loke as well as my children Sathya and Shivani for their love and support. Finally I want to extend a massive thank you to Phil Xiu for taking a chance on me and for providing this great opportunity.

Priya Sriskandarajah

I would like to thank Dr Mehra for giving me the opportunity to be part of this new edition. It has been an incredible experience as a junior doctor. Massive thanks and congratulations to my fellow authors, Priya, Ioanna and Michael, for their hard work! Phil Xiu and the *Crash Course* team have also been such an invaluable support. My contributions are dedicated to my parents Ahsan and Hina, and my brother Daniyal.

Maheen Ahsan

I would like to thank Priya, Varun, Phil Xiu and the *Crash Course* team for the opportunity to contribute to this new edition and for their support throughout this process.

Michael Lim

I would like to thank Phil Xiu and the *Crash Course* team for their great support and professionalism throughout this process. Special thanks to Dr Varun Mehra, who has given me the opportunity to contribute to this new edition. I have really enjoyed the whole journey and I am grateful to my fellow authors Priya, Maheen and Michael for the collaboration and support and their hard work. My contribution is dedicated to my husband Constantinos and my son Stavros.

Ioanna Lazana

Series editor's acknowledgement

We would like to express our sincere gratitude to those who have provided their support and expertise in preparing this sixth edition of the *Crash Course* series. Our junior doctor contributors' participation in crafting the manuscript has been indispensable. Their first-hand experience and current medical knowledge have infused realism and practicality into our content.

Our faculty editors deserve a special note of thanks. They have extensively validated the correctness of the information, ensuring that the content is not just accurate but also contemporaneous, credible and aligns with the latest medical standards.

We extend our heartfelt thanks to our publisher, Elsevier. Their staff have demonstrated an unwavering commitment to quality, maintaining the high standards set since the first edition. Their insights have routinely enriched the content and process alike.

Our Commissioning Editor, Jeremy Bowes, deserves a special mention for his consistent support and guiding hand throughout the development process. His directions and advice have bettered this edition and spurred us on our quest for excellence.

We are greatly indebted to Alex Mortimer for her wisdom, practical insights and valuable guidance. A big thank you to our Content Strategists, Trinity Hutton and Cloe Holland-Borosh, who need special acknowledgement for meticulously outlining the direction and scope of the content. They've managed to mix details with a strategic plan, keeping our readers in mind.

Lastly, much gratitude is owed to our Content Product Managers, Taranpreet Kaur, Ayan Dhar, Shivani Pal and Tapajyoti Chaudhuri, who have juggled the numerous day-to-day tasks with utmost dedication and perseverance. Despite the ever-approaching deadlines, they have shown remarkable patience and steadfast determination, ensuring that each step of the book's development was accomplished seamlessly.

In conclusion, we sincerely thank each of these wonderful people for their outstanding contributions and support, without which this work wouldn't have been achieved. Their passion, commitment and collaborative effort have helped us bring this edition together.

Philip Xiu

Rapid MLA Index

The MLA Curriculum Conditions Priority levels have been based on the below:

Level 1: Conditions that a newly qualified doctor should have a good knowledge of and be able to recognise and manage.
Level 2: Conditions requiring knowledge for recognising and confirming diagnosis and planning first–line management in straightforward cases.
Level 3: Conditions where recognition of clinical presentation and describing principles of management are important.

Table 1 MLA Conditions and Where to Find Them

Priority	MLA Conditions	Chapter	Page
2	Adverse drug effects	Chapter 1: Principles of haematology Chapter 3: Red blood cell disorders Chapter 6: Haemostasis	10 , 35, 43, 78, 79
1	Allergic disorder	Chapter 12: Immune dysfunction	156
1	Anaemia	Chapter 3: Red blood cell disorders	25
1	Anaphylaxis	Chapter 12: Immune dysfunction	105-106, 158
1	Arterial thrombosis	Chapter 5: Haematological malignancies Chapter 6: Haemostasis	55, 89
3	Contact dermatitis	Chapter 12: Immune dysfunction	163
1	Deep vein thrombosis	Chapter 6: Haemostasis	91
3	Disseminated intravascular coagulation	Chapter 6: Haemostasis	80, 86
1	Epistaxis	Chapter 6: Haemostasis	87
3	Haemochromatosis	Chapter 2: Red blood cells and haemoglobin	17
2	Haemoglobinopathies	Chapter 3: Red blood cell disorders	38
2	Haemophilia	Chapter 6: Haemostasis	87
1	Human immunodeficiency virus	Chapter 12: Immune dysfunction	171
1	Hypercalcaemia of malignancy	Chapter 5: Haematological malignancies	67
3	Hyposplenism/splenectomy	Chapter 1: Principles of haematology	8
2	Leukaemia	Chapter 5: Haematological malignancies	59, 61
1	Lymphoma	Chapter 5: Haematological malignancies	64
3	Malaria	Chapter 3: Red blood cell disorders Chapter 11: The functioning immune system	38, 153
1	Malnutrition	Chapter 3: Red blood cell disorders	170
1	Multiple myeloma	Chapter 5: Haematological malignancies	67
3	Myeloproliferative disorders	Chapter 5: Haematological malignancies	55
2	Pancytopenia	Chapter 3: Red blood cell disorders Chapter 4: White blood cells Chapter 5: Haematological malignancies Chapter 6: Haemostasis	36, 43, 53, 179
1	Pathological fracture	Chapter 5: Haematological malignancies	67

continued

Table 1 MLA Conditions and Where to Find Them—cont'd

Priority	MLA Conditions	Chapter	Page
3	Patient on anti-coagulant therapy	Chapter 6: Haemostasis	84, 89, 91, 92
3	Patient on anti-platelet therapy	Chapter 6: Haemostasis	35, 77
3	Polycythaemia	Chapter 3: Red blood cell disorders	22, 44
3	Postpartum haemorrhage	Chapter 7: Blood transfusion	98
1	Pulmonary embolism	Chapter 6: Haemostasis	39, 56, 91
1	Sepsis	Chapter 4: White blood cells Chapter 9: The innate immune system	31, 59, 104, 116, 123
2	Sickle cell disease	Chapter 3: Red blood cell disorders	8, 38
1	Spinal cord compression	Chapter 5: Haematological malignancies	65, 68
3	Spinal fracture	Chapter 5: Haematological malignancies	68
3	Toxic shock syndrome	Chapter 10: The adaptive immune system	143
1	Transfusion reactions	Chapter 7: Blood transfusion	100, 105-106
1	Tuberculosis	Chapter 11: The functioning immune system	147, 152
3	Urticaria	Chapter 12: Immune dysfunction	15,51,56,158
3	Vitamin B12 and/or folate deficiency	Chapter 3: Red blood cell disorders	27-29, 147
3	VTE in pregnancy and puerperium	Chapter 6: Haemostasis	90

Table 2 MLA Presentations and Where to Find Them

MLA Presentations	Chapter	Page
Allergies	Chapter 12: Immune dysfunction	155
Anaphylaxis	Chapter 12: Immune dysfunction	105-106,158
Bleeding antepartum	Chapter 6: Haemostasis Chapter 7: Blood transfusion	101, 107
Bleeding from lower GI tract	Chapter 6: Haemostasis Chapter 7: Blood transfusion	89, 92, 94, 108
Bleeding from upper GI tract	Chapter 6: Haemostasis Chapter 7: Blood transfusion	89, 92, 94, 108
Bleeding postpartum	Chapter 6: Haemostasis Chapter 7: Blood transfusion	98, 101, 107
Bone pain	Chapter 5: Haematological malignancies	67
Bruising	Chapter 6: Haemostasis	78-79, 87, 180
Fatigue	Chapter 3: Red blood cell disorders Chapter 5: Haematological malignancies	25, 57, 59, 120
Fever	Chapter 4: White blood cells Chapter 5: Haematological malignancies	36, 55, 120, 143
Haemoptysis	Chapter 6: Haemostasis	91
Jaundice	Chapter 3: Red blood cell disorders	17, 30, 33, 35, 100, 106
Limb weakness	Chapter 5: Haematological malignancies	68, 166
Lump in groin	Chapter 5: Haematological malignancies	8-10, 63
Lymphadenopathy	Chapter 5: Haematological malignancies	8-10, 63
Massive haemorrhage	Chapter 7: Blood transfusion	108

Table 2 MLA Presentations and Where to Find Them—cont'd

MLA Presentations	Chapter	Page
Neck lump	Chapter 5: Haematological malignancies	8-10, 63
Night sweats	Chapter 5: Haematological malignancies Chapter 11: The functioning immune system	1,48,153
Organomegaly	Chapter 1: Principles of haematology Chapter 5: Haematological malignancies	8-10, 63
Painful swollen leg	Chapter 6: Haemostasis	89
Pallor	Chapter 3: Red blood cell disorders	59, 106
Petechial rash	Chapter 5: Haematological malignancies Chapter 6: Haemostasis	78, 79
Postpartum haemorrhage	Chapter 7: Blood transfusion	98
Purpura	Chapter 6: Haemostasis	78, 80, 108
Stridor	Chapter 5: Haematological malignancies	65, 106, 158
Vaccination	Chapter 13: Medical intervention	129, 175
Weight loss	Chapter 5: Haematological malignancies	26, 55, 64
Wheeze	Chapter 12: Immune dysfunction	1,55,157

Contents

Principles of haematology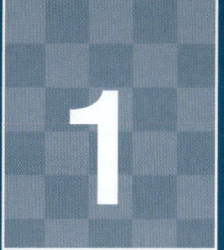

1

PRINCIPLES

Haematology is the medical specialty concerned with the study, diagnosis, treatment and prevention of diseases related to blood and is the subject of the first part of this book. This chapter discusses blood cells, their production (haematopoiesis), bone marrow and the spleen.

BLOOD

Blood is the fluid contained within the heart, arteries, veins and capillaries of the circulatory system. It delivers oxygen and nutrients to organs and tissues and carries carbon dioxide and metabolic 'waste' products to excretory organs such as the kidneys, liver and lungs.

Blood consists of several components:

- Plasma
- Cells (red cells, white cells, platelets)
- Electrolytes (e.g., Na^+, K^+, Ca^{2+})
- Proteins (including enzymes, hormones and immunoglobulins)
- Lipids
- Glucose

The cellular components of blood are synthesized in the bone marrow in a process called 'haematopoiesis'.

BLOOD CELLS

This section discusses mature blood cells found in the bloodstream.

Red blood cells

Red blood cells ('erythrocytes') are derived from the erythroid burst-forming unit (BFU-E) progenitor cell. Red cells lack a nucleus and have a biconcave discoid shape.

Their primary role is the transportation of oxygen (from lung to tissue) and carbon dioxide (from tissue to lung). They contain haemoglobin, a specialized molecule that avidly binds these gases under conditions of high partial pressure and releases them under conditions of low partial pressure, thus allowing bulk transport of oxygen and carbon dioxide to proceed in the appropriate direction. Red blood cells are discussed in further detail in Chapter 2.

Platelets

Like red cells, platelets lack nuclei. Platelets (thrombocytes) are derived from megakaryocytes, which derive from the colony-forming unit megakaryocyte (CFU-Meg) progenitor cell. They play a pivotal role in haemostasis (Chapter 6).

White blood cells

White blood cells (leucocytes) are large unpigmented cells with primarily immune roles. They are also found in the bloodstream, along with red blood cells and platelets. Leucocytes are further classified into granulocytes, monocytes/macrophages and lymphocytes. Each group fulfils different immunological roles, participating in immune defences against infection.

Granulocytes

'Granulocytes' is the collective term for white blood cells with granules in their cytoplasm. The term encompasses neutrophils, eosinophils and basophils. The specific chemical content of the granules (and thus the cell's function role) varies according to subtype. Note that some clinicians misleadingly use the term 'granulocytes' for neutrophils, which can cause confusion.

Neutrophils

Neutrophils (aka 'polymorphs') have multilobed nuclei. Neutrophils (diameter 12–14 μm) comprise ~60% of the bloodstream white cell population. They leave the bone marrow, where they are synthesized, and circulate in the bloodstream for ≤10 hours before entering tissues.

Neutrophils are an essential component of the innate immune system, due to their ability to phagocytose (engulf) microorganisms and kill them by releasing cytotoxic molecules from their granules. Once they arrive at the site of an infection or inflammation, they also recruit further immune cells with chemotactic mediators (see Chapter 9: Neutrophils). Neutrophils therefore represent a key component of the first-line defence against bacterial infections.

Eosinophils

Eosinophils (diameter 12–17 μm) have bilobed nuclei. They stain strongly with acidic dyes (pink appearing cytoplasm) and comprise ~1% to 6% of the bloodstream white cell population. Like other granulocytes, eosinophils release specific cytotoxic and messenger molecules. These are released directly into the extracellular space by degranulation. Note how eosinophils differ in this respect from neutrophils, which phagocytose pathogens *before* releasing cytotoxic molecules. Eosinophils migrate into areas of inflammation or infection, particularly infection with multicellular parasites, e.g., helminths (worms). They are also important in both innate (see Chapter 9: Eosinophils) and adaptive immunity and allergic responses.

Basophils

Basophils (diameter 14–16 μm) have bilobed nuclei and granular cytoplasm, like eosinophils, but stain strongly with basic dyes (blue-appearing cytoplasm). Basophils represent ≤1% of the bloodstream's white cell population. In concert with eosinophils and mast cells, they contribute strongly to innate and adaptive immunity. Physiological histamine is derived in part from basophilic granules.

Monocytes/macrophages

Monocytes and macrophages are larger than granulocytes (diameter ≤25 μm). They have a large eccentrically placed reniform (kidney-shaped) nucleus. In the bloodstream, they are called monocytes and account for ~2% to 10% of the white cell population. They circulate for 1 to 3 days, then leave the circulation and enter the tissues, where they differentiate further, developing into macrophages.

Macrophages comprise the reticuloendothelial system and are found in tissues throughout the body. They phagocytose cellular debris and pathogens and produce various cytokines. They also process and present antigens to lymphocytes as part of the adaptive immune response (see Chapter 10: MHC processing).

Lymphocytes

These white blood cells are small and have a relatively large, round nucleus relative to their nongranular, basophilic cytoplasm volume. They all originate from the lymphoid lineage.

B lymphocytes

These small lymphocytes (diameter 6–9 μm) express the B-cell receptor. They secrete immunoglobulins (antibodies). A large proportion of B lymphocytes reside in lymph node germinal centres, where they are known as memory B cells. Some B lymphocytes also mature further into plasma cells.

Plasma cells are larger than B lymphocytes and have a strongly basophilic cytoplasm and an eccentric round nucleus. They are mainly seen in the bone marrow, but a few may be seen circulating in the peripheral blood.

T lymphocytes

These small lymphocytes (diameter 6–9 μm) express the T-cell receptor. T cells are subclassified by type of surface glycoproteins they express, indicated by the CD prefix. Cytotoxic T cells (CD8 + ve) mediate destruction of cells infected by intracellular organisms, while T-helper cells (CD4 + ve) release cytokines to regulate and assist in the adaptive immune response (Chapter 10).

Natural killer cells

These large granular lymphocytes are also cytotoxic lymphocytes, like T cells, but natural killer (NK) cells are larger. Their behaviour differs from that of T cells in that they do not require major histocompatibility complex (MHC) or antibody-bound antigen complexes to recognize and destroy foreign or infected cells. They are thus prominent in the innate immune response (Chapter 9).

HAEMATOPOIESIS

Haematopoiesis is the formation and development of blood cells. The haematopoietic system is composed of the bone marrow, spleen, liver, lymph nodes and thymus.

Pluripotent haemopoietic stem cells

All blood cells originally derive from a population of pluripotent, CD34 + ve haemopoietic stem cells, residing in haematopoietic tissues. These stem cells may either:

- Remain as pluripotent stem cells, dividing to form identical daughter cells, maintaining the haemopoietic population
- Differentiate into specific progenitor cells, which ultimately develop into specific cellular components of blood

After initially differentiating into either a myeloid or lymphoid progenitor cell, further developmental changes follow. As cells progress down their respective development pathways, they sequentially acquire characteristic receptors and functions, ultimately forming a mature blood cell (Fig. 1.1) with characteristics specific to the cell type.

Progenitor cells

The pluripotent stem cells can differentiate into one of the two multipotent progenitors:

- Myeloid lineage progenitor cell
- Lymphoid lineage progenitor cell

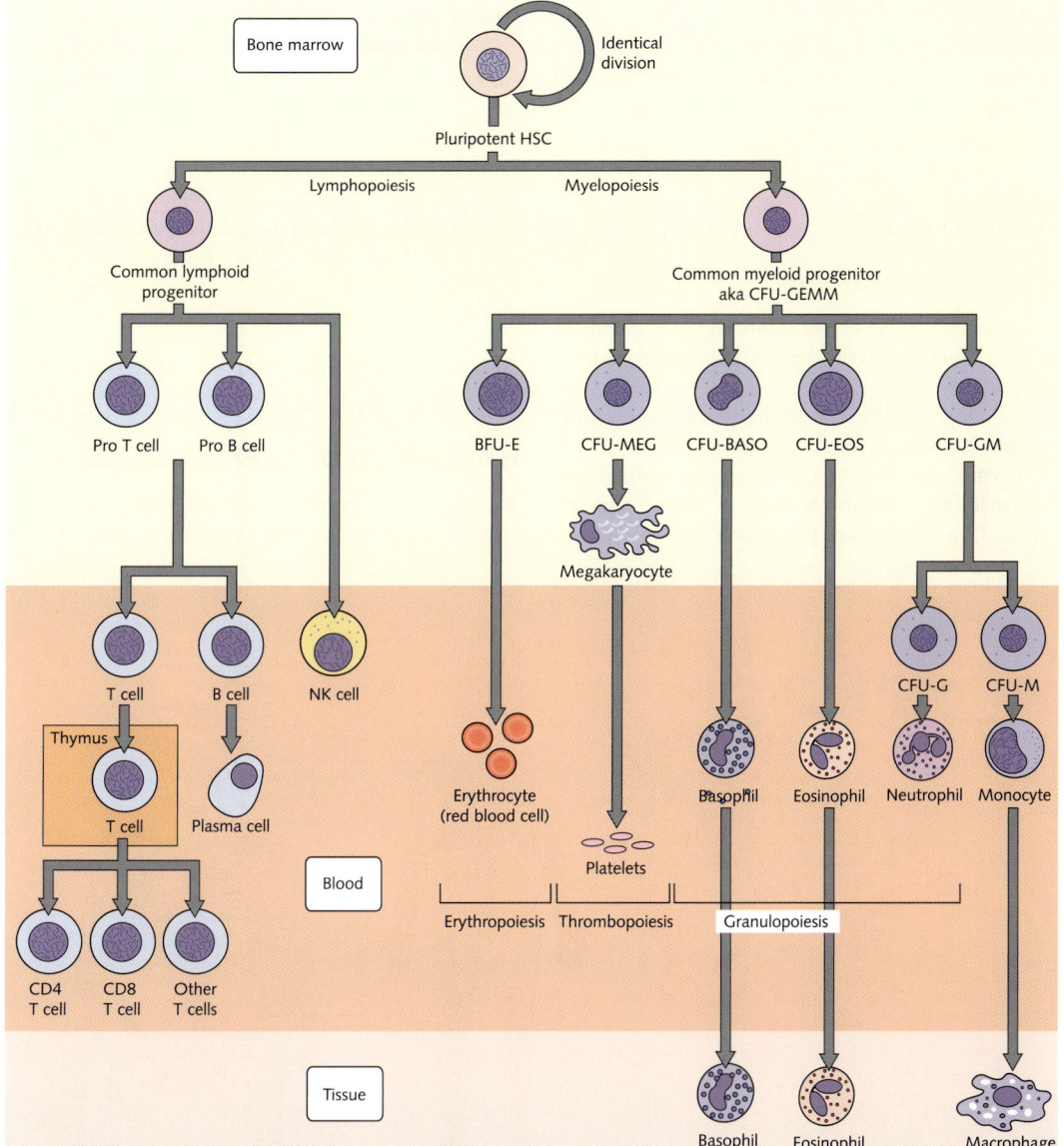

Fig. 1.1 Overview of haemostasis. All blood cells are derived from the pluripotent CD34+ve haematopoietic cells within the bone marrow (*yellow* area of figure). The progenitor cells are not typically found in the blood, including megakaryocytes. These progenitors subsequently produce the white cells, red cells and platelets which are typically found in the blood (*peach* area of figure).

Myeloid lineage multipotent progenitor cell

The CFU-generating myeloid cells (CFU-GEMM) multipotent stem cell subsequently further differentiates into either:

- Red cell progenitor (BFU-E)
- Platelet progenitor (CFU-Meg)
- Eosinophil progenitor (CFU-Eos)
- Basophil progenitor (CFU-Baso)
- Neutrophil/monocyte progenitor (CFU-GM)

HINTS AND TIPS

COLONY-FORMING UNITS (CFU)

CFU describes a progenitor cell committed to the development of a particular blood cell. For example, CFU-Baso is a progenitor cell that ultimately develops into a basophil.

Lymphoid lineage multipotent progenitor cell

The common lymphoid progenitor may further differentiate into one of the following:

- Pre-B cell (B-cell precursor)
- Pre-T cell (T-cell precursor)
- NK cell precursor

Sites of haematopoiesis

The location of haematopoiesis differs according to developmental stage (Fig. 1.2). Table 1.1 lists the various haematopoiesis locations in health.

In certain pathological situations, the bone marrow becomes unable to maintain a sufficient rate of haematopoiesis. If this scenario persists chronically, the liver and spleen may resume haematopoietic capability. This is known as extramedullary haematopoiesis. Two classic examples where this is seen are thalassaemia major (see Chapter 3: Thalassaemia) and primary myelofibrosis (see Chapter 5: Primary myelofibrosis).

Table 1.1 Sites of haemopoiesis according to developmental stage

Developmental stage	Site
Conception to 6 weeks' gestation	Foetal yolk sac
6 to 26 weeks' gestation	Foetal liver Foetal spleen
26 weeks to childhood	Bone marrow of most bones
Adult	Bone marrow of axial skeleton Bone marrow of proximal long bones

Regulation of haemopoiesis

The presence of growth factors promotes cell division. Growth factors are glycoproteins produced in the bone marrow, liver and

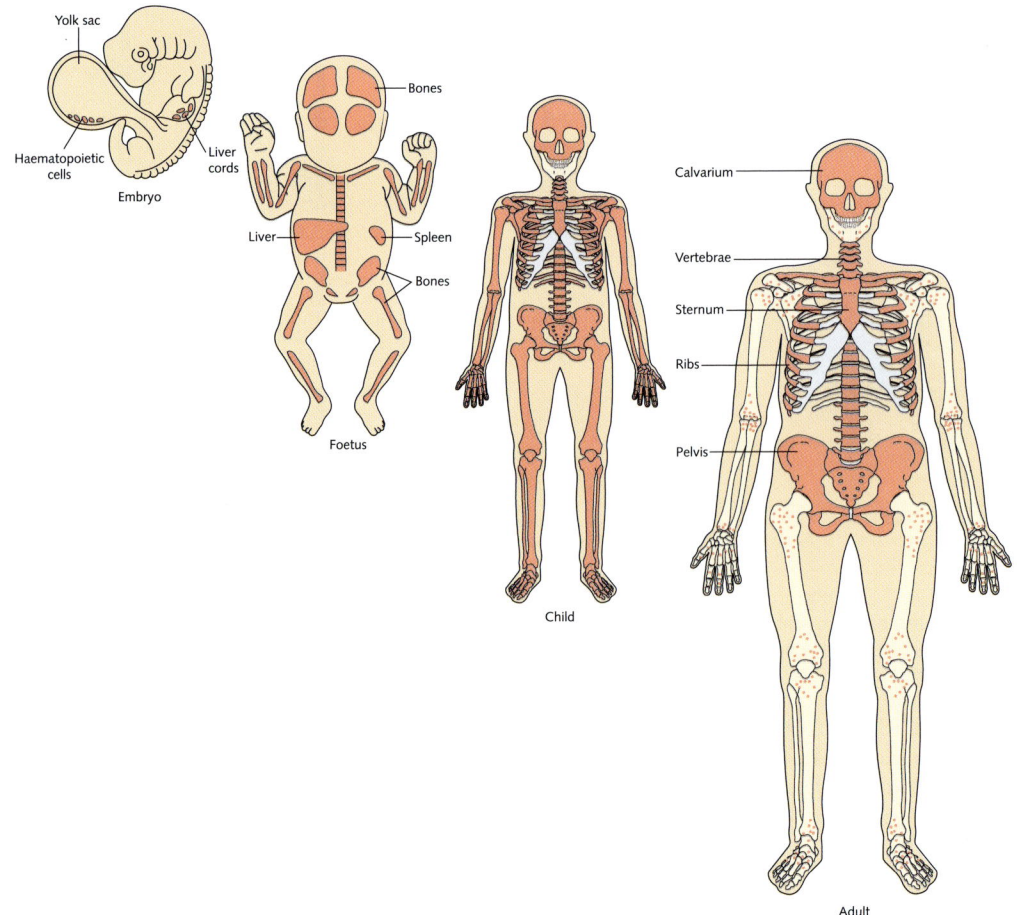

Fig. 1.2 Sites of haemopoiesis (see also Table 1.1).

kidneys. They bind to surface receptors on haemopoietic cells and can trigger replication, differentiation or functional activation, depending on the particular growth factor and the physiological context. In the absence of protective growth factor stimulation, cells undergo apoptosis (regulated cell death of old or dysfunctional cells). Specific growth factors and their respective responsive cells are indicated in Table 1.2. Note that some growth factors are used clinically.

CLINICAL NOTES

CLINICAL USE OF GROWTH FACTORS

Recombinant growth factors may be used clinically to increase the synthesis of a specific blood cell and compensate for a cytopenia. As an example, erythropoietin is used to increase red cell synthesis in the context of insufficient endogenous erythropoietin (such as in chronic end-stage renal disease). G-CSF stimulates the CFU-GM progenitors to differentiate into mature neutrophils. It is used when neutrophil count is dangerously low, for example, following chemotherapy. Eltrombopag and romiplostim stimulate platelet synthesis via stimulation of the thrombopoietin (TPO) receptor on megakaryocytes. They are used to increase platelet counts in immune thrombocytopenic purpura (ITP).

BONE MARROW

Bone marrow is the major haematopoietic organ in adults, producing ~500 billion cells daily and accounting for ~5% of body weight. It is divided into red marrow and yellow marrow. Red marrow is red due to haematopoiesis and yellow marrow is yellow due to fat. In situations where the existing red marrow is unable to perform haematopoiesis at a rate sufficient for normal physiological function, yellow marrow retains the ability to resume haematopoiesis, in which case it becomes red marrow.

Structure

Bone marrow tissue lies within central cavities of bones, supported by a matrix of bony trabeculae. Red marrow provides an optimal microenvironment for haematopoietic stem cell growth and development. It has two main components: haematopoietic parenchyma (developing blood cells) and supporting stromal tissue.

Stroma

In red marrow, stroma consists of vascular sinusoids and specialized fibroblasts. Vascular sinusoids consist of blood-filled spaces, fed by arterioles and interconnected by multiple fenestrated capillaries. Sinusoids ultimately drain (radially) into a large central vein from whence they enter the venous

---

Table 1.2 Growth factors

Growth factor	Source	Cellular target	Action
Erythropoietin	Kidneys	BFU-E and CFU-E	Stimulates the BFU-E and CFU-E to progress down the differentiation pathway of red cell precursors, ultimately forming mature red cells
Thrombopoietin	Liver	CFU-Meg, megakaryocytes	Enhancement of basal production rate of megakaryocytes (from CFU-Meg) and platelets (from megakaryocytes)
G-CSF	Endothelial cells, macrophages, lymphocytes	CFU-G	Differentiation into mature neutrophils
GM-CSF	Macrophages, T cells and mast cells	CFU-GM	Granulocyte and monocyte precursor growth and differentiation
Interleukin 2	Activated T cells, NK cells, macrophage	Pre-T cell	T-cell growth and differentiation
Interleukin 3	T cells, thymic epithelium	CFU-GEMM	Haematopoiesis
Interleukin 5	T cells, mast cells, eosinophil	CFU-Eos	Eosinophil growth and differentiation
Interleukin 6	T cells, macrophages, some B cells	Activated B cells, plasma cells, T cells, macrophages	Inflammatory cytokine that induces acute-phase response

BFU-E, Erythroid burst-forming unit; CFU, colony-forming unit; CFU-Eos, CFU eosinophil progenitor; CFU-G, CFU neutrophil precursor; CFU-GEMM, CFU generating myeloid cells; CFU-GM, CFU granulocyte-myeloid precursor (the neutrophil/monocyte precursor); G-CSF, granulocyte-colony stimulating factor; GM-CSF, granulocyte-macrophage colony-stimulating factor; NK, natural killer.

circulation. The fenestrations allow passage of matured blood cells out of the marrow and into the bloodstream by this route. Specialized fibroblasts (adventitial reticular cells) secrete reticulin (a subtype of collagen) fibres, which form a supportive mechanical framework for the haematopoietic tissue.

Haemopoietic tissue

Also known as 'haematopoietic islands' or 'haematopoietic cords', the synthetic tissue of red marrow contains stem cells, progenitors, precursors and mature blood cells. This haematopoietic tissue fills the area between the vascular sinusoids. Anatomical compartmentalization occurs according to the type of blood cell being synthesized (e.g., red cell synthesis occurring in erythroblastic islands, megakaryopoiesis occurring in zones adjacent to the sinusoids).

Haematopoietic cord macrophages

Macrophages, full of iron-rich stores of ferritin and haemosiderin, are centrally located within each cluster of haematopoietic synthesis. They have three main functions:

1. Provision of an iron supply for developing erythroblasts (for haemoglobin synthesis)
2. Phagocytosis of the cellular debris associated with haematopoiesis
3. Contributing to the cellular regulation of haematopoiesis

Lymphocyte differentiation

Bone marrow synthesizes lymphocytes and is thus termed a 'primary' lymphoid organ.

B-cell differentiation

B-cell development is dependent on bone marrow stroma. As B-cell precursors develop, they migrate towards the central axis of the marrow cavity and become less reliant on stromal support. Any developing B cells that demonstrate binding to self-antigens are destroyed at this stage. The surviving B cells enter the circulation, travelling to the spleen/lymph nodes for final maturation.

T-cell differentiation

T-lymphocyte precursors leave the bone marrow earlier in their development. They enter the circulation and travel to the thymus for maturation.

Natural killer cell differentiation

NK cells undergo initial development in the bone marrow but ultimately deploy to secondary lymphoid tissue (tonsils, lymph nodes and spleen) for further maturation.

THE SPLEEN

The spleen is the largest secondary lymphoid organ (primary lymphoid organs being the bone marrow and thymus). In some ways, it may be thought of as a very large and sophisticated lymph node. The spleen is responsible for the following physiological roles:

- Removal of particulate matter from the bloodstream (e.g., opsonized bacteria, antibody-coated cells)
- Destruction of elderly and poorly deformable erythrocytes
- Initiation of the immune response to blood-borne antigens
- A storage zone for platelets (approximately one-third of the platelet population is found in the spleen)
- Foetal haematopoiesis

Embryology

The spleen originates as a mesodermal proliferation from the primitive gut during the fifth week of foetal development.

Anatomy

The spleen is an intraperitoneal organ, measuring between 6 cm and 13 cm when healthy. It is wrapped in a dense fibroelastic capsule that protrudes conspicuously into the organ, subdividing it. Blood supply to the spleen is via the splenic artery, which enters at the hilus. Venous drainage via the splenic vein also leaves via the hilus, ultimately entering the portal vein via the superior mesenteric vein. It is connected to the body wall by the lienorenal ligament and to the stomach by the gastrolienal ligament.

It is anatomically related to:

- Stomach, tail of pancreas, left colic flexure (anteriorly)
- Left kidney (medially)
- Diaphragm, ribs 9–11 (posteriorly)

There are two types of functional tissue: red pulp and white pulp. These are separated by the marginal zone.

Red pulp

Red pulp is a 3D meshwork of splenic cords (connective tissue) and numerous blood-filled sinusoids. Blood cells are extravasated into splenic cord filtration beds where lattice-like networks of connective tissue and macrophages perform the mechanical filtration function of the spleen, removing antigens, microorganisms, senescent blood cells and blood-borne particulate matter. Once through the filtration bed, cells return to the circulation via the sinusoids, which drain into the venous system.

White pulp

White pulp consists of B-cell follicles and periarteriolar lymphoid sheaths (PALS), which protrude into the red pulp. PALS are dense areas of lymphatic tissue, mainly consisting of T cells, wrapped around splenic arterioles. The B-cell follicles are continuous with the PALS.

Marginal zone

This region (histologically considered white pulp) delineates red pulp and white pulp. Some resident macrophages and marginal zone B cells are permanent features. Other B cells and T cells are only present temporarily, in transit between the circulation and their splenic domains (follicles or PALS, respectively). This makes the marginal zone an optimal site for antigen processing and presentation and lymphocyte/dendritic cell interaction.

Disorders of the spleen

Splenomegaly

Enlargement of the spleen (splenomegaly) may arise in many different disorders, as illustrated in Table 1.3. Clinically palpable splenomegaly must be accurately assessed with appropriate imaging.

Table 1.3 Causes of splenomegaly

System/mechanism	Specific causes
Infection: bacterial	Tuberculosis Salmonella Brucella Syphilis Infective endocarditis
Infection: viral	Epstein-Barr virus[a] Hepatitis Cytomegalovirus HIV
Infection: parasitic	Malaria Toxoplasmosis Schistosomiasis Visceral leishmaniasis Trypanosomiasis
Inflammation/immune	Sarcoidosis Rheumatoid arthritis Systemic lupus erythematosus
Haematological malignancy (Chapter 5)	Lymphomas Leukaemias Myeloproliferative disorders (especially primary myelofibrosis)
Nonmalignant haematological causes	Haemoglobinopathies Haemolytic anaemia
Congestive (portal hypertension)	Liver cirrhosis[a] Right ventricular failure[a] Thrombosis of portal, hepatic or splenic veins
Trauma	Splenic intracapsular haematoma
Infiltrative	Lipid deposition disorders (e.g., Gaucher disease) Niemann-Pick disease Amyloidosis Glycogen storage disorders

[a]Most common causes for splenomegaly in the United Kingdom.

CLINICAL NOTES

SPLENOMEGALY

The spleen must increase significantly in size in order for it to be palpated below the costal margins; so a palpable splenic edge always indicates splenomegaly. How far below the costal margin the spleen is palpable can help grade the degree of splenomegaly:

- Mild: 1–3 cm below the costal margin
- Moderate: 4–8 cm below the costal margin (in between the costal margin and umbilicus)
- Massive: >8 cm below the costal margin (crosses the midline of abdomen and umbilicus)

HINTS & TIPS:

If someone has massive splenomegaly, think haematological disorders (chronic myeloid leukaemia, myelofibrosis, splenic marginal zone lymphoma) or parasitic infections (malaria, leishmaniasis).

Hypersplenism

Irrespective of the underlying cause of a splenomegaly, the enlarged spleen filters out more cells, resulting in excessive clearance of cells from the bloodstream. This reduces circulating numbers and results in cytopenias, leading to the release of immature blood cells into the bloodstream from functionally normal bone marrow. This phenomenon is called hypersplenism and should be identified, because the effective treatment of the underlying cause of the splenomegaly can improve blood cell counts without resorting to a splenectomy.

Splenic infarction

Splenic infarction is the ischaemic death of splenic tissue due to occlusion of the arterial supply. It may affect part (partial infarction) or all (complete infarction) of the spleen. Emboli (secondary to atrial fibrillation) are the most common cause, but locally formed thrombi within the splenic artery or its major branches (associated with sickle cell disease and myeloproliferative disorders) can also be responsible.

Following complete infarction (autosplenectomy), patients are rendered functionally asplenic and require asplenic management.

Rupture of the spleen

The spleen may rupture secondary to abdominal trauma, certain infections (e.g., Epstein-Barr virus; see Clinical notes) or disorders of haematopoiesis (e.g., primary myelofibrosis).

Splenectomy

Indications for splenectomy (surgical removal of the spleen) include:

- Severe splenic trauma causing uncontrollable bleeding
- Splenic lymphoma
- Immune cytopenias (autoimmune haemolytic anaemia, immune thrombocytopenia)
- Nonimmune haemolysis when secondary to splenic RBC destruction (thalassaemia major, hereditary spherocytosis)
- Splenic cysts (only rarely)

Autosplenectomy refers to the hyposplenism that develops when the spleen is rendered nonfunctional by disease. Splenic artery thrombosis is an illustrative example. Sickle cell disease is one of the most common causes in infancy, due to cumulative localized small-vessel thrombosis. Coeliac disease is another well-known cause of autosplenectomy, although the exact mechanism is unclear.

Congenital abnormalities

Congenital asplenia (absent spleen) is rare and usually associated with other congenital abnormalities. Conversely, ~10% of people have accessory spleens (additional small areas of splenic tissue).

Management of the hyposplenic patient

Regardless of the cause of their hyposplenism, asplenic and hyposplenic patients are at an increased risk of infection, particularly infection by encapsulated bacteria (e.g., *Neisseria meningitides, Streptococcus pneumoniae, Haemophilus influenzae*). This is primarily because the spleen, being the largest lymphoid organ, is the major site for immunoglobulin synthesis, including IgM. IgM is necessary for opsonization (tagging of pathogens for elimination by phagocytes) of encapsulated organisms. For further details, see Chapter 9: The innate immune system. Macrophages lining the meshwork of the red pulp also ingest and remove unopsonized bacteria. In the absence of a spleen, both these functions are lost. The clinical consequence is a patient with lifelong susceptibility to overwhelming postsplenectomy infections (OPSI).

To reduce the chance of OPSI, several interventions are required in asplenic/hyposplenic patients:

1. Vaccinations (courses to be completed >2 weeks prior to splenectomy or initiated >2 weeks postsplenectomy). The first three vaccines must be protein conjugate vaccines, which are more effective than plain polysaccharide vaccines:
    - Pneumococcal vaccine (with boosters every 5–10 years afterward)
    - Haemophilus influenzae vaccination course
    - Meningococcal vaccines
    - Influenza vaccination (repeated annually lifelong)
2. Lifelong prophylactic daily oral antibiotics: Penicillin V (clarithromycin if penicillin-allergic). Many patients unfortunately stop taking their daily antibiotics after a few years, only to die of overwhelming sepsis.
3. Clear advice regarding the need for urgent medical review if patients develop symptoms of infection (e.g., sore throat/fever/productive cough/lethargy/diarrhoea/vomiting).
4. Medical alert bracelets, to ensure it can be highlighted that patient has had a splenectomy, if they ever become so unwell that they cannot communicate.

It is of paramount importance that patients repeat the above vaccinations as required for the rest of their lives, as well as continue to take their daily prophylactic antibiotics.

LYMPHADENOPATHY

Enlarged lymph nodes (lymphadenopathy) are normal when occurring in response to infection or inflammation. However, in the absence of these factors, lymphadenopathy may be an important indicator of neoplastic disease. An illustration showing the main groups of lymph nodes is given in Fig. 1.3. Acute, localized tender/painful lymphadenopathy is generally a helpful indicator of infection in the area drained by the enlarged nodes. Insidious, painless, nontender generalized (involving >1 anatomical region) node enlargement is more likely to be due to malignancy (see Chapter 5: Lymphadenopathy red flags) but may be due to a nonmalignant pathology. Examples are detailed in Table 1.4.

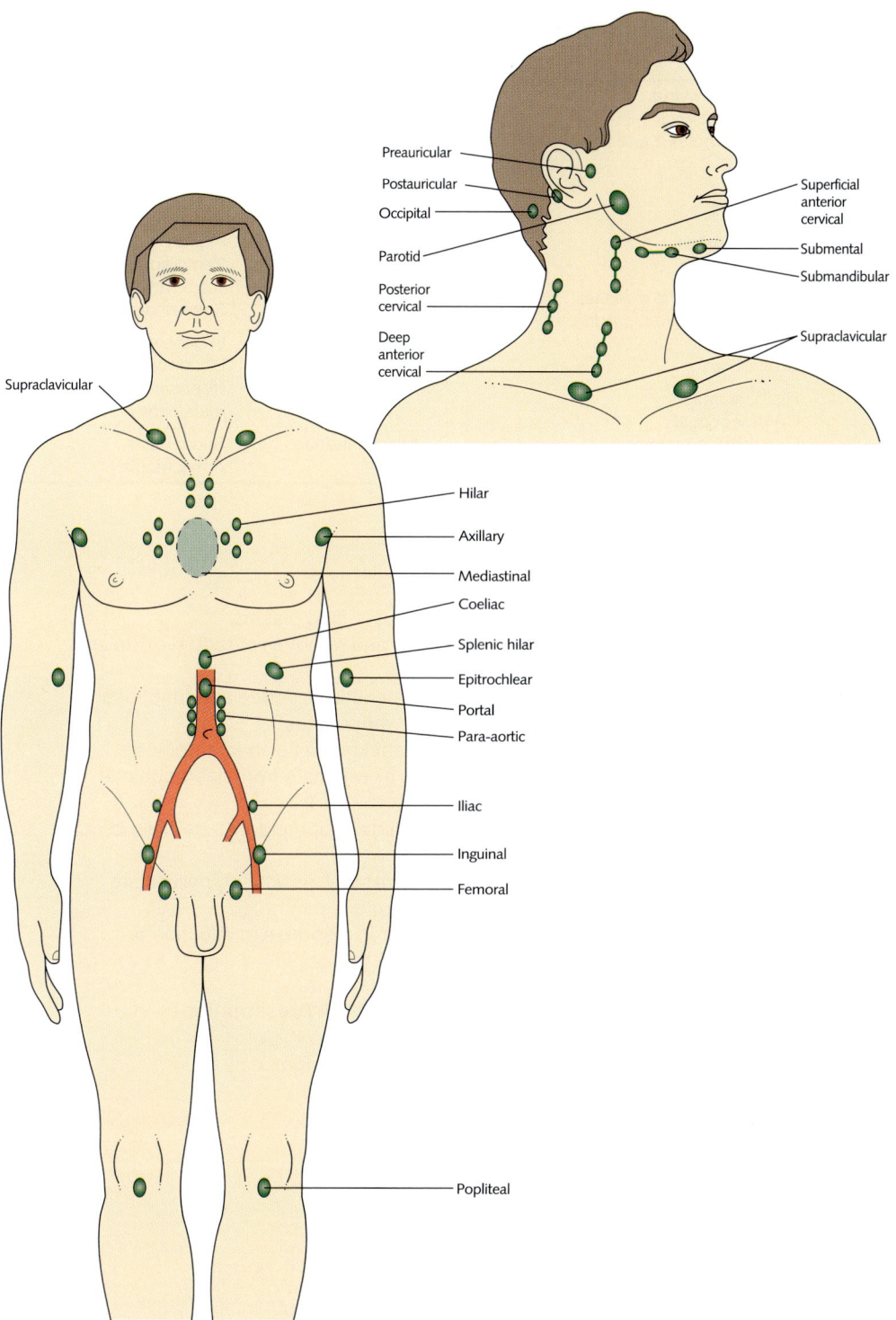

Fig. 1.3 Lymph node locations. *Solid circles* represent palpable lymph node(s), *unfilled circles* represent impalpable or internal lymph nodes. Note that the popliteal lymph nodes are palpable in the popliteal fossa on the posterior surface of the leg.

Table 1.4 Causes of generalized lymphadenopathy

Mechanism	Examples	Mechanism	Examples
Infection: viral	Epstein-Barr virus Cytomegalovirus Herpes simplex 1 and 2 Rubella Measles Hepatitis B	Connective tissue disease	Rheumatoid arthritis Systemic lupus erythematosus Churg-Strauss syndrome Dermatomyositis
Infection: protozoal	Toxoplasmosis Leishmaniasis	Drugs	Phenytoin Isoniazid Aspirin Penicillins Tetracyclines Sulphonamides
Infection: bacterial	Borreliosis (Lyme disease) Leptospirosis (Weil syndrome) Tularaemia Brucellosis	Neoplasia	Leukaemias Lymphomas Nonhaematological metastatic malignancy
Infection: fungal	Histoplasmosis Cryptococcosis Coccidioidomycosis	Miscellaneous	Sarcoidosis Amyloidosis

Chapter summary

- Blood consists primarily of different cell types suspended in fluid plasma.
- Blood delivers oxygen and nutrients to cells of the body and removes carbon dioxide and waste products.
- There are several types of blood cells, each with characteristic structure and functions: erythrocytes, platelets, lymphocytes, granulocytes and monocytes.
- Blood cells are synthesized via a process of development known as haematopoiesis.
- Different development pathways for different cell types all originate from haemopoietic stem cells.
- Haematopoiesis occurs in different tissues according to developmental stage. This takes place in the bone marrow in adults.
- The spleen plays several important immunological roles as well as filtering particulate matter and removing aged red cells from the bloodstream.
- Lymph node enlargement (lymphadenopathy) may occur in response to infection or malignancy.

MLA Conditions
Adverse drug effects
hyposplenism/splenectomy

MLA Presentations
Lump in groin
Organomegaly

Red blood cells and haemoglobin

2

ERYTHROCYTES

Erythrocytes are mature red cells. Their average lifespan is 120 days. The normal concentration of erythrocytes in the blood is $3.9–6.5 \times 10^{12}$/L.

Structure

A typical red cell has an average diameter of 7.2 μm. Their three-dimensional shape is a biconcave discoid (Fig. 2.1), offering a high surface area:volume shape, which is optimal for gas exchange (the primary function of the red cell). It also facilitates rapid, reversible cellular deformation, necessary for squeezing through microvasculature where vessel diameter may be as small as 3 μm.

Contents

Erythrocytes have no nuclei or organelles. Instead, they are packed with haemoglobin, the oxygen-carrying, haem-containing metalloprotein, which gives blood its familiar red colour.

Function

The primary function of erythrocytes is gas exchange. In mammals, oxygen is transported from the lungs to peripheral tissues and carbon dioxide from the tissues to the lungs.

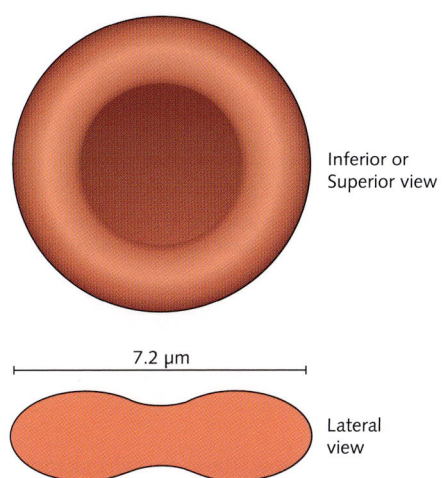

Inferior or Superior view

7.2 μm

Lateral view

Fig. 2.1 Erythrocyte three-dimensional shape.

Oxygen transport

The vast bulk of oxygen transported from the lungs to the tissues travels bound to red cell haemoglobin; only a minute fraction is dissolved in solution in blood. Oxygen carriage by haemoglobin varies according to several variables:

- Haemoglobin concentration
- Haemoglobin affinity for oxygen (varies according to environmental factors such as pO_2, pCO_2)
- Haemoglobin saturation (determined by the arterial partial pressure of oxygen [pO_2])

Carbon dioxide transport

Carbon dioxide is a product of respiration (aerobic and anaerobic). Blood pCO_2 is tightly regulated by changes in ventilation. Carbon dioxide is carried in the blood in three forms:

- Bicarbonate ions (~90%). Functioning as a biochemical carbon dioxide reservoir, these play a significant role in blood pH buffering
- Direct solution (~5%)
- Carb-amino compounds (~5%): Carbon dioxide combines with protein amino groups, primarily those of haemoglobin

Secondary functions

Haemoglobin is also a key blood pH buffer, due to its ability to bind H^+ ions. The H^+ ions associated with haemoglobin are derived from bicarbonate generation and carb-amino compound formation (Fig. 2.2).

Another important (but secondary) erythrocyte role is vasodilation. This is mediated by release of biomediators including adenosine triphosphate (ATP), S-nitrosothiols, nitric oxide (NO) and hydrogen sulphide. This is triggered by red cell shear stress from collision with vessel walls, which occurs more in vasoconstricted vessels.

ERYTHROPOIESIS

Erythropoiesis (Fig. 2.3) is red blood synthesis, starting with the CFU-GEMM myeloid lineage progenitor (see Chapter 1, Fig. 1.1). Erythropoiesis occurs in erythroblastic islands within bone marrow. Macrophages situated here supply iron (needed for haemoglobin synthesis) to the surrounding developing cells. It takes ~1 week for a stem cell to differentiate fully into a mature erythrocyte.

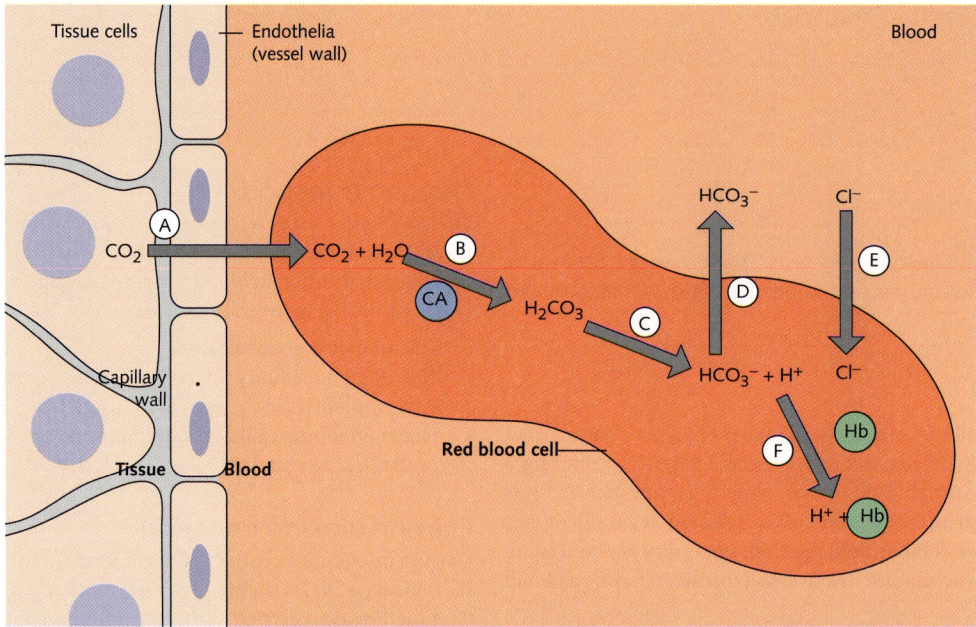

Fig. 2.2 Carbon dioxide transport in blood. (A) Carbon dioxide travels down the partial pressure gradient (respiring cells → blood). (B) Red cell carbonic anhydrase enzyme catalyzes the formation of carbonic acid (H_2CO_3) from H_2O and CO_2. (C) H_2CO_3 dissociates into protons (H^+) and bicarbonate ions ($HCO3^-$). (D) Bicarbonate ions diffuse down their concentration gradient into the plasma. (E) Chloride ions (Cl^-) enter the cell to maintain electroneutrality (the chloride shift). (F) H^+ (produced as a result by dissociation of H_2CO_3) bind to imidazole groups on the amino acids comprising haemoglobin. *CA*, Carbonic anhydrase.

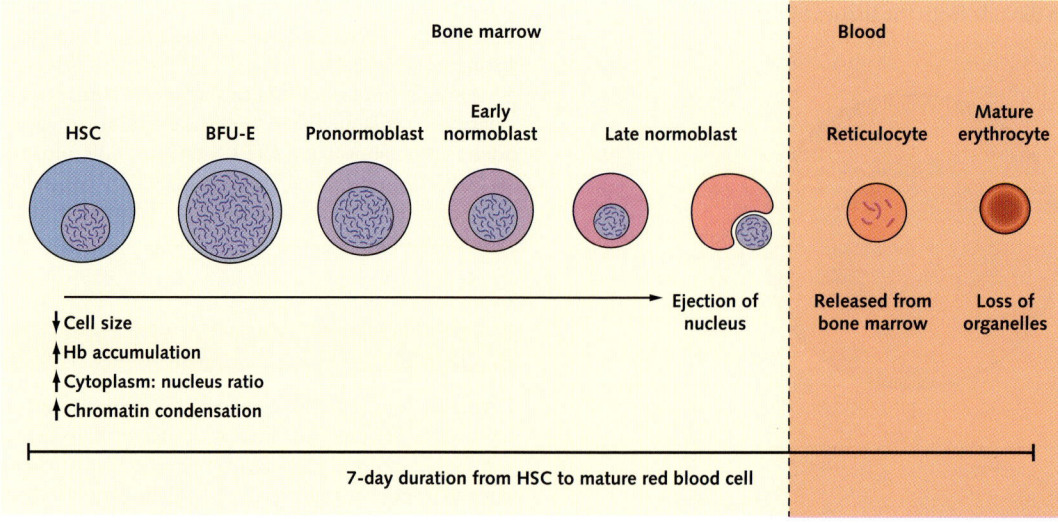

Fig. 2.3 The sequence of erythropoiesis takes place within erythroblastic islands in bone marrow. These contain macrophages, which supply iron to the surrounding erythroid progenitor cells. For intervening stages between the haematopoietic stem cell and BFU-E, please see Fig. 1.1. *HSC,* Haematopoietic stem cell; *BFU-E,* burst-forming unit-erythroid.

Sequence of erythropoiesis

Maturation is characterized by the following key stages:

- Erythroid burst-forming units (BFU-E): colony-forming unit generating myeloid cells (CFU-GEMM) differentiation to a BFU-E commits to the erythrocyte development pathway.
- Pronormoblast: haemoglobin is absent, organelles are still present and the nucleus is large relative to cytoplasm volume.
- Early, intermediate and late normoblasts: Overall cell size and nuclear size (relative to cytoplasm) decrease. Haemoglobin accumulates and the nucleus is ejected from the late normoblast to form a reticulocyte.
- Reticulocyte: These are released from bone marrow into the bloodstream. Some ribonucleic acid (RNA) is still present and the shape remains rounded.
- Erythrocyte: The biconcave discoid shape defines the mature erythrocyte. Intracellular organelles have been lost.

In a healthy person, bone marrow erythrocyte production rate is approximately matched by splenic erythrocyte removal rate. The total erythrocyte population therefore remains approximately constant.

An imbalance developing due to excessive destruction of red cells (e.g., acute haemolysis) can be compensated by an increase in erythropoiesis, so the red cell count remains constant. Enhanced erythropoiesis is suggested by the (abnormal) presence of nucleated precursors in peripheral blood (i.e., on a blood film) or an increased reticulocyte count.

Regulation of erythropoiesis

The principal factor promoting erythropoiesis is a hormone called erythropoietin.

Erythropoietin

Erythropoietin (EPO) is a heavily glycosylated polypeptide, 165 amino acids in length with molecular weight $\sim$30,400 kDa. It is secreted by:

- Peritubular capillary endothelial cells (renal cortex; 90%)
- Kupffer cells and hepatocytes (liver; 10%)

Control of erythropoietin secretion

Hypoxia (low intracellular pO_2) is the main stimulus for EPO synthesis and secretion. Hypoxia is defined by insufficient oxygen delivery to meet cellular requirements. Hypoxia may arise due to a multitude of causes (Fig. 2.4). Most causes can ultimately be categorized within one of the following underlying mechanisms:

- Reduction in the oxygen-carrying capacity of blood
- Impaired oxygenation at the pulmonary alveolar-arteriole interface

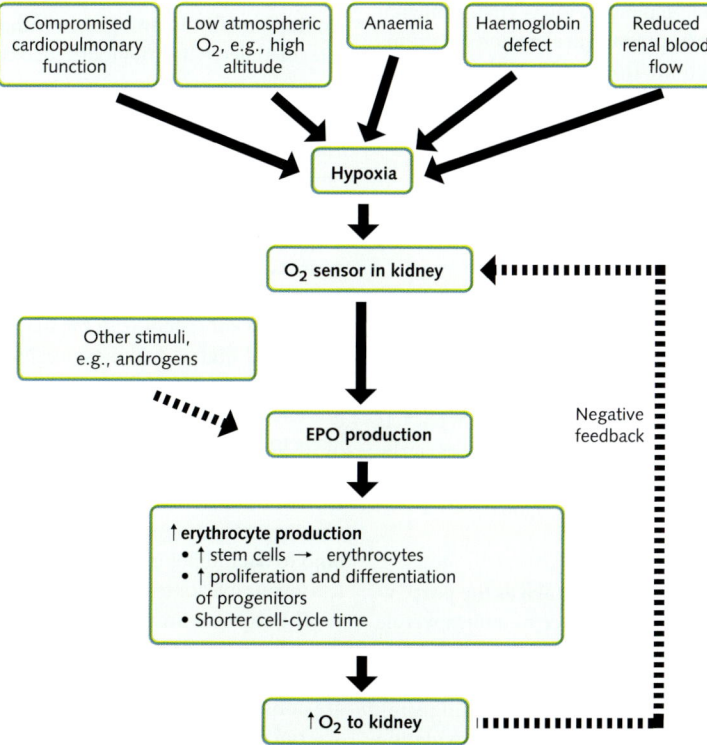

Fig. 2.4 Regulation of erythropoietin (EPO) synthesis.

- Compromised tissue perfusion (i.e., oxygen delivery, which may be local or global)

A loss of functional renal tissue, for example, nephrectomy or renal disease, will also result in decreased EPO production with the physiological consequence of anaemia. Conversely, renal cell carcinomas can produce excessive levels of EPO, resulting in a pathological increase in red cell production. Chronically raised EPO levels can also lead to extramedullary haematopoiesis (see Chapter 1).

Clinical indications for erythropoietin

Recombinant EPO (produced in animal cells) is used to increase the red cell count in specific anaemia scenarios, that is, where the underlying pathology is due to a failure of serum (EPO) to increase appropriately in response to anaemia, for example,

- Anaemia secondary to chronic renal failure
- Some specific cases of anaemia of chronic disease, for example, congestive heart failure
- Postchemotherapy
- Certain subtypes of myelodysplastic syndromes (MDS), where EPO may be combined with granulocyte-colony stimulating factor (G-CSF)
- To boost the red cell count prior to autologous blood transfusions or for those where blood transfusion is contraindicated (e.g., Jehovah's Witness)

Altitude training

Athletes training at high altitude exploit the lower environmental pO_2 (due to reduced atmospheric pressure at elevation) to stimulate endogenous EPO production. This increases their red cell counts and thus the oxygen-carrying capacity of their blood, theoretically improving athletic performance. Synthetic EPO may be illegally administered with the same intention.

HAEMOGLOBIN

Structure

A haemoglobin molecule consists of four globin chains united by noncovalent interactions (Fig. 2.5). Each globin features a haem pocket, a hydrophobic crevice containing the haem moiety. Each haem group can bind one molecule of oxygen. Since there are four haem pockets (one per globin chain), a maximum of four oxygen molecules can be transported per haemoglobin molecule. Normal adult haemoglobin (HbA) is tetrameric, consisting of two α and two β globins.

Haem (Heme)

Haem belongs to a family of compounds known as the porphyrins, which are characterized by the presence of a tetrapyrrole ring. The haem group consists of an Fe^{2+} (ferrous) ion at the centre Each ferrous ion is bonded to four N atoms, one from each pyrrole ring. The ferrous ion acts as an oxygen-binding site). Importantly, the iron ion remains in the ferrous 2+ oxidation state, regardless of whether oxygen is bound or not.

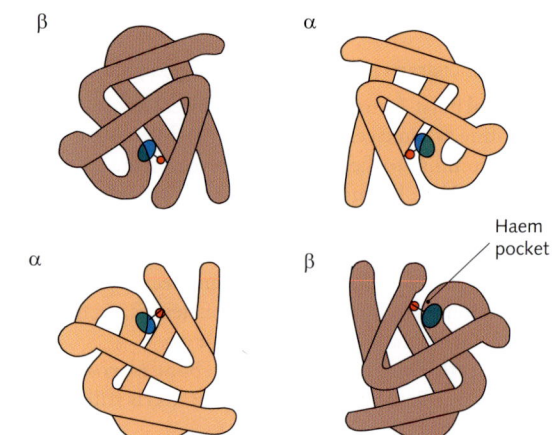

Fig. 2.5 Structure of adult haemoglobin. α polypeptides (globins) are 141 amino acids, whilst β polypeptides (globins) are 146 amino acids in length. Note the haem pocket featuring in each globin.

Physiological properties of haemoglobin

Each Hb molecule is capable of binding four molecules of oxygen, one at each haem site.

Haemoglobin: deoxyHb and oxyHb

Haemoglobin with ≥1 haem-bound oxygen is termed oxyhaemoglobin (oxyHb). Haemoglobin without any haem-bound oxygen is termed deoxyhaemoglobin (deoxyHb).

Haemoglobin: tense versus relaxed

The haemoglobin molecule may exist in two structural configurations: relaxed (R-Hb) and taut (T-Hb). In the R-Hb state, there is increased mobility between globin chains compared with the T-Hb state. Oxygen molecules can more easily access the haem pockets and therefore the R-Hb state has a greater affinity for oxygen (holds onto oxygen more).

Factors consistent with the tissue environment (low pH, high pCO_2 and high 2,3-diphosphoglycerate [2,3-DPG]) favour the T-Hb conformation, which exhibits reduced oxygen affinity. In the presence of these environmental factors, bound oxygen is more likely to dissociate from T-Hb. This is ideal, since in the environment of respiring cells, oxygen offloads readily in environments where it is most needed. The mechanism underlying the variable affinity is that H^+ ions, carbon dioxide and 2,3-DPG covalently bind to haemoglobin, imposing conformational changes that are less favourable for the oxygen–haemoglobin association.

The converse scenario (high pH, low pCO_2 and low 2,3-DPG) favours the relaxed conformation R-Hb, which has increased oxygen affinity and thus binds oxygen more avidly. These factors are consistent with the gas exchange surface (i.e., the alveolar-arterial surface in the lungs), where it is physiologically advantageous for haemoglobin to bind oxygen avidly.

Cooperation

The binding of an oxygen molecule increases the haemoglobin molecule's binding affinity for any subsequent oxygen molecules. Thus the fourth oxygen molecule binds much more readily than the first. Conversely, unloading of oxygen from one haem group facilitates oxygen offloading from the other haem groups. This property accounts for the characteristic sigmoidal (S-shaped) shape of the oxygen dissociation curve (Fig. 2.6).

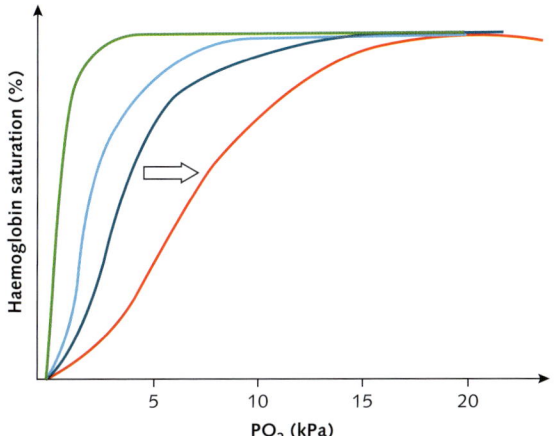

Fig. 2.6 The Oxygen disassociation curve. This plots pO_2 on the X-axis against the haemoglobin oxygen saturation on the y-axis. Haemoglobin's affinity for oxygen increases as successive molecules of oxygen bind until the maximum amount has been reached. When this limit is met, no further oxygen can bind and the curve levels out as the haemoglobin is now saturated with oxygen. This produces the characteristic sigmoid curve. In the figure, normal adult haemoglobin is shown as the dark blue curve. Several factors can shift the curve including temperature, 2,3-DPG, pCO_2 and pH, which affects the binding (i.e. affinity) between haemoglobin and oxygen. When shifted to the left, this is in keeping with haemoglobin having higher O_2 affinity (light blue curve) so this is not released easily. However, when shifted to the right, the haemoglobin has lower O_2 affinity (red curve) and therefore oxygen is released easily. Typically fetal haemoglobin has a higher O_2 affinity (i.e. similar to the light blue curve).

The oxygen dissociation curve

The oxygen dissociation curve is a plot of pO_2 (*x*-axis) against haemoglobin oxygen saturation (*y*-axis). Elevated pCO_2, 2,3-DPG, H^+ and temperature shift the curve to the right, that is, reducing the affinity for oxygen and promoting oxygen offloading. These conditions are consistent with respiring tissues. For a given pO_2 value, the right-shifted curve exhibits a lower haemoglobin saturation.

Due to the sigmoidal nature of the curve, as the pO_2 falls, there is initially little change in the oxygen affinity and therefore haemoglobin saturation. However, below a certain pO_2 there is a sharp drop in oxygen affinity and therefore Hb saturation, resulting in greater release of oxygen as pO_2 lowers.

Foetal haemoglobin

Foetal Hb (HbF) is distinguished from adult Hb (HbA) by the substitution of two γ globins for the two β globins. HbF has greater affinity for oxygen than HbA. This ensures that even at very low pO_2 (such as the gas exchange surfaces of the placenta), where HbA would offload its oxygen cargo, HbF still binds oxygen avidly. The oxygen dissociation curve for HbF is shifted to the left (Fig 2.6). HbF is the predominant haemoglobin in foetuses and newborns until 6 months at which point HbA takes over. Once babies reach 12 months age, HbF reduces to very low levels (<1%). Table 2.1 highlights the different types of haemoglobin molecules at different developmental stages.

Haemoglobin variants

Different variants of haemoglobin exhibit variable oxygen affinities and thus have their own characteristic oxygen dissociation curves. Sickle haemoglobin (HbS) is a pathological form of haemoglobin, where a point mutation distinguishes it structurally and functionally from normal HbA.

Under normal pO_2 conditions, HbS and HbA have similar oxygen affinities. At low pO_2, HbS does exhibit a lower oxygen affinity than normal HbA. Importantly, however, the rightward shift in the dissociation curve that characterizes HbS is not solely due to this affinity variance at low pO_2. It is also due to abnormal HbS polymerization at low pO_2, causing structural distortion and vaso-occlusion. Occluded, ischaemic cells increase their

Table 2.1 Haemoglobin types present at different developmental stages

Developmental stage	Haemoglobin type	Globin components	Specific
Embryonic	Hb Gower I Hb Gower II Hb Portland	$\zeta_2\varepsilon_2$ $\alpha_2\varepsilon_2$ $\zeta_2\gamma_2$	From conception to 2nd trimester of foetal life
Foetal	Hb F	$\alpha_2\gamma_2$	From 2nd trimester of pregnancy to 12 weeks age
Adult	Hb A Hb A2	$\alpha_2\beta_2$ $\alpha_2\delta_2$	The primary type of Hb Typically represents ≤2% of Hb

Hb, Haemoglobin

anaerobic activity, elevating the 2,3-DPG, which shifts the oxygen dissociation curve rightwards for HbS.

Haemoglobin genetics

The genes encoding the ϵ, γ, δ and β globins are found on chromosome 11. The ζ- and two copies of the α-chain genes are found on chromosome 16. Each globin gene consists of three exons, each separated by an intron. Different globins are separately synthesized before uniting in various combinations to form a functional Hb tetramer.

MYOGLOBIN

The other major haem-containing protein in humans is myoglobin, which consists of a single globin with a single haem group. Myoglobin is found principally in muscle, where it only releases bound oxygen at extremely low pO_2, effectively functioning as an oxygen reservoir when oxygen demand exceeds delivery.

IRON AND HAEM METABOLISM

Total body iron is $\sim$4 g, distributed as shown in Table 2.2. Dietary iron occurs as haem iron or nonhaem iron.

Iron metabolism

Absorption of haem iron

Dietary haem iron is almost exclusively derived from animal tissue such as meat or offal. In haem iron, the iron ion in the +2 (ferrous) oxidation state is incorporated in the haem group. This form of dietary iron is more completely and easily absorbed, since a receptor-mediated endocytosis absorbs the iron intact within the haem structure. The iron is intracellularly dismantled from the haem group within the enterocyte. Extrusion into the portal circulation from the enterocyte basal surface is via a common iron exporter.

Absorption of nonhaem iron

Dietary nonhaem iron is obtained from dark leafy green vegetables. In nonhaem iron, the iron ion is in the +3 (ferric) oxidation state and is usually protein-associated. Nonhaem iron is less easily absorbed, since it must be divorced from its associated protein and then be reduced to the ferrous state prior to absorption across the enterocyte. This preabsorption processing confers sensitivity to the chemical properties of coingested foods. Acid and reducing agents, for example, ascorbic acid (vitamin C), increase absorption of ferric (nonhaem) iron by promoting the $Fe^{3+} \rightarrow Fe^{2+}$ reduction. The ferrous (Fe^{2+}) iron ions then enter enterocytes via the H^+/Fe^{2+} symport.

Transport in the circulation

Once in the serum, ferrous ions (Fe^{2+}) oxidize, becoming ferric (Fe^{3+}) ions. In this form, they bind to transferrin, a transport protein. This delivers the iron to cells possessing transferrin receptors, including:

- Erythroblasts (within bone marrow) for incorporation into haemoglobin during erythropoiesis
- The liver and reticuloendothelial macrophages, where it is incorporated into ferritin or haemosiderin for storage
- Muscle, where it is incorporated into myoglobin

Ferritin and haemosiderin

Both ferritin and haemosiderin function as iron storage proteins, storing iron in the (Fe^{3+}) ferric form. Ferritin is a water-soluble compound of protein and iron. Haemosiderin is insoluble and consists of aggregates of ferritin that have partially lost their protein component.

Regulation of iron absorption

As there is no specific physiological iron excretion mechanism, iron levels in the body can only be regulated by variation of dietary iron absorption. This is mediated by hepcidin, a protein synthesized by the liver. Hepcidin binds to and internalizes (removes) the iron exporter from the basolateral enterocyte surface, limiting the iron's access to the circulation.

Excretion

Since a specific mechanism for excess iron excretion is absent, iron loss from the body can only take place via:

- desquamation of keratinocytes
- sloughed mucosal cells – most commonly in the gastrointestinal tract
- blood loss

Table 2.2 Physiological distribution of iron. Total body iron = 5 g	
Total body iron (%)	**Location**
70	Component of haem moiety of haemoglobin
25	Reticuloendothelial macrophages, usually incorporated into iron storage proteins such as ferritin and haemosiderin
4.9	Component of iron-containing enzymes and proteins
0.1	In plasma, typically bound to transferrin

Iron overload

Excess iron is deposited in the tissues, where it results in organ damage. The heart, liver and endocrine organs are particularly susceptible. Due to the lack of an iron excretion mechanism, iron overload is a significant hazard of iron administration or abnormally increased gastrointestinal iron absorption.

Increased absorption

Increased absorption may result from the following:

- Primary haemochromatosis (see 'Haemochromatosis' section below): normal amount of iron available for absorption, but excessive proportion absorbed
- Iron-containing supplement overdose: normal proportion of iron absorbed, but increased iron available
- High levels of ineffective erythropoiesis (e.g., as seen in thalassaemia)

Iatrogenic causes of excess iron intake

- Multiple blood transfusions (1 unit of blood contains ~200–250 mg iron)
- Inappropriate or excessive oral or parenteral iron therapy

Treatment of iron overload

It is important to start therapy as soon as possible to prevent irreversible organ damage. Options include:

- Dietary advice (decrease iron intake, increase intake of natural chelators, e.g., tea)
- Venesection (1 mL blood represents 0.5 mg iron)
- Chelation therapy: desferrioxamine is an iron-chelating agent that is administered subcutaneously or intravenously. Deferiprone and deferasirox are oral iron-chelating alternatives

Haemochromatosis

This autosomal recessive disorder of iron metabolism arises from the failure of hepcidin synthesis due to human haemochromatosis (HFE) gene (chromosome 6) mutations. This results in a dramatic and pathological increase of enterocyte-absorbed dietary iron into the circulation (hepcidin usually *reduces* iron export from enterocytes to the circulation). Although a normal amount of iron may be ingested, a much higher proportion accesses the circulation.

Epidemiology

Around 0.5% of the population are homozygous for various HFE mutations. However, clinical penetrance shows considerable heterogeneity: only ~5% of homozygotes present symptomatically. Males present more commonly than females. Alcohol may enhance disease presentation.

Clinical features

Clinical features arise from inappropriate iron deposition in the relevant organs and include:

- Bronze skin pigmentation (skin)
- Hepatomegaly and/or cirrhosis (liver)
- Diabetes mellitus (pancreas)
- Cardiomyopathy, cardiac arrhythmias (heart)
- Arthritis (iron deposition in joints)

Management includes venesection, chelation with desferrioxamine and ultimately transplantation if cirrhotic failure is acute. Genetic testing of first-degree relatives is also advisable.

HAEMOGLOBIN METABOLISM

Haemoglobin consists of globin chains and haem groups that consist of ferrous iron complexed to a protoporphyrin ring.

Haemoglobin biosynthesis

Protoporphyrin biosynthesis occurs in the mitochondria of developing erythroblasts in the bone marrow (Fig. 2.7). The iron ion (derived from transferrin or ferritin) is integrated into the protoporphyrin in the cytoplasm, forming haem.

Globins are translated in the cytoplasm in the typical manner of protein synthesis. Each haem moiety is integrated into a globin and tetramerization results in a functional haemoglobin molecule.

Haemoglobin breakdown

Degradation of senescent erythrocytes occurs in the macrophages of the spleen, liver and reticuloendothelial system. The haemoglobin is dismantled to component haem and globins (Fig. 2.8).

Haem breakdown

Haem is further degraded to protoporphyrin and iron components as described in Fig 2.8.

Bilirubin:

If bilirubin is generated at a rate exceeding the liver's conjugation capacity, serum (bilirubin) increases. This is hyperbilirubinaemia, which may be clinically apparent as jaundice of the sclera, mucosal membranes and skin. This scenario occurs where red cell breakdown is excessive, that is, haemolysis of any cause.

Unconjugated hyperbilirubinaemia may also occur where the liver's conjugation capacity is impaired, so even where bilirubin production rate is normal, unconjugated hyperbilirubinaemia occurs. Such conditions include Crigler-Najjar syndrome, Gilbert syndrome and physiological neonatal jaundice.

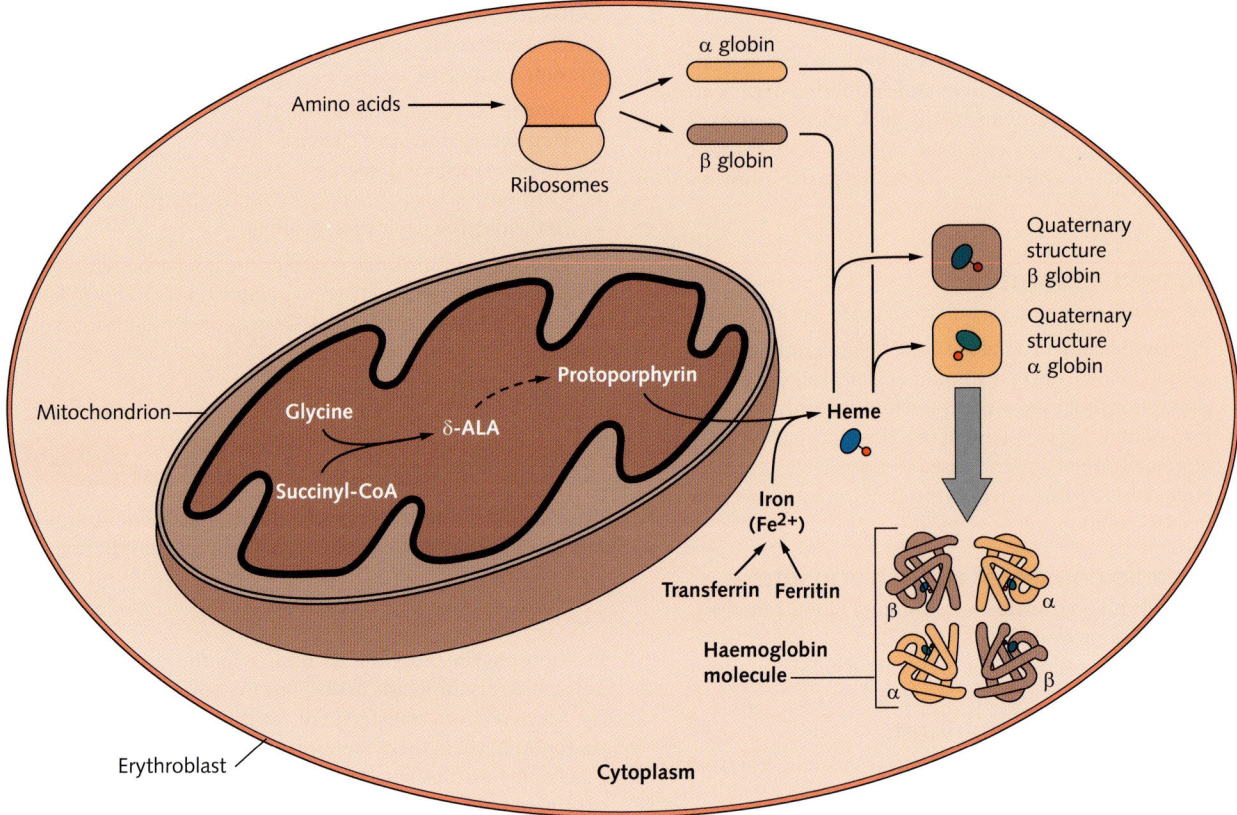

Fig. 2.7 Haemoglobin synthesis in erythroblasts. Within the mitochondria, glycine and succinyl CoA combine to form δ-aminolaevulinic acid (δ-ALA). This step is catalyzed by δ-ALA synthase/coenzyme vitamin B_6. δ-ALA is converted to protoporphyrin (*dashed line*) via multiple intermediates; not shown for simplicity. Protoporphyrin then exits the mitochondria and incorporates a ferrous iron to form haem. The iron may be derived from either ferritin or transferrin. Each haem molecule then combines with a globin chain (α or β) and tetramerization occurs to form the haemoglobin molecule. Please note the mitochondrion is not to scale relative to the cell.

RED CELL CYTOSKELETON

Structure

The erythrocyte plasma membrane is supported internally by a dense, fibrillar, protein shell—the cytoskeleton. The cytoskeleton:

- Maintains resting cell three-dimensional shape
- Confers the erythrocyte membrane with structural flexibility, allowing rapid and reversible deformity during passage through the microvasculature

The proteins of the plasma membrane are important constituents of the cytoskeleton (Fig. 2.9) and are categorized as integral or peripheral. Band numbers refer to the protein's electrophoretic mobility.

Integral proteins

Integral proteins span the cell membrane bilayer and are closely associated with it. These include band 3 protein and glycophorins.

Peripheral proteins

Peripheral proteins are loosely attached to the lipid bilayer and include spectrin, ankyrin, band 4.1 protein and actin. Dysfunction within the peripheral proteins is the basis of some inherited diseases that result in anaemia. The two most common are hereditary spherocytosis and hereditary elliptocytosis.

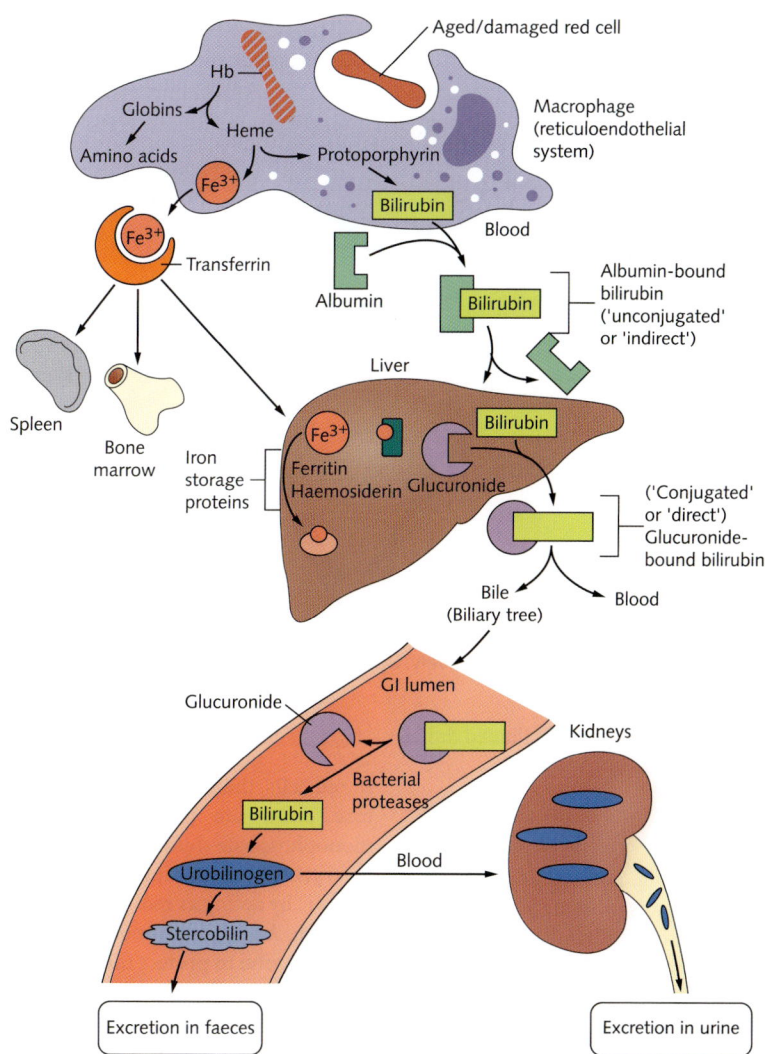

Fig. 2.8 Haemoglobin catabolism. Haemoglobin is separated into haem and globin components. Haem is broken down into iron and protoporphyrin. Iron is transported by transferrin to the bone marrow for erythropoiesis or to the liver for storage. Protoporphyrin is degraded to bilirubin, which is insoluble and bound to albumin in the blood (described as unconjugated bilirubin). On reaching the liver, bilirubin is conjugated to glucuronide before being excreted in bile into the gastrointestinal (GI) lumen. Bilirubin is oxidized to urobilinogen in the GI lumen, which may be reabsorbed and excreted in the urine or further oxidized to stercobilin and excreted in the faeces.

Surface proteins

There are numerous proteins projecting from the surface of the red cell. Many are anchored by the glucosyl phosphatidylinositol (GPI) molecular anchor. Somatic mutations in the gene for phosphatidylinositol glycan protein A (PIG-A) result in the condition, paroxysmal nocturnal haemoglobinuria (see Chapter 3: Paroxysmal nocturnal haemoglobinuria).

RED CELL METABOLISM

As red cells lack mitochondria, they cannot oxidize metabolic substrates aerobically. Anaerobic glycolysis is the primary ATP-generating pathway in red cells, while the pentose phosphate pathway is the main generator of the NADPH + H$^+$ needed for glutathione regeneration. Glucose is therefore the principal

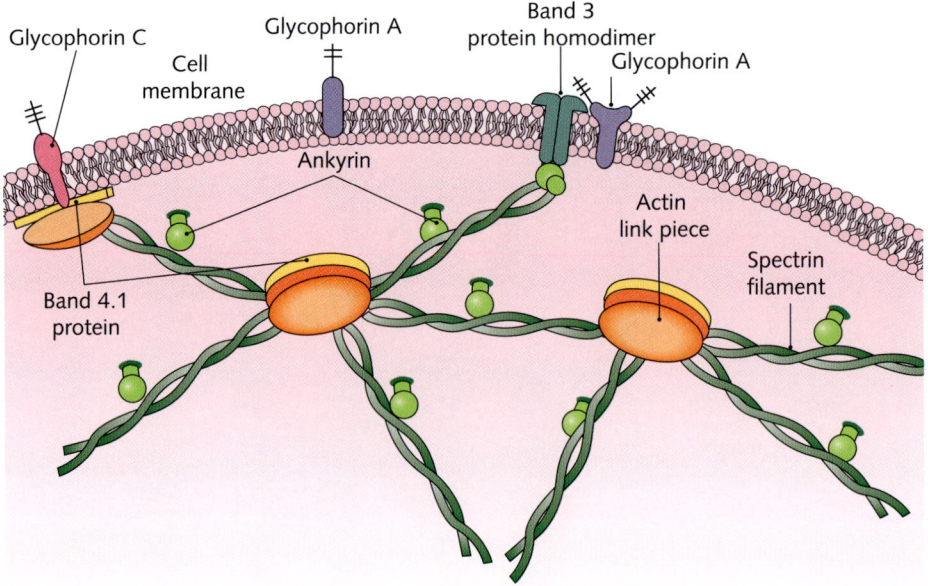

Fig. 2.9 Components of the cytoskeleton. The spectrin lattice is anchored to glycophorin C or band 3 protein dimers studding the red cell membrane by band 4.1 protein and ankyrin, respectively. Spectrin is the primary structural component of the cytoskeleton.

metabolic substrate for red cells. It is taken up by facilitated diffusion in an insulin-independent fashion.

Glycolysis

Glycolysis occurs in all living cells (Fig. 2.10). The fate of pyruvate, the end-product of the pathway, is ultimately determined by whether both oxygen and mitochondria are present. In aerobic conditions (where oxygen is available), pyruvate is converted to acetyl CoA and enters the TCA cycle within the mitochondrial matrix. Reducing equivalents generated by the TCA cycle then participate in oxidative phosphorylation, generating large amounts of ATP. However, in anaerobic conditions or cells lacking mitochondria (such as the red cell) pyruvate is metabolized to lactate with a net yield of two ATP molecules.

$$glucose + 2P_i + 2ADP \rightarrow 2\,lactate + 2ATP + 2H_2O$$

Defects of the glycolytic enzymes are rare. Approximately 95% are associated with pyruvate kinase and their consequences are largely restricted to red blood cells. Within erythrocytes, one of the earliest casualties of restricted intracellular ATP is the structural integrity of the cytoskeleton. The outcome of this is an overly fragile red cell with a shortened life span. The most overt clinical manifestation relates to anaemia secondary to haemolysis (see Chapter 3: Enzyme defects).

Pentose phosphate pathway

In red cells, the supply of NAPH + H^+ is generated by the pentose phosphate pathway (PPP), also called the hexose monophosphate shunt. NADPH + H^+ (reduced $NADP^+$) is vital in erythrocytes because it regenerates oxidized glutathione (GSSG) by acting as redox partner for the necessary reduction reaction. An available pool of intracellular reduced glutathione (GSH) is vital to protect the red cell membrane and intracellular proteins (including Hb) from oxidative damage. Defects in PPP enzymes (see Chapter 3: Glucose-6-phosphate dehydrogenase deficiency) may also manifest with shortened red cell lifespan.

METHAEMOGLOBINAEMIA

When the iron ion (within the haem component of haemoglobin) is oxidized ($Fe^{2+} \rightarrow Fe^{3+}$), Hb becomes methaemoglobin (metHb). Typically, ≤1% of a person's Hb is in this oxidized form. A higher proportion (≥1%) is known as methaemoglobinaemia. Levels >10% lead to a progressive blueish discolouration of mucosal membranes and skin. Levels >20% cause symptoms related to hypoxia. Treatment is oxygen supplementation and methylene blue. Pulse oximetry is unreliable in the context of methaemoglobinaemia.

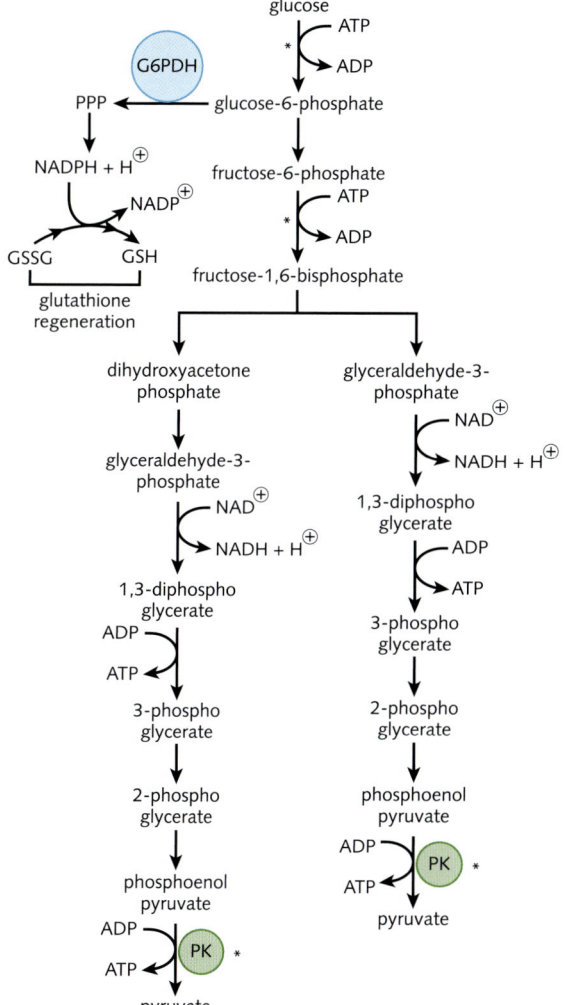

Fig. 2.10 Glycolysis. Starred arrows represent the rate-limiting steps.
ADP, Adenosine diphosphate; *ATP*, adenosine triphosphate, *G6PDH*, glucose-6-phosphate dehydrogenase; *NAD⁺/NADH + H⁺*, nicotinamide adenine dinucleotide/reduced nicotinamide adenine dinucleotide; *NADPH + H⁺/NADP⁺*, nicotinamide adenine dinucleotide phosphate/reduced nicotinamide adenine dinucleotide phosphate; *PK,* pyruvate kinase.

Methaemoglobinaemia is dangerous, because MetHb is useless in terms of oxygen delivery, but more seriously the presence of MetHb shifts the normal Hb's dissociation curve to the left, that is, rendering intact Hb less likely to appropriately offload its oxygen cargo at a given pO₂. This impairs oxygen delivery to the tissue on two levels. An NADH + H⁺-dependent enzyme (methaemoglobin reductase) is usually responsible for returning the ferric (3+) ion to the ferrous (2+) state.

Causes

Elevated methaemoglobin may arise due to:

- Exposure to certain substances (see Box 2.1 below)
- Structurally abnormal haemoglobins rendering the ferric ion resistant to normal enzymatic reduction (e.g., HbM)
- Nicotinamide adenine dinucleotide (NADH) methaemoglobin reductase deficiency
- Glucose-6-phosphate dehydrogenase deficiency (see Chapter 3: Glucose-6-phosphate dehydrogenase deficiency)

BOX 2.1

- Anaesthetics (Benzocaine; Lidocaine; Phenazopyridine)
- Anti-Malarials (Primaquine; Chloroquine)
- Herbicides and Insecticides (Paraquat; Nitrites/Nitrates)
- Methylene blue
- Antibiotics (Sulfonamides)
- Dapsone
- Metoclopramide
- Recreational drugs (Cocaine; Phenylamine)

CLINICAL NOTES

DRUGS KNOWN TO CAUSE METHAEMOGLOBINAEMIA

This category includes prilocaine, benzocaine, primaquine, chloroquine, nitroprussin, nitroglycerin, glyceryl trinitrate, amyl nitrite, dapsone and sulphonamides.

Amyl nitrite – commonly seen recreational drug overdose in A&E, be aware of patients reporting they took 'poppers'.

FULL BLOOD COUNT AND RETICULOCYTE COUNT

Blood samples are collected in EDTA-lined sample tubes (see Chapter 6: Calcium chelation for samples). The samples are tested by an automated analyzer, which provides the following parameters:

- Hb concentration, haematocrit, red cell count, mean cell volume (MCV), mean cell haemoglobin (MCH) and mean cell haemoglobin concentration (MCHC)
- Red cell distribution width (RDW): a measure of size variability of the sampled population of red cells
- Total white cell count with differential
- Platelet count

Red cell parameters and the description terms used to describe abnormalities of the full blood count are given in Table 2.3. When interpreting results, be aware that the normal range will usually vary slightly depending on the population subgroup and the assessing laboratory.

PERIPHERAL BLOOD FILM

Examination of a peripheral blood film is a simple haematological investigation, which can provide an enormous amount of diagnostic information (Table 2.4). The blood sample is evenly spread across a glass slide, forming a film of blood on the glass. This is then dried and stained, usually with a Romanowsky stain. The blood film allows assessment of the morphology of blood cells and can show intracellular inclusions. A normal peripheral blood film is shown in Fig 2.11. A film stained with supravital stain (which precipitates intracellular RNA) is used to identify reticulocytes, which retain RNA (in contrast to mature red cells).

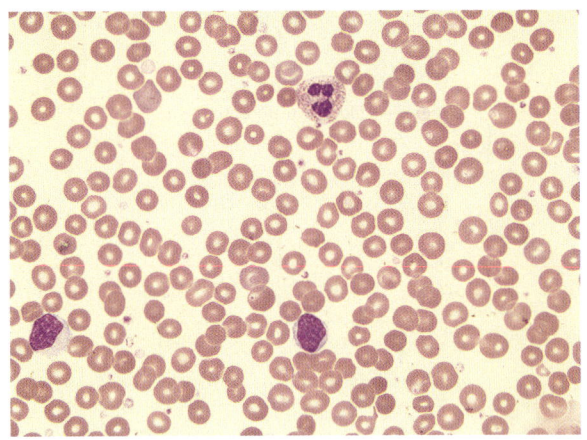

Fig. 2.11 Normal peripheral blood film (Romanowsky stain).

Table 2.3 Red cell parameters: diagnostic inference

Parameter	Normal range (adult male)	Elevation/reduction nomenclature
Red cell count	4.4–5.8 × 10^{12}/L	↑ Polycythaemia ↓ Anaemia
Haemoglobin concentration	13–17 g/dL (130–170 g/L)	↑ Polycythaemia ↓ Anaemia
Haematocrit (packed cell volume; Hct)	40%–51%	↑ Polycythaemia ↓ Anaemia
Mean cell volume (MCV)	80–100 fL	↑ Macrocytic ↓ Microcytic
Mean corpuscular haemoglobin (MCH)	27–32 pg	↓ hypochromic
Reticulocyte count	10–100 × 10^9/L 1%–2% of red cell population	↑ reticulocytosis ↓ reticulocytopenia

Table 2.4 Description of abnormalities of red cells that may be seen on the peripheral blood film

Abnormality	Description	Diagnostic inference
Anisocytosis	Increased variation in size, accompanied by increased RDW	Coexistence of microcytic and macrocytic with normal red cell populations. Combination of >1 disease process, marrow dysplasia
Poikilocytosis	Increased variation in shape	Variable, depending on the specific features of the poikilocyte
Spherocyte	Small, spherical cells (no area of central pallor discernible)	Hereditary spherocytosis, warm autoimmune haemolytic anaemia
Elliptocyte	Elliptically shaped cell	Hereditary elliptocytosis
Echinocyte	Cell with regular long outward projections from the surface	Renal disease
Acanthocyte	Cell with irregular outline	Liver disease, postsplenectomy, abetalipoproteinaemia, pyruvate kinase deficiency
Target cells	Central and peripheral dark staining zones seen separated by a paler area	Thalassaemia, sickle cell disease, iron deficiency (see Chapter 3), liver disease
Teardrop cells	Teardrop-shaped cells	Primary myelofibrosis (see Chapter 5), extramedullary haemopoiesis

Table 2.4 Description of abnormalities of red cells that may be seen on the peripheral blood film—cont'd

Abnormality	Description	Diagnostic inference
Schistocytes	Small fragments of nonintact cells	DIC, microangiopathic haemolytic anaemia (see Chapter 6), mechanical cardiac valve replacement
Polychromasia	Large blueish cells	Reticulocytosis
Rouleaux	Stacks of red cells (similar to piles of coins)	Multiple myeloma, Waldenström macroglobulinaemia (see Chapter 5), any cause of raised globulins
Heinz bodies	Precipitates of oxidized, denatured haemoglobin	Glucose-6-phosphate dehydrogenase deficiency (see Chapter 3)
Howell-Jolly bodies	Small nuclear inclusions	Hyposplenism, postsplenectomy
Basophilic RBC stippling	Small dots of rRNA at periphery. Sign of accelerated erythropoiesis of defective Hb.	Lead poisoning, megaloblastic anaemia, liver disease, myelodysplasia, haemoglobinopathies
Leucoerythroblastic (nucleated RBCs)	Nucleated RBCs, often with seen with primitive WBCs	Marrow infiltration (i.e., myelofibrosis, malignancy)
Reticulocytes	Immature RBCs, more visible with methylene blue stains on film	Normal range 0.5%–2.5% in adults. ↑ in haemolytic anaemias. ↓ with chemo or in aplastic anaemia
Stomatocytes	Central pallor of RBC is a rod-like shape	Hereditary stomatocytes, high alcohol intake or liver disease

DIC, Disseminated intravascular coagulation; Hb, haemoglobin; RBC, red blood cell; RDW, red cell distribution width; rRNA, ribosomal ribonucleic acid; WBC, white blood cell.

● Chapter summary

- Red blood cells (erythrocytes) have a biconcave discoid three-dimensional structure.
- This shape increases their surface area, optimizing them for their primary function of gas transfer.
- The protein haemoglobin allows binding of both oxygen and carbon dioxide with release at appropriate locations (peripheral tissues and the lungs, respectively).
- Haemoglobin contains haem as a component of its quaternary structure. Haem contains ferrous iron (Fe^{++}) and therefore iron metabolism has important consequences for red cell haemoglobin.
- Anaemia describes the clinical consequences of deficient haemoglobin concentration in the blood. Characteristic manifestations are related to reduced oxygen delivery to tissues, but also include skin, hair and nail abnormalities.
- The binding haemoglobin and oxygen alters at different environmental partial pressures of oxygen. This relationship is described by the oxygen dissociation curve.
- Erythropoiesis (development of erythrocytes from the haemopoietic stem cell) develops via several stages and is promoted by erythropoietin. Disorders of erythropoiesis occur in iron deficiency.
- The full blood count gives information about red cell concentration, size and haemoglobin concentration.
- A peripheral blood film identifies particular structural abnormalities associated with specific disease states and is a key diagnostic investigation in various red cell disorders as well as generalized systemic disorders.
- Red blood cells lack mitochondria, rendering their intracellular milieu anaerobic. They therefore rely on glycolysis as the sole metabolic pathway for ATP generation. Disorders of glycolysis enzymes therefore prominently affect red cell survival.

MLA Conditions
Haemochromatosis

MLA Presentations

ANAEMIA

Introduction

The term anaemia refers to a low level of haemoglobin (Hb) in the blood. This is defined as <130 g/L (males) or <120 g/L (females). As [Hb] falls, additional symptoms appear and become more severe. Symptoms arise due to impaired oxygen delivery to respiring tissues. This is because a reduced [Hb] results in a decrease in the oxygen-carrying capacity of the blood. Anaemia is caused by one or more of the following factors:

- Reduced or impaired red cell production
- Increased or accelerated red cell destruction
- Blood loss (acute or chronic)

CLINICAL NOTES

SYMPTOMS AND SIGNS OF ANAEMIA

Symptoms include fatigue, exertional breathlessness, palpitations, presyncope/syncope and headache. Signs include skin, conjunctival and mucous membrane pallor. A hyperdynamic cardiovascular response develops in response to the impaired oxygen delivery imposed by the overall reduction in oxygen carriage, typically seen in cases of a resting tachycardia and a new cardiac flow murmur.

Anaemia affects up to one-third of the global population. Specific underlying causes reflect local disease patterns, but the most common cause of anaemia (worldwide and in the UK) is iron deficiency. However, in the UK hospital population, anaemia secondary to chronic disease predominates. In developing countries, hookworm infestation-induced iron deficiency, malaria, human immunodeficiency virus (HIV) and tuberculosis (TB) are the most important causes.

Classification of anaemia

Mean cell volume

Types of anaemia are classified by the mean cell volume (MCV) of red cells, which is an important parameter within the full blood count. The MCV may be:

- Microcytic (MCV <80 fL) (Table 3.1)
- Normocytic (MCV 80–100 fL)
- Macrocytic (MCV >100 fL)

Mean cell haemoglobin

The mean cell haemoglobin (MCH) parameter quantifies the average mass (per red cell) of haemoglobin. It is calculated by dividing the total sample mass of Hb by the number of red cells in the sample. The normal range is 27 to 31 pg (per cell). Note that the value is usually given in pg, assuming that 'per cell' is intuitively understood.

The MCH usually correlates to the MCV, since a low volume (microcytic cell) typically contains a lower mass of Hb. The suffix 'chromic' is a semiquantitative descriptive term referring to the MCH. <27 pg/cell is hypochromic, 27 to 31 pg/cell is normochromic and >31 pg/cell is hyperchromic.

ANAEMIA SECONDARY TO HAEMATINIC DEFICIENCY

Haematinics is the descriptive term for nutrients required for normal synthesis and development of blood cells. Iron, folate and B12 are the most clinically significant haematinics; deficiency of any of these micronutrients results in anaemia. Common causes of haematinic deficiency are discussed in the following sections.

Iron-deficiency anaemia

If iron loss/utilization exceeds iron intake, iron stores are ultimately depleted, resulting in a microcytic (MCV <80 fL), hypochromic (MCH <27 pg) anaemia.

Iron deficiency may be caused by:

- Inadequate dietary iron intake (see Chapter 2: Iron metabolism)
- Impaired iron absorption (e.g., high intake of dietary iron-absorption inhibitors or a loss of parietal cell mass, e.g., postgastrectomy; see Chapter 2: Iron absorption)
- Loss of iron, for example, heavy menstrual periods and gastrointestinal (GI) bleeding

A relative iron deficiency may develop with normal iron intake and intact absorption when iron requirements are increased, for example:

- Growth (childhood and adolescence)
- Pregnancy
- Lactation

Symptoms and signs specifically associated with iron deficiency anaemia (IDA) include: angular stomatitis, diffuse hair loss/thinning, nail abnormalities (classically koilonychias:

Table 3.1 Diagnostic features of microcytic anaemia

FBC parameter	Iron deficiency	Anaemia of chronic disease	Thalassaemia	Sideroblastic anaemia
MCV	Reduced	Normal (2/3) Reduced (1/3)	Reduced (often disproportionately to the degree of ↓[Hb])	Low (congenital) Raised (acquired)
MCH	Reduced	Normal/mildly reduced	Normal	Raised
TIBC	Raised	Reduced/Normal	Normal	Normal
Serum (ferritin)	Low	Normal/raised	Normal	Raised
Transferrin saturation	Reduced	Reduced	Increased	Increased
Serum (transferrin)	Raised	Normal/low	Variable	Normal
Bone marrow iron stores	Absent	Present	Present	Increased

FBC, Full blood count; MCH, mean cell haemoglobin; MCV, mean cell volume; TIBC, total iron binding capacity.

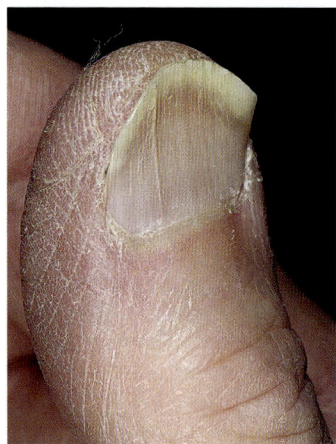

Fig. 3.1 Koilonychia – abnormally thin nails in IDA, which lose their convexity. (From Habif TP, ed. *Clinical Dermatology*, 4th ed. Philadelphia: Mosby; 2004:885.)

concavity of the nail plate) Fig. 3.1, neurocognitive and/or neuropsychiatric impairment, for example, depression.

IDA occurs frequently in females of reproductive age, due to menstrual blood loss. However, the other very important cause of iron deficiency is chronic blood loss from an insidious bleed inside the GI tract. Since 1 mL blood contains ~0.5 mg iron, it is easy to appreciate how an iron-deficient state could swiftly develop.

A slow bleeding ulcer of polyp in the GI tract can be concerning for GI malignancy (i.e., stomach or colon cancer), especially in the older male population. Therefore, it is very important to establish if a patient presenting with IDA has any overt signs of GI bleeding (such as a change in bowel habit, melaena or fresh per-rectum bleeding) as well constitutional symptoms of weight loss, loss of appetite, chronic fevers and night sweats.

Melaena refers to dark, sticky, almost tar-like stool which is associated with an upper GI bleed (oesophagus, stomach, small intestine). Its characteristic appearance and odour are a result of haemoglobin being digested and altered by GI enzymes as it travels through the GI tract.

CLINICAL TIP

BOWEL CANCER SCREENING

Bowel cancer is the fourth most common form of cancer and early diagnosis significantly improves survival outcomes. In the UK, we have a bowel cancer screening programme through faecal immunochemical testing (FIT). The public receive a home collection kit when they reach applicable age and can send back a small sample of their stool to be tested for small traces of blood. If they are FIT positive (blood was found in the stool), they will be highlighted for further investigations. Currently, those aged 60 to 74 are eligible for bowel cancer screening, with the NHS expanding this to include over 50s by 2025.

Haematological findings of iron deficiency

- [Hb] <130 g/L (male) or <120 g/L (female)
- Microcytic (↓ MCV), hypochromic (↓ MCH) red cells (Fig. 3.2)
- ↓ serum [iron] and [ferritin]
- ↑ serum [transferrin] and total iron-binding capacity
- ↓ plasma transferrin saturation
- Bone marrow smear shows absent iron stores
- Microcytic, hypochromic cells will be seen on a blood film. Pencil cells, elliptocytes and target cells may also be present (Fig. 3.2).

Management of iron deficiency anaemia

The underlying cause must be identified and treated in addition to providing iron supplementation.

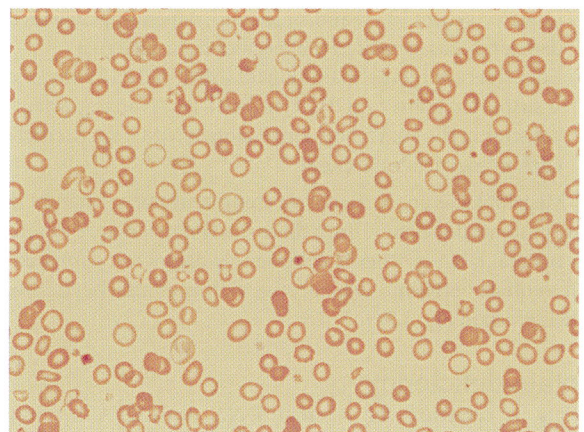

Fig. 3.2 Iron deficiency anaemia: blood film appearance. Notice overall reduction in concentration of red cells compared to normal blood film in Chapter 2, Fig. 2.11. Additionally, there is increased central pallor due to decreased Hb and more oddly shaped cells.

If there is suspicion of GI malignancy (either through signs and symptoms or via FIT test), further investigation is required to examine the GI tract for the site of bleeding. Patients will be offered a colonoscopy and/or gastroscopy – endoscopic camera tests. Gastroscopy (or OGD as commonly shortened to) visualizes the oesophagus, stomach up to the duodenum), whereas a colonoscopy examines the large bowel. If an abnormality is found (such as an ulcer or polyp), this can be biopsied (or resected in the case of polyps) for histological analysis for a definitive diagnosis. In some cases, patients are not suitable for the invasive nature of endoscopic procedures (i.e., frailty) in which instances clinicians may prefer to start with computed tomography (CT) alternatives.

Females presenting with IDA due to heavy or prolonged menstrual flow (menorrhagia) will likely require referral to gynaecology to ensure there is no additional underlying pathology (such as uterine fibroids or endometriosis). They may benefit from regulation of their menses through the oral contraceptive pill, however, this will require careful discussion of the associated benefits as well the side effect risks for the individual. Tranexamic acid (an antifibrinolytic) can also be used in short courses for menorrhagia.

Oral administration of iron is in the form of ferrous sulphate, fumarate or gluconate tablets. These must be taken every day for ≥3 months to replenish fully the body iron stores. Common side effects of oral iron supplementation include constipation, diarrhoea, abdominal cramps and dark faeces. Vitamin C is a strong enhancer of iron absorption and is recommended to be taken in conjunction with oral iron supplementation for maximum efficacy. Parenteral iron may be used if the patient has impaired GI absorption or is very intolerant to oral iron. This can be given in the form of iron infusions.

CLINICAL TIP

IV IRON

Dosage which is dependent patient weight, starting Hb and on the specific formulation of IV iron (there are three common forms in the UK: iron sucrose, iron dextran and ferric carboxymaltose). Care has to be taken not administered to pregnant females in the first trimester, those with active infections, or those without diuretic cover in fluid-restricted cardiac or renal failure patients. Side effects of IV iron include anaphylaxis, hypophosphatemia and nonanaphylactic hypersensitivity reactions (described as Fishbane reactions – these settle with stopping or slowing down of the infusions)

Megaloblastic anaemia

In megaloblastic anaemia, impaired DNA synthesis in erythroblasts manifests with abnormal maturation of the developing red cell precursors. These abnormal erythroblasts, situated in the bone marrow, are called megaloblasts. They are very large cells with retarded nuclear maturation. Megaloblasts are:

- Unable to generate sufficient mature red cell progeny (like normal erythroblasts)
- Destroyed by bone marrow macrophages

Overall, this results in ineffective erythropoiesis. The red cell progeny they do manage to create are macrocytic.

COMMON PITFALLS

MEGALOBLASTIC VERSUS MACROCYTIC ANAEMIA

Although megaloblastic anaemia is macrocytic (MCV >100 fL), the two terms have different meaning. Macrocytes are red cells with volume >100 fL. Megaloblasts are abnormal, giant red cell precursors with disproportionately large, immature nuclei, located in the bone marrow. All causes of megaloblastic anaemia will cause macrocytosis, but not all causes of macrocytic anaemia are due to megaloblastosis.

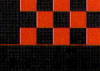

RED FLAG

FOLATE AND B12 COSUPPLEMENTATION

Folate and B12 supplements are coadministered. This is because without B12, all tetrahydrofolate eventually becomes trapped as a nonfunctional methylated compound. This compound cannot participate in the usual reactions and thus symptoms of folate deficiency manifest, even where folate intake and absorption are adequate! All B12 deficiency will therefore cause a functional folate deficiency, even if folate intake is sufficient. Replacement of folate in isolation without B12 coadministration will correct the megaloblastic anaemia but will allow neurological damage secondary to B12 deficiency to progress and become irreversible.

Haematological findings of megaloblastic anaemia

Haematological findings particular to megaloblastic anaemia include:

- Macrocytic anaemia (MCV >100 fL)
- Hypersegmentation of neutrophil nuclei (right shift)
- Megaloblasts visible on a bone marrow smear
- Coexisting leucopoenia +/− thrombocytopenia in severe cases
- Low red cell [folate] (in both B12 and folate deficiencies)

- Lowered serum [B12] and/or [folate], depending on which deficiency has provoked the megaloblastic anaemia
- Raised serum methylmalonic acid (MMA) if B12 deficiency is suspected but serum B12 is normal. B12 is an important cofactor in the enzymatic conversion of MMA to succinyl-CoA in the metabolic chain.

Megaloblastic anaemia is most commonly due to vitamin B12 and/or folate deficiency. Both these micronutrients are required for normal DNA synthesis. An example diagnostic approach to differentiate between the respective causes of macrocytic anaemia is given in Fig. 3.3.

Folate deficiency

Folate is required for normal DNA and RNA synthesis. Tetrahydrofolate (THF) is the bioactive form of folate. THF is required for purine and pyrimidine synthesis and thus for RNA and DNA synthesis. Since the requirement for THF is greatest in rapidly dividing cells, where the greatest rate of DNA replication and protein synthesis occurs, this population of cells is the first to manifest the consequences of deficiency.

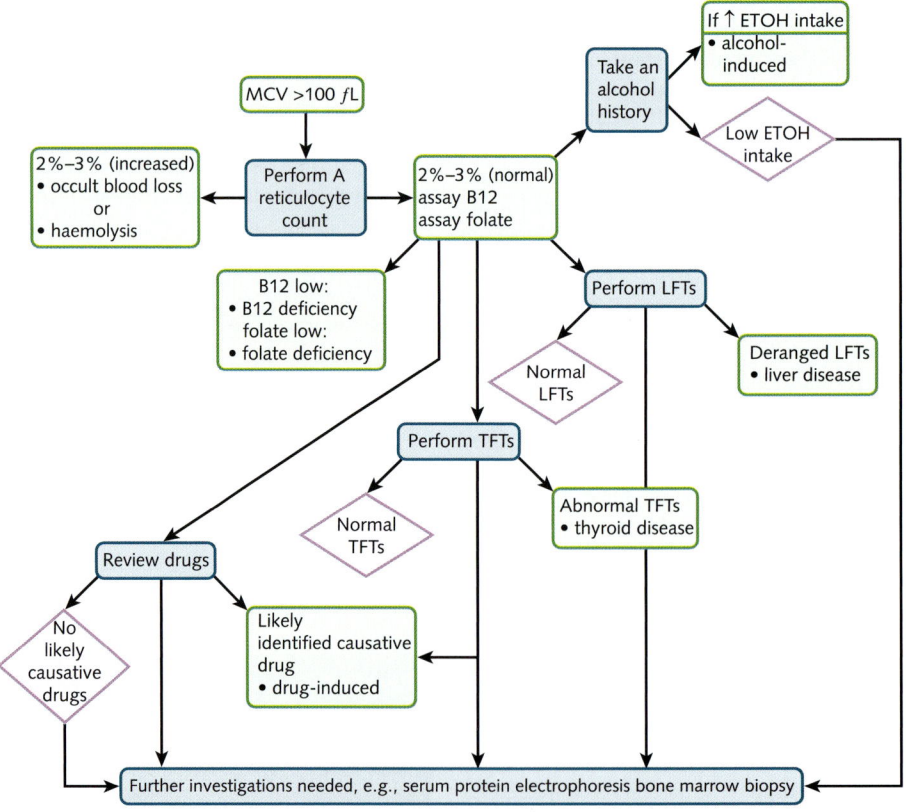

Fig. 3.3 Diagnostic approach to macrocytic anaemia (MCV >100 fL). *ETOH*, Ethanol; *LFTs*, liver function tests; *MCV*, mean cell volume; *TFTs*, thyroid function tests.

Early symptoms of folate deficiency are related to the macrocytic anaemia, which is also megaloblastic. In addition, angular stomatitis, glossitis and neuropsychiatric deficits are reported in severe, prolonged deficiency. Serum [folate] or red cell [folate] are used as biomarkers of folate status, the latter being more representative of long-term status. However, serum [folate] is the more discriminating investigation, since red cell [folate] is lowered in B12 deficiency even if folate stores are replete. Folate deficiency is treated with oral folate supplementation accompanied by B12 supplements.

Folate metabolism

Folate (vitamin B9) is a water-soluble vitamin that is abundant in a wide variety of foods. It is stored in the liver and absorption occurs in the duodenum and jejunum. Unlike vitamin B12, vitamin B9 stores are small relative to daily requirements. Megaloblastic anaemia therefore develops more rapidly (within a few months) of sustained inadequate folate intake.

Causes of folate deficiency can be grouped into: insufficient intake, excessive loss, abnormal THF activation or increased folate demand (rendering a normally sufficient intake insufficient) (Table 3.2). Alcohol excess is particularly effective at inducing folate deficiency, since all the risk factors for deficiency typically coexist in alcoholics.

Vitamin B12 deficiency

The bioactive vitamin B12 derivatives are 5′-deoxyadenosylcobalamin and methylcobalamin.

Table 3.2 Folate deficiency: causative mechanisms

Mechanism	Examples
Decreased folate intake	Decreased dietary intake of folate (usually due to generalized malnutrition) Impaired GI absorption due to diseases of malabsorption Impaired GI absorption due to drugs (e.g., phenytoin)
Increased loss	Haemodialysis
Increased folate requirement due to high rates of cell division: a usually adequate intake is insufficient in these contexts	Growth (childhood and adolescence) Pregnancy and lactation Cancer Haemolytic anaemia
Abnormal bioactivation of folate: despite adequate intake/absorption, THF formation is impaired with all the functional consequences of folate deficiency	Vitamin B12 deficiency Dihydrofolate reductase inhibitors: trimethoprim, methotrexate Antifolate metabolites: sulphasalazine

GI, Gastrointestinal; THF, tetrahydrofolate.

Methylcobalamin

In B12 deficiency, there will always be a functional folate deficiency, even if total body folate stores are replete. This phenomenon arises because the regeneration of THF, the bioactive form of folate, is reliant on a B12-dependent enzyme (methionine synthase).

5′-deoxyadenosylcobalamin

Vitamin B12 is also essential for normal fatty acid synthesis. Odd-chain fatty acid synthesis requires 5′-deoxyadenosylcobalamin as a cofactor. Neuronal myelination demands a continuous supply of fatty acids to maintain the myelin sheath integrity (due to constant myelin turnover). Disintegration of the myelin sheath therefore occurs in the context of reduced availability of 5′-deoxyadenosylcobalamin (secondary to B12 deficiency). This mechanism accounts for the neurological symptoms associated with B12 deficiency. These neurological features usually manifest insidiously and much later than the symptoms and signs of the megaloblastic anaemia. They include:

- Peripheral paraesthesia and numbness
- Myelopathy: ascending distal motor weakness, gait disturbance
- Progressive cognitive deficit, depression

The combination of neurological symptoms due to degeneration of the posterior and lateral columns within the spinal cord is termed 'subacute combined degeneration of the spinal cord'. Patients can recover remarkably with adequate B12 replacement, however, prolonged deficiency can lead to irreversible damage.

Nonneurological symptoms include anorexia, glossitis, angular stomatitis and constipation. Treatment is with oral or parenteral vitamin B12.

Causes of B12 deficiency include:

- Inadequate dietary intake – dietary vitamin B12 is almost exclusively obtained from animal-derived food products, thus veganism confers a risk of deficiency if appropriate supplements are not taken regularly
- Inability to separate B12 from its protein-bound dietary form (food cobalamin malabsorption)
- IF deficiency (congenital, pernicious anaemia or postgastrectomy)
- Intestinal malabsorption, particularly if affecting the terminal ileum (where the bulk of IF-bound B12 is absorbed)
- Blind loop or diverticulae in the small bowel, which breed bacteria that avidly consume B12

Alcohol excess and dependence can often result in B12, folate and other vitamin deficiencies due to the relative lack of normal diet.

Because endogenous B12 stores are sizable and urinary/faecal daily loss is small, the symptoms/signs of deficiency may occur up to 2 years after dietary intake becomes inadequate.

Pernicious anaemia

Pernicious anaemia is the most common cause of nondietary B12 deficiency. It is an autoimmune phenomenon, typically secondary to antibody-mediated gastric parietal cell destruction (causing failure of intrinsic factor secretion, which is the enzyme responsible for binding and internalizing B12 from the gut lumen), but the cellular B12 transporter (cubilin) or transcobalamin-bound B12 are also potential auto-antibody targets.

Classically, in addition to the anaemic, neurological and mucosal symptoms, premature greying/whitening of the hair is seen when B12 deficiency arises due to pernicious anaemia and a lemon-yellow pallor is used to describe the combination of mild jaundice (ineffective erythropoiesis→increased red cell fragility and haemolysis) and anaemia-induced pallor.

Current diagnosis of pernicious anaemia

Historically pernicious anaemia was investigated with the Schilling test, in which radiolabelled B12 was injected and consumed and subsequently measured in the urine. However, due to the obvious hazard of using radioactive materials, it is no longer used.

In clinical practice, the diagnosis is made if specific autoantibodies (anti-IF or antiparietal cell antibodies) are present where serum [B12] is reduced. Be aware, however, that despite high specificity, the sensitivity of the IF autoantibody test is only ~70%. Antiparietal cell autoantibodies have even lower sensitivity and are also poorly specific, since they are often raised in gastritis.

Food cobalamin malabsorption

This is a common cause of B12 deficiency in the elderly. Many varied causes leading to achlorhydria such as drugs (antacids, H2 receptor blockers, proton pump inhibitors), *Helicobacter pylori* infection or atrophic gastritis render the gastric luminal pH too high for effective protease action. Dietary B12 thus remains complexed with dietary protein and cannot be absorbed. Pancreatic insufficiency of any cause leads to failure of protease secretion, with the same effect. Note that oral B12 supplementation corrects B12 deficiency secondary to food cobalamin malabsorption, since the downstream processes following protease-mediated separation of B12 from dietary protein are intact.

Metformin use

Chronic biguanide (e.g., metformin) use in type 2 diabetics is a known cause of B12 deficiency. Biguanides interfere with the calcium-dependent absorption of the B12-IF complex at terminal ileal enterocytes.

ANAEMIA OF CHRONIC DISEASE

This is the most common type of anaemia seen in hospital patients and in the elderly. It is associated with chronic inflammatory and malignant disease. The mechanism underlying the anaemia of chronic disease is complex, but it is believed to include:

- Inflammatory cytokine-induced (e.g., interleukin 1, TNF) suppression of erythropoietin (EPO)-mediated erythropoiesis.
- Inflammatory increase in hepcidin. Hepcidin decreases iron exporter expression, impairing the release of iron stores (necessary for erythropoiesis) by bone marrow macrophages, causing functional iron deficiency (which can be corrected with IV iron).

Whatever the mechanism, anaemia of chronic disease results in reduced red cell production. Two-thirds of cases are normocytic and normochromic, although approximately one-third of cases exhibit instead a microcytic hypochromic anaemia. The anaemia is unresponsive to iron therapy and is corrected only by treatment of the underlying cause. EPO can in some cases help to increase erythrocyte production (but it is rarely used).

Chronic renal failure

Chronic renal failure is almost always associated with anaemia. A decrease in functional renal tissue results in reduced EPO synthesis, EPO being produced by interstitial cells in the renal cortex. The anaemia is typically normochromic and normocytic. It is treated with regular EPO injections, and IV iron is often of benefit to treat functional iron deficiency.

ANAEMIA DUE TO BLOOD LOSS

Like the anaemia of chronic disease, anaemia secondary to blood loss may be normocytic or microcytic.

Acute blood loss

Common causes of acute blood loss include trauma, surgery, obstetric haemorrhage and GI, urinary or pulmonary tract loss.

The plasma lost during haemorrhage is typically restored within ~48 hours. Initially, restoration is due to redistribution of extracellular fluid intravascularly and later increased fluid intake and endocrine homeostasis. However, it takes several weeks for the lost red cells (and therefore the [Hb]) to be replaced to normal levels.

Haematological findings in acute blood loss include:

- Normocytic, normochromic anaemia
- Reticulocytosis, peaking 1 to 2 weeks post haemorrhage
- ↑ platelet and neutrophil counts
- Following significant haemorrhage, neutrophil precursors are seen in peripheral blood (left shift)

It is important to appreciate that during or immediately after blood loss, parameters such as the red cell count (which is expressed as a concentration) will be normal. This is because both plasma and red cells have been lost in the same proportions as they are present in the blood. Do not be falsely reassured by a normal [Hb] in the context of known or likely blood loss. The levels will not fall until significant early intravascular volume restoration occurs, since the readings show actual concentrations rather than absolute levels. For details on management of acute blood loss, see Chapter 7: Transfusion – Massive haemorrhage.

MICROCYTIC ANAEMIA: OTHER CAUSES

Fig. 3.4 provides a diagnostic approach to microcytic anaemia. Rare causes of microcytic anaemia include:

- Thalassaemia. These defects of globin synthesis are discussed in the later sections on types of thalassaemia.
- Sideroblastic anaemia (hereditary or acquired). This is a hypochromic anaemia characterized by the presence of ring sideroblasts and increased iron stores in the bone marrow. Ring sideroblasts are abnormal red-cell precursors with a halo of iron granules around the nucleus. Some subtypes respond to vitamin B6 supplementation (B6 is a cofactor for ferrochelatase, which mediates the final iron-incorporation reaction of haem synthesis). Fig. 3.5M
- Lead poisoning, which inhibits both haem and globin synthesis. It may cause a baffling array of diverse symptoms and signs accompanied by a microcytic anaemia. Basophilic stippling of red cells on the peripheral blood film is seen in lead poisoning. Fig. 3.5E.

MICROCYTIC ANAEMIA

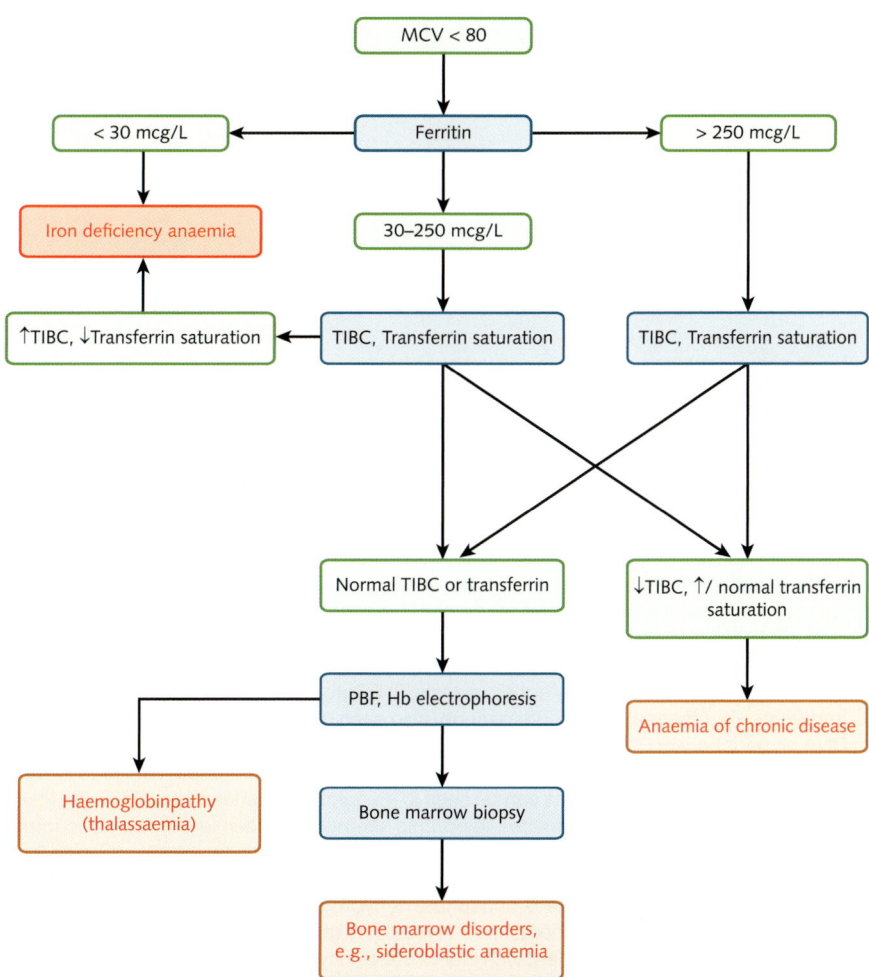

Fig. 3.4 Diagnostic approach to microcytic anaemia (MCV <80 fL). *MCV,* Mean cell volume; *TIBC,* total iron binding capacity.

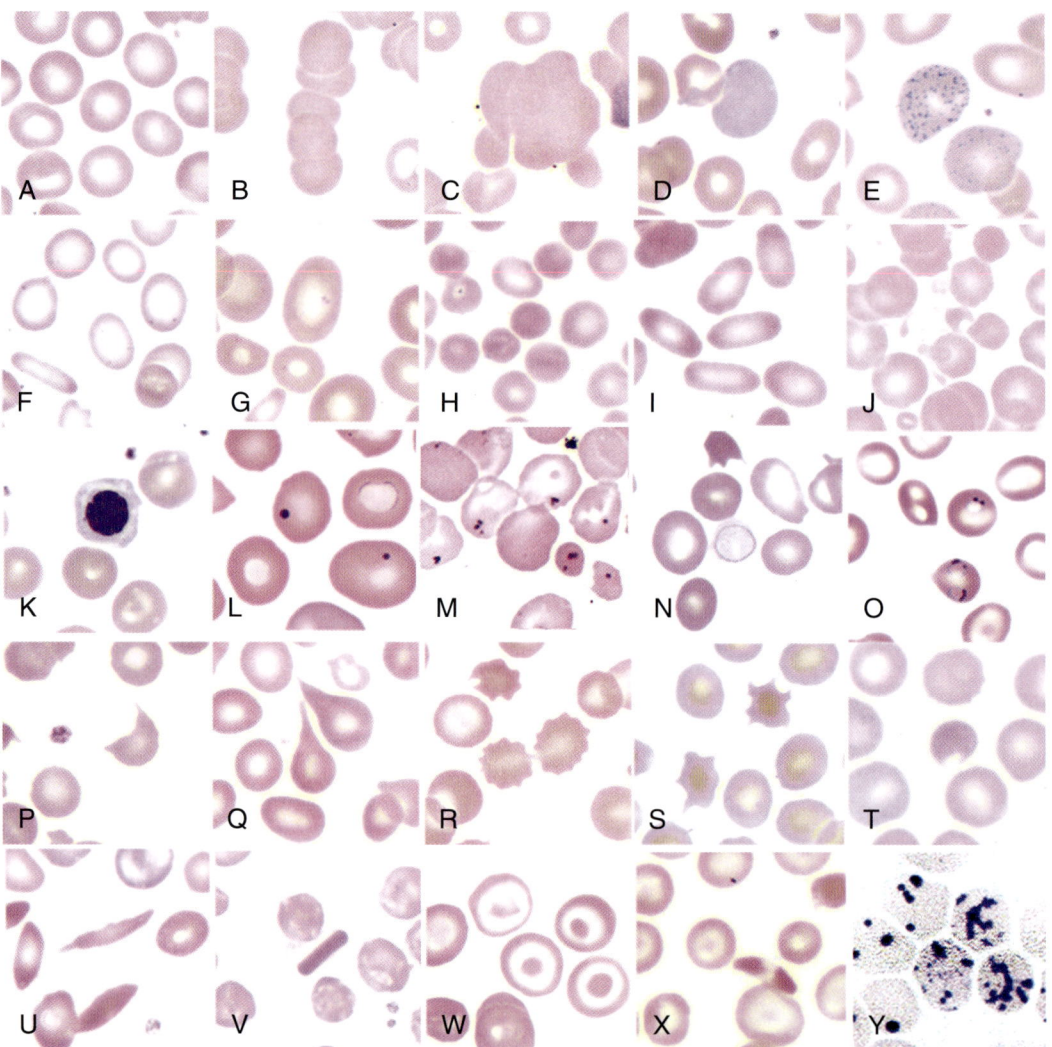

Fig. 3.5 Useful peripheral blood and red blood cell features in the evaluation of anaemia. (A) Normal red blood cells (RBCs). (B) Rouleaux formation, seen in states of increased plasma protein such as myeloma. (C) Agglutination as seen in antibody-mediated process such as cold agglutinin disease. (D) Polychromatophilic cell. The grey–blue colour is attributable to RNA and the cell is equivalent to a reticulocyte. (E) Basophilic stippling, deposits of denatured RNA remnants, seen in lead toxicity. (F) Hypochromic microcytic cells, typical of iron-deficiency anaemia. (G) Macroovalocyte, seen in either megaloblastic anaemia or myelodysplastic syndrome. (H) Microspherocytes as seen in hereditary spherocytosis. (I) Elliptocytes as seen in patients with hereditary elliptocytosis. (J) RBC fragments from thermal injury (burn patient), also seen in haemolysis. (K) Nucleated RBC. (L) Howell-Jolly bodies, single body of DNA on periphery of RBC. Usually cleared by the spleen, hence seen in splenic dysfunction or postsplenectomy. (M) Pappenheimer bodies from a patient with sideroblastic anaemia. Appear similar to Howell-Jolly bodies, but are abnormal iron granules, not DNA. (N) Cabot ring, as can be seen in megaloblastic anaemia or MDS. (O) Malarial parasites (*Plasmodium falciparum*). (P) Schistocyte typical of a microangiopathic haemolytic anaemia. (Q) Tear-drop form indicates marrow fibrosis and extramedullary haematopoiesis. (R) Echinocyte (Burr cell) with rounded edges. (S) Acanthocyte (spur cell) with more irregular pointed ends. Can be seen in pyruvate kinase deficiency. They can also be seen in patients with liver disease and lipid abnormalities. (T) 'Bite' cell from a patient with glucose-6-phosphate dehydrogenase (G6PD) deficiency. (U) Sickle cell, from a patient with homozygous sickle cell disease. (V) Haemoglobin C crystal. (W) Target cells, seen in iron deficiency anaemia. (X) Haemoglobin C disease. (Y) Heinz bodies, in a patient with G6PD deficiency. (From Hoffman R. *Hematology: Basic Principles and Practice*. 7th ed. Philadelphia, PA: 2018; Elsevier.)

HAEMOLYTIC ANAEMIA

Haemolytic anaemia occurs when red cell lifespan is shortened due to accelerated destruction. Low [Hb] leads to tissue hypoxia, provoking an increase in EPO synthesis (up to sevenfold!). This promotes a compensatory accelerated erythropoiesis. This may succeed in restoring and maintaining a normal [Hb]; as long as the increased destruction is matched by the increased synthesis, anaemia is prevented and symptoms do not develop.

Causes of haemolysis

A shortened lifespan (<120 days) may arise due to intrinsic defects (typically hereditary) of erythrocyte structure or function. Alternatively, several particular environmental conditions (extracorpuscular features) may result in premature destruction of the red cells. Table 3.3 gives various examples, categorized by underlying causative mechanisms, that is, intrinsic or extracorpuscular.

Laboratory findings in haemolysis

Haemolysis is suggested by:

- ↑ serum bilirubin (unconjugated) – and consequent jaundice
- ↑ urinary urobilinogen and faecal stercobilinogen
- ↑ serum lactate dehydrogenase

Table 3.3 Examples of specific causes of haemolytic anaemia classified by underlying mechanism

Main mechanism	Submechanism
Intrinsic erythrocyte defects	**Defective metabolism:** G6PD deficiency, PK deficiency **Defective membrane structure:** Hereditary spherocytosis, hereditary elliptocytosis **Defective haemoglobin structure:** Sickle cell disease, thalassaemia
Environmental (extracorpuscular) causes	**Immune:** Haemolytic transfusion reactions, haemolytic disease of the newborn Autoimmune: (warm or cold) haemolytic anaemia, drug-induced immune haemolysis **Infectious:** Falciparum malaria, clostridia species, generalized septicaemia **Mechanical:** Mechanical cardiac valves, MAHA, extreme repetitive impact exercise Hypersplenism: (see Chapter 1: Hypersplenism) **Drug-related:** Dapsone, sulfasalazine

G6PD, Glucose-6-phosphate dehydrogenase (see Glucose-6-phosphate dehydrogenase deficiency section); MAHA, microangiopathic haemolytic anaemia (see Microangiopathic haemolysis section); PK, pyruvate kinase (see Pyruvate kinase deficiency section).

- ↓ or absent haptoglobins
- Reticulocytosis on blood film (apparent ↑ MCV on full blood count). The film may also show polychromasia (in keeping with reticulocytosis), spherocytes (in immune-mediated haemolysis) or schistocytes (in microangiopathic haemolysis) (Fig. 3.5D)
- Folate deficiency (excessive folate consumption due to DNA synthesis during rapid cell division of upregulated erythropoiesis)
- Erythroid hyperplasia (within bone marrow) → marrow cavity expansion

Classification of haemolysis

Haemolysis is typically classified into intravascular and extravascular, depending on the physiological location of the haemolysis.

Extravascular haemolysis

Extravascular haemolysis refers to an enhanced rate of the normal red cell breakdown process, that is, by reticuloendothelial macrophages (in the spleen, bone marrow and liver). Extravascular haemolysis tends to be less severe and progress more gradually than intravascular haemolysis.

Intravascular haemolysis

Intravascular haemolysis is the destruction of red cells within the circulatory system. Intravascular haemolysis exhibits all the laboratory findings listed above (in common with extravascular haemolysis), but in addition:

- Free serum Hb is elevated (haemoglobinaemia) with the following clinical consequences:
  - Hb appears in the urine once serum Hb exceeds renal tubular resorption capacity
  - Haemosiderin (an iron storage protein) appears in the urine
- Methaemalbuminaemia: free Hb is oxidized (→MetHb) and binds to serum albumin

ANTIBODY-MEDIATED HAEMOLYSIS

The following sections describe antibody-mediated mechanisms responsible for haemolytic anaemia.

Autoimmune haemolytic anaemia

In autoimmune haemolytic anaemia (AIHA), antibodies against red cell antigens result in the haemolytic destruction of red cells bearing the relevant antigen. A positive direct antigen test (DAT or Coombs test) is seen. There are three types of AIHA:

1. Warm AIHA, where haemolysis usually occurs at body temperature

2. Cold AIHA, where haemolysis usually occurs below core body temperature
3. Paroxysmal cold haemoglobinuria

Warm AIHA

Warm AIHA may be idiopathic or secondary to autoimmune disease or malignancy. Particular diseases carrying a high probability of secondary warm AIHA include systemic lupus erythematosus (SLE), leukaemia and lymphomas. Certain drugs are known to provoke warm AIHA (e.g., mefenamic acid). In addition to the usual anaemia and jaundice associated with haemolysis, mild splenomegaly frequently occurs.

The underlying cause (if identified) should be treated, in addition to the management of the haemolysis itself. Patients generally respond well to steroids (which require slow tapering over months) but other immunosuppressive therapies such as the monoclonal antibody rituximab (anti-CD20, see Chapter 5 for details) or splenectomy are beneficial in relapsing cases. Severe warm AIHA of acute onset, may require IV steroids with additional intravenous immunoglobulin (IVIG).

Cold AIHA

Cold AIHA may be idiopathic or secondary to lymphoma, leukaemia or infection. Certain infections (e.g., mycoplasma pneumonia, Epstein-Barr virus) are particularly likely to provoke a cold AIHA. The clinical features, which are exacerbated by cold temperatures, include:

- Raynaud phenomenon (peripheral localized vasospasm, which may lead to ischaemic damage of tissues)
- Acrocyanosis (purplish discolouration of the skin) due to vascular sludging secondary to red-cell agglutination

Treatment involves avoidance of cold environments, as well as aggressive management of the underlying provoking disease (if identified). Unlike warm AIHA, steroids are ineffective in Cold AIHA. Rituximab is effective in idiopathic cold AIHA and cold AIHA associated with B-lymphoproliferative diseases. Rituximab may be combined with cytotoxic agents to reduce the likelihood of relapse. Unlike warm AIHA, cold AIHA largely causes intravascular haemolysis (Table 3.4) driven by complement activation. Eculizumab, C5 inhibitor, has shown efficacy in cold AIHA and may be seen more widely in the clinical setting.

Cold AIHA – transfuse blood using a blood warmer system, otherwise cold blood from the fridge will only lead to more haemolysis!

Paroxysmal cold haemoglobinuria

Paroxysmal cold haemoglobinuria (PCH) is a rare condition, usually presenting with acute haemolysis in childhood following a viral infection. It is a subset of cold AIHA. However, while haemolysis occurs at body temperature, the antibody–red cell interaction only occurs at cold temperatures in vitro. This antibody behaviour is diagnostic (the Donath-Landsteiner test). PCH is usually self-limiting, but in cases of life-threatening haemolysis supportive red cell transfusion (via a blood warmer) is employed. The patient should be kept warm, preferably at an ambient temperature of 37°C. Table 3.4 details the laboratory findings associated with the various AIHAs.

Drug-induced immune haemolytic anaemia

Certain drugs (e.g., penicillin, cephalosporin and fludarabine) are established precipitants of haemolysis. Individual specific mechanisms vary with the precipitant.

Alloimmune haemolytic anaemia

Alloimmune haemolytic anaemia is caused by a reaction between the patient's antibodies and donor blood cells following transfusion or transplant, for example:

- Transfusion of ABO-incompatible blood (typically IgM-mediated)
- Transfer of maternal antibodies across the placenta to the foetus (haemolytic disease in newborn)
- Allogeneic transplantation (including stem cell or organ transplants)

Refer to Chapter 7: Transfusion products for more details.

Table 3.4 Laboratory findings in autoimmune haemolytic anaemia

	Warm AIHA	Cold AIHA	PCH
Antibody type	IgG	IgM	IgG
Antigen targeted	Rh factor	L or I antigens	P antigen
Antibody binding temperature	37°C	<32°C	<32°C
Red cell agglutination	No	Yes	Yes
Complement fixation	No	Yes	Yes
Haemolysis mechanism	Mainly extravascular	Mainly intravascular	Mainly intravascular
Direct antigen test (Coomb test)	+ ve for IgG and complement	+ ve for complement	+ ve for IgG and complement

AIHA, Autoimmune haemolytic anaemia; Ig, immunoglobulin; PCH, paroxysmal cold haemoglobinuria; Rh, Rhesus.

INTRINSIC RED CELL DEFECTS CAUSING HAEMOLYSIS

Defects intrinsic to red cell structure or metabolism can lead to haemolysis and characteristic morphological abnormalities are often apparent on the blood film.

Cytoskeletal defects

Hereditary spherocytosis

Hereditary spherocytosis (HS) is an autosomal dominant disorder with variable penetrance. Clinical presentation ranges from asymptomatic to significant jaundice at birth. A typical disease course would be a low-grade anaemia with fluctuating haemolysis and jaundice. Splenomegaly may be present.

HS is relatively common (prevalence 1:2000 in Northern Europeans). A defective cytoskeletal protein, most commonly spectrin, impairs membrane integrity. This causes progressive spherification of the red cell, with marked reduction in flexibility. The spherocytes are visible on a blood film (Fig. 3.5H) and classically demonstrate increased osmotic fragility in hypotonic solutions (the historical osmotic fragility membrane test). The haemolysis of HS is defined as extravascular, since premature removal of spherocytic red cells occurs in the spleen, where the microcirculation is too tortuous for poorly flexible cells to successfully pass through.

Hereditary elliptocytosis

This autosomal dominant disorder arises as a result of an abnormality of the spectrin protein, which impedes normal tetramer formation from spectrin dimers. Clinical and laboratory findings are as for HS, however the film appearance differs (elliptocytes have a more elongated appearance), Fig. 3.5I. However, patients with elliptocytosis typically experience less severe symptoms. Membrane disorders are now diagnosed with EMA (eosin 5′ maleimide) binding test.

Enzyme defects

Pyruvate kinase deficiency

This rare autosomal recessive condition impairs glycolysis, which represents the sole source of adenosine triphosphate (ATP) synthesis in red cells. The earliest manifestation of insufficient ATP is structural rigidity, which significantly increases the probability of red cell removal by the spleen as they traverse the splenic filtration beds. The haemolysis of pyruvate kinase (PK) is thus designated as extravascular. Splenectomy improves the anaemia by removing the main mechanism of red cell destruction. PK-induced anaemia varies widely in severity and thus depending upon the severity, affected individuals may be asymptomatic or present with jaundice at birth. Diagnosis is suggested by the film appearance (poikilocytosis and acanthocytes are seen) and confirmed by direct enzyme assay (Fig. 3.5S).

Glucose-6-phosphate dehydrogenase deficiency

Glucose-6-phosphate dehydrogenase (G6PD) deficiency is an X-linked disorder affecting the pentose phosphate pathway. There are numerous variants of G6PD deficiency, two of which account for the vast majority of cases: the African and Mediterranean subtypes. Of these two, the Mediterranean type is clinically more serious, because the abnormal enzyme's functional impairment is more extreme. Patients with G6PD deficiency usually remain asymptomatic unless exposed to oxidative stress, for example:

- Infection
- Acidosis, for example, critical illness, diabetic ketoacidosis
- Certain drugs
- Broad (fava) beans: favism (Mediterranean subtype only)
- Moth balls

Such oxidant stresses increase red cell reliance on $NADPH + H^+$ to ensure adequate glutathione regeneration. However, in G6PD deficiency intracellular $[NADPH + H^+]$ is reduced, as a result of failure of the pentose phosphate pathway. Oxidative damage accumulates more rapidly, shortening the lifespan of the cell.

Haemolysis of G6PD deficiency is primarily intravascular. During oxidative stress-induced haemolysis, Heinz bodies (precipitates of oxidized, denatured Hb) form intracellularly; see Fig. 3.5Y The spleen usually removes Heinz bodies, leaving structural damage to the red cell (bite or blister cells). Heinz bodies and bite/blister cells are apparent on a blood film; however, the film can be normal in an asymptomatic patient. Direct enzyme assay is diagnostic, but cautious interpretation is necessary if samples are taken during or immediately after a haemolytic crisis when reticulocytosis will confound the assay (reticulocytes have much higher enzyme levels than mature erythrocytes). Avoidance or prompt treatment of any precipitating factors (with red cell transfusion and circulatory support if necessary) is the priority in treating a haemolytic crisis in these patients. There is no specific curative treatment. All patients with haemolysis should be commenced on folic acid supplementation.

CLINICAL TIP

COMMON DRUGS THAT CAUSE OXIDATIVE STRESS AND CAN TRIGGER A HAEMOLYTIC CRISIS IN G6PD DEFICIENCY

- Aspirin – analgesic and antiplatelet liberally used in treatment and prevention of ischaemic heart disease and ischaemic strokes.

- Primaquine – be aware of those on malaria treatment or travellers on prophylaxis.
- Dapsone – antibiotic used in the treatment of dermatitis herpetiformis (be aware of those with celiac disease) and leprosy.
- Sulphonamides – antimicrobials such as sulphamethoxazole (second component alongside trimethoprim in co-trimoxazole, commonly used to treat *Pneumocystis* pneumonia.

Other enzyme defects

Several other defects have been identified in enzymes involved in erythrocyte metabolism. They are very rare and include hexokinase and glutathione synthetase deficiencies.

OTHER CAUSES OF HAEMOLYSIS

Various additional causes of haemolysis exist. A useful diagnostic approach to haemolysis is given in Fig. 3.6.

Microangiopathic haemolysis

Microangiopathic haemolytic anaemia (MAHA) occurs when fibrin is deposited in small vessels. Red cell haemolysis occurs due to shearing and collision with obstructing fibrin strands. The traumatic red cell destruction provides a pathognomonic blood film appearance with red cell fragments (schistocytes). Occurrence of MAHA usually indicates a serious underlying disorder. Common causes include haemolytic uraemic syndrome (HUS), thrombotic thrombocytopenic purpura (TTP), disseminated intravascular coagulation (DIC) of any cause (septicaemia, disseminated carcinoma), malignant hypertension and preeclampsia/eclampsia microangiopathic haemolytic anaemia later in this chapter. Rarely, MAHA is seen in patients with metallic heart valves, where it may indicate valvular dysfunction. These conditions are covered later in detail in Chapter 6: Haemostasis.

Infections

Falciparum malaria may cause both intravascular and extravascular haemolysis, because parasitized red cells are both destroyed within the circulation and removed by the spleen. Blackwater fever is the term used to describe acute kidney injury secondary to haemoglobinaemia in the context of falciparum malaria. The term refers to passing of very dark/black urine secondary to haemoglobinuria.

Mechanical

Physical trauma to red cells within the circulation may cause traumatic destruction of red cells. Mechanical cardiac valves are the classic cause.

Toxins

Copper toxicity in Wilson disease may provoke haemolytic anaemia. Lead, chloral and arsine cause severe haemolysis. Certain drugs (e.g., dapsone and sulphasalazine) cause oxidative damage resulting in haemolysis.

Burns

Severe, extensive burns lead to red cell damage in the disrupted burn zone microvasculature. Acanthosis and spherocytosis may be seen on the blood film.

Exercise

March haemoglobinuria is caused by damage to red cells in the feet during long periods of repetitive weight-bearing exercise, for example, walking or running. The blood film does not show fragments, spherocytes or pathognomonic abnormalities.

Paroxysmal nocturnal haemoglobinuria

Paroxysmal nocturnal haemoglobinuria (PNH) is an acquired bone marrow stem cell disorder caused by expansion of an abnormal haemopoietic stem cell clone harbouring the phosphatidylinositol glycan protein A (PIG-A) mutation on the X chromosome. Mutant PIG-A leads to absent/deficient glycosyl phosphatidylinositol (GPI) synthesis. GPI plays an important role: it anchors immunoprotective proteins (e.g., CD55 and CD59 proteins) to the cell membrane. These proteins normally protect the red cell from complement-induced cell lysis. Absence of surface CD55 and CD59 results in a chronic, intravascular red cell haemolysis with constant haemosiderinuria, anaemia, jaundice and fatigue. Secondary iron deficiency requiring supplementation often occurs.

Since the abnormality is present in a haemopoietic cell, complications related to cytopenia of other cell lineages derived from the same clone (e.g., leucopoenia and thrombocytopenia, pancytopenia, aplastic anaemia) may also occur in addition to the haemolytic anaemia.

Several other features also characterize PNH:

- Morning haemoglobinuria – intravascular haemolysis especially at night.
- Recurrent thrombosis: both arterial and venous including at unusual sites (despite a typically low platelet count). This warrants lifelong anticoagulation and is a key feature of the disease.
- Renal impairment: this may be due to renal vein thrombosis or acute tubular necrosis (secondary to haemoglobinuria).
- Budd-Chiari syndrome – liver enzyme derangement, abdominal pain, ascites and hepatomegaly due to thrombosis and occlusion of hepatic veins.

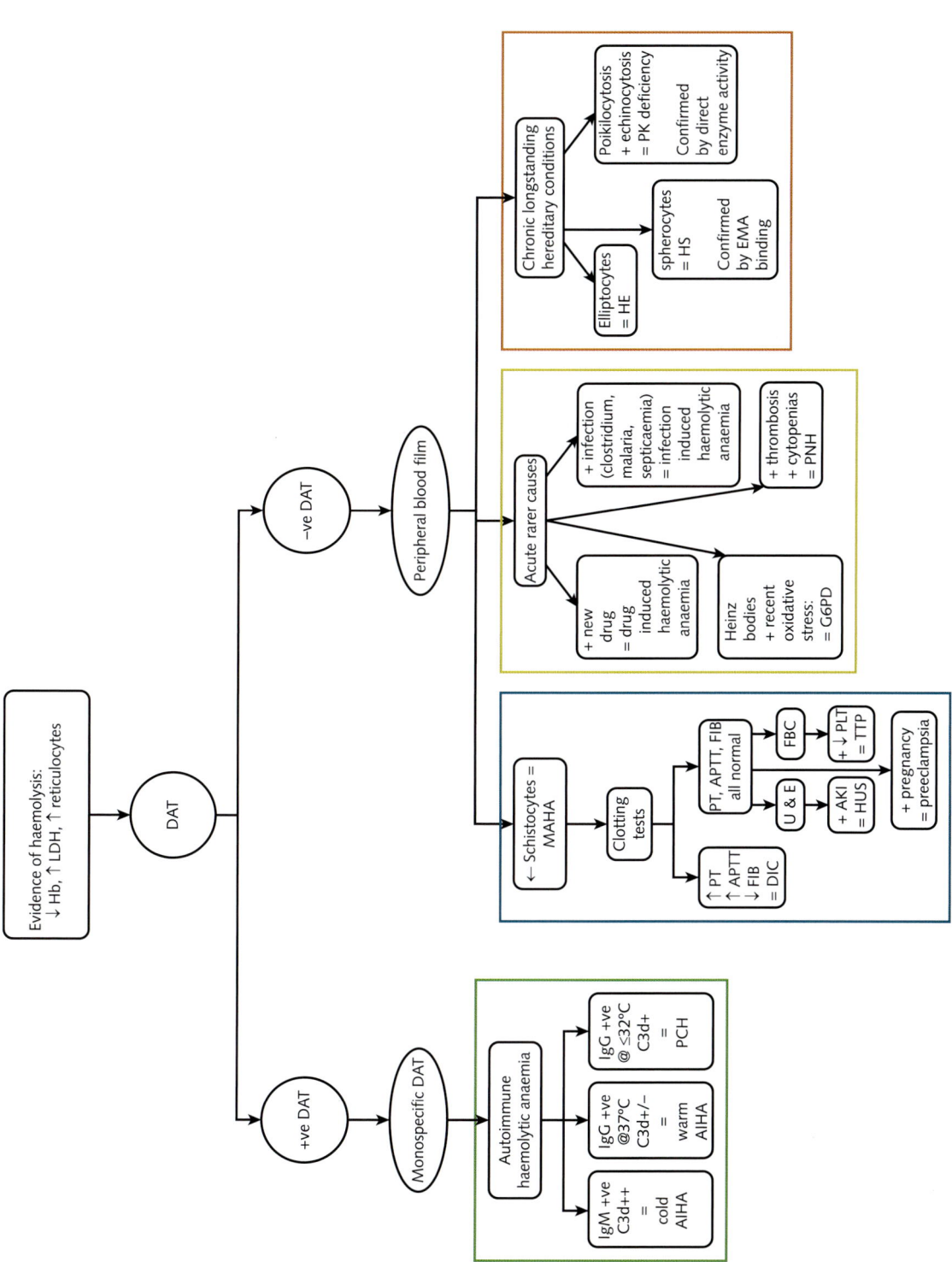

Fig. 3.6 Diagnostic approach to haemolytic anaemia.

AIHA, Autoimmune haemolytic anaemia; *APTT*, activated partial thromboplastin time; *DAT*, direct antigen test; *DIC*, disseminated intravascular coagulation; *EMA* binding, eosin 5′ maleimide binding; *FIB*, fibrinogen (see Chapter 6: Fibrinogen); *G6PD*, glucose-6-phosphate dehydrogenase; *HE*, hereditary elliptocytosis; *HS*, hereditary spherocytosis; *HUS*, haemolytic uraemic syndrome; *Ig*, immunoglobulin; *MAHA*, microangiopathic haemolytic anaemia (see Chapter 6: Platelet consumption by microthrombi); *PCH*, paroxysmal cold haemoglobinuria; *PK*, pyruvate kinase (all discussed earlier in this chapter); *PT*, prothrombin time; *TTP*, thrombotic thrombocytopenic purpura.

- Smooth muscle abnormalities: the presence of free haemoglobin in the circulation depletes nitric oxide, dysregulating normal smooth muscle tone, which manifests as dysphagia, odynophagia, erectile dysfunction and ileus.
- Pulmonary hypertension: likely secondary to nitric oxide depletion.

HAEMOGLOBINOPATHIES

Abnormalities of haemoglobin (haemoglobinopathies) may result from:

- Abnormal haemoglobin (e.g., sickle cell anaemia). Abnormal structure leads to abnormal function and behaviour, resulting in disease.
- Reduced synthesis of normal haemoglobin (thalassaemia) Reviewing structural features of the haemoglobin molecule (see Chapter 2: Structure) may facilitate understanding of this section.

Sickle cell disease

In sickle variant haemoglobin, a single base-pair substitution in the gene coding for the β globin on chromosome 11 results in a valine substitution for glutamic acid. This single amino acid substitution has immense structural and functional consequences for haemoglobin incorporating this abnormal beta globin (βS), which is known as HbS (sickle variant haemoglobin). At low pO$_2$, de-oxy HbS polymerizes into long intracellular fibres (tactoids). This elongation deforms the red cell into an inflexible sickle shape (Fig. 3.7). Initially, reoxygenation in conditions of high pO$_2$ will reverse the sickle deformation, but after several recurrences the shape becomes irreversibly sickled. This inflexibility of sickled red cells causes capillary occlusion with distal tissue

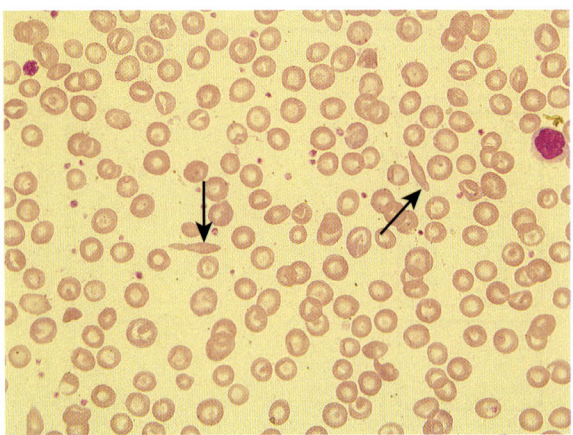

Fig. 3.7 Blood film in sickle cell anaemia.

hypoxia. Chronically, recurrent hypoxic injury and structural vascular damage accumulate with time and cause irreparable damage to organs such as the spleen, accounting for the bulk of the long-term morbidity of sickle cell anaemia. Acute episodes (sickle cell crises) are due to the same underlying mechanisms. Sickle cell crises manifest with severe pain from ischaemic tissue distal to vessels occluded by sickled cells.

Persistence of the sickle gene

The HbS gene is prevalent in tropical Africa and parts of the Mediterranean, Middle East and India. In some areas, up to 40% of the population are heterozygous (HbA/HbS). Sickle-cell heterozygosity confers protection against *Plasmodium falciparum* (the protozoan responsible for severe malaria) parasitization of red cells, perhaps accounting for the persistence of the genotype in malaria-endemic areas.

Sickle cell anaemia

If an individual possesses two copies of the β^S gene (i.e., a homozygous genotype: β^S/β^S), their phenotype is sickle cell anaemia. This disease carries significant morbidity due to the extensive complications it presents to sufferers. Table 3.5 lists the main complications with discussion of the underlying mechanisms.

Diagnosis

Hb is typically 60 to 90 g/L. It is typically a normochromic, normocytic anaemia with reticulocytosis (due to the chronic haemolytic anaemia). Sickle cells and target cells are seen on blood film. Hb electrophoresis shows HbS, variable amounts of HbF and absent HbA in homozygous patients.

Long-term management

These patients are managed by haematologists, who oversee outpatient management and inpatient crises. Treatment goals include maintaining a stable Hb, prompt management of acute crises, preventing infections and trying to minimize the numerous long-term complications of the disease.

- Haemoglobin levels may be maintained with top-up transfusions as needed or regular exchange transfusions. Iron status must be monitored to avoid iron overload.
- Influenza, pneumococcal, meningococcal and *Haemophilus influenzae* type B (Hib) vaccination is mandatory, as is oral daily antibiotic prophylaxis (due to functional hyposplenism or asplenia if the spleen has been resected). Prompt, aggressive treatment of infection is essential.
- Folate supplements reduce the likelihood of a folate deficiency-induced aplastic crisis.
- Patients must be effectively counselled as to lifestyle habits to minimize their exposure to factors known to provoke infarctive crises (dehydration, cold, etc.). It is also very important to ensure they understand how to self-care appropriately in mild self-limiting crises scenarios as well as

providing a clear escalation plan for medical intervention if self-care is not sufficient.

- Hydroxycarbamide stimulates the production of HbF ($\alpha 2\gamma 2$), which can limit the impact of sickle cell disease for patients with moderate-to-severe recurrent episodes of vaso-occlusive crises. Unfortunately, not all patients respond.
- Stroke prevention with regular exchange transfusions to maintain HbS <30% – a large randomized controlled trial found significant benefit in stroke prevention in children with sickle cell anaemia with high-risk intracranial arterial flow (measured by doppler).
- Preoperative transfusion if undergoing medium-/high-risk surgery.
- Iron chelation therapy (either desferrioxamine or deferasirox) for those at risk of iron overload.

Bone marrow (or hematopoietic stem cell) transplantation is the only potential cure. Due to the high risk of this procedure, it is only performed for selected individuals.

CLINICAL NOTES

TRANSFUSION IN SICKLE CELL ANAEMIA

As well as ABO compatibility (as always), donor transfusions should have full extended matching for Rh and Kell antigens and sickle negative. A history of red cell antibodies should be excluded and, if present, appropriately antigen-negative donor transfusion products must be used instead.

CLINICAL NOTES

EXCHANGE TRANSFUSIONS (OR RED CELL EXCHANGE)

This technique describes removal of a unit of the patient's blood followed by replacement with the same volume of donor red cells. The aim is to reduce the proportion of abnormal HbS to ≤30%.

Indications for emergency exchange transfusion in sickle cell: severe or worsening acute chest crisis, acute ischaemic stroke, acute sickle hepatopathy (acute liver injury), severe sepsis and multiorgan failure.

Acute management of sickle crises

Prompt treatment of any reversible precipitating factors is a priority. Aggressive rehydration and antibiotics (intravenous if necessary), adequate analgesia, supplemental oxygen (to increase oxygen saturation and thus delivery capacity of intact haemoglobin) and

warming are important components of supportive treatment. Incentive spirometry is encouraged to prevent complications from or development of acute chest crisis. Patients do slow, deep expiration exercises via a hand-held mechanical breathing device. Simple transfusion or exchange transfusion may be necessary. A haematologist should be consulted when possible for guidance as to target Hb parameters. Inpatient venous thromboprophylaxis is necessary as sickle patients have higher risk of venous thromboembolism (VTE). This can be pharmacological in the form of low-molecular-weight heparin (LWMH) or if contraindicated, mechanical with lower limb compression stockings/boots.

CLINICAL NOTES

ADEQUATE ANALGESIA IN SICKLE CRISES

Paracetamol, nonsteroidal antiinflammatory drugs and opiates are the mainstay. Be aware that these patients may have extremely high opiate requirements due to tolerance acquired from analgesia needed during multiple historic painful crises. Seek anaesthetic/pain specialist advice if assistance is needed to attain adequate analgesia. If known to a haematologist or haematology centre, most patients should have an established crisis care plan to guide emergency clinicians on first line and subsequent analgesic regimes for that individual patient.

Acute chest crisis

For symptoms/signs, please refer to Table 3.5. An acute chest crisis is a life-threatening complication and remains the most common cause of death in young patients with sickle cell anaemia. It can be triggered by infection or simply vaso-occlusion of the pulmonary vasculature. It should be managed with sufficient intravenous analgesia, antibiotics (including antivirals if influenza suspected), rehydration and incentive spirometry. Particular caution is needed to avoid exacerbating pulmonary oedema while attempting to restore intravascular volume. A bronchodilator should be used if there is evidence of bronchospasm or coexisting asthma. Early haematology advice regarding therapeutic simple (see earlier Clinical notes: Transfusion in sickle cell anaemia) or exchange transfusion (see earlier Clinical notes: Exchange transfusions) is necessary because appropriate transfusion reduces the chance of progressive deterioration. Continuous oximetry as a minimum is appropriate and regular arterial blood gases advisable. Rapid respiratory decompensation is not unusual and this requires early involvement of the critical care team and mechanical ventilation if indicated. CT is not usually helpful in the acute setting of an acute chest crisis, unless a pulmonary embolism is suspected.

Table 3.5 Complications of sickle cell disease

Clinical feature	Causative mechanism
Chronic haemolytic anaemia	Poorly deformable red cells are removed from the circulation, shortening their lifespan to 10–20 days (compared with the normal 120-day red cell lifespan).
Haemolytic crises	Often accompanying an infarctive crisis, an acute worsening of haemolysis is accompanied by an acute fall in Hb and red cell count. Reticulocytosis increases in an attempt to compensate.
Painful infarctive crises	Vaso-occlusive crises are the hallmark of sickle cell disease. These are acute episodes of pain, usually in the lower back, pelvis, legs but also sometimes abdomen and chest. Painful infarctive crises are the most common reason for hospital admissions in this patient population. Infection, acidosis, dehydration, cold and hypoxia predispose to infarcts in areas of complete ischaemia distal to occluded microvasculature. In many cases, no specific precipitating factor can be identified. Any organ or tissue may be affected, sometimes irreversibly.
Aplastic crises	These may be provoked by folate deficiency or parvovirus B19 infections. The abrupt fall in Hb of an aplastic crisis is differentiated from that in an acute haemolytic crisis by absence of reticulocytes.
Splenic complications	The tortuous microvasculature of the splenic filtration beds is a prime zone of susceptibility for sickling vaso-occlusion. Repeated micro-infarctions lead to destruction and atrophy of splenic tissue (hyposplenism). Acute splenic sequestration refers to sudden, rapid spleen engorgement with trapped blood. It presents with abdominal pain, acute splenomegaly and a falling Hb level.
Infection susceptibility	Hyposplenic patients are susceptible to infections, which may be catastrophic. Susceptibility to encapsulated microorganisms is particularly high.
Acute chest syndrome	This diagnosis is defined by fever, dyspnoea, low arterial pO_2, chest pain and clinical and radiographic evidence of pulmonary oedema.
Cerebrovascular ischaemia	Intracerebral vaso-occlusion of brain microvasculature may cause complications ranging from transient (TIA) to irreversible ischaemic events (stroke).
Other complications	Other phenomena (secondary to microvasculature occlusion) particularly associated with sickle cell anaemia include priapism (prolonged and painful erections), skin ulceration and proliferative retinopathy.

Hb, Haemoglobin; TIA, transient ischaemic attack.

Sickle cell trait

This heterozygous (genotype β^S/β) condition is typically benign and asymptomatic, even though up to 45% of Hb may be HbS. Sickling in this context occurs only at extremely low pO_2 and rarely occurs in vivo. Pregnancy, labour, altitude and anaesthesia may, however, cause increased risk. Both HbA and HbS are present on electrophoresis. Heterozygous patients are carriers and can pass the HbS gene on to their children.

Sickle cell/haemoglobin C disease

This condition is defined by heterozygosity of the β globin gene; one copy is the β^S and the other is β^C (forming haemoglobin C). β^C has an amino acid substitution (GLU→LYS) at the same site as the responsible substitution in the β^S mutant gene with similar abnormal aggregation under conditions of low pO_2. Both HbC and HbS are present on electrophoresis. Compared with sickle cell anaemia (β^S/β^S), these patients typically have milder anaemia and complications with greater life expectancy. However, they have a greater risk of thrombotic complications, particularly during pregnancy.

Sickle cell beta thalassaemia

This condition is also defined by heterozygosity of the β globin gene; one copy is the β^S, while the other copy carries the β thalassaemia variant of the globin gene. The MCV and MCH are significantly lower than the relatively normal values seen in sickle cell anaemia (β^S/β^S).

Iron overload

Repeated blood transfusions in patients over time can lead to accumulation and excess of iron in the body. This is an important complication to avoid both in sickle cell anaemia and thalassaemia. Excess iron can have devastating impact on organs such as liver cirrhosis and cardiomyopathies. As discussed in Chapter 2: Iron and Haem metabolism, iron-chelating medications are utilized to prevent this complication.

Red cell alloimmunization

Sickle cell patients can develop alloantibodies to red blood cells, more so than otherwise well patients. This can lead to an increased risk of haemolytic transfusion reactions. These patients will require increasingly specific extended matched blood, which can cause delays in an acute situation. It is suggested that the free haem from chronic haemolysis in sickle cell causes general inflammation in the body, prompting the immune system to produce these allo-antibodies.

Hyperhaemolysis syndrome

Similarly, hyperhaemolysis syndrome (HHS) is a rare haemolytic transfusion reaction with rapid and severe progression. Features are: lower Hb than pretransfusion, pain, fever and laboratory findings of haemolysis (discussed earlier in this chapter). It is a rare complication that you would not be expected to manage alone. If you come across a sickle cell patient who reports they have had HHS, do not administer blood transfusion without careful discussions with a haematologist. They will likely require steroids and IVIG to cover while transfused. Unlike AIHA, HHS is a DAT-negative haemolysis but there are similar agents used in management such as rituximab and eculizumab.

Future of SCA treatment

There is current research on potential management for sickle cell anaemia. Pharmacological therapies targeting various stages of polymerization and cell adhesion are being trialled. Notably, the hopeful future of curative options is going to be gene therapy, where viral vectors can be built to deliver a normal haemoglobin gene to stem cells. These are currently in phase 1 and 2 trials. Further rigorous research is needed to establish safety profiles and true efficacy.

Thalassaemia

Thalassaemia arises from mutations in the genes coding for the α or β globin protein component of haemoglobin. They are accordingly classified as α or β thalassaemia, depending on which gene is mutated. The mutation gives rise to abnormality of the corresponding globin in terms of both structure and function. Each type of thalassaemia results in a surfeit of unpaired normal globins (α globins in β thalassaemia, β globins in α thalassaemia). These unpartnered globins precipitate within red cell precursors, causing ineffective or abortive erythropoiesis and predisposing precursors to phagocytosis by bone marrow macrophages. Red cells that reach the circulation haemolyze easily and therefore have a shortened lifespan.

HINTS AND TIPS

DIFFERENCE BETWEEN THALASSAEMIA AND SICKLE CELL SYNDROMES

Thalassaemia is characterized by a deficiency of either α- or β globins. Sickle-cell syndromes are due to abnormal β globin chains only.

Beta thalassaemia

β Thalassaemia is much more frequent in individuals originating within a broad geographical band starting in the Iberian Peninsula and ending in the Philippines in Southeast Asia.

A partial (β⁻) or complete (β⁰) failure of β globin synthesis arises from a wide array of possible mutations, ranging from single base changes to deletions, aberrant splicing, premature truncations and frameshifts. The severity of disease depends on the particular mutation and whether one or both copies of the β globin gene are affected.

If both copies of the β globin gene are affected (homozygosity), the disease is called β thalassaemia major. A single affected copy (heterozygosity) is called β thalassaemia trait.

CLINICAL NOTES

β THALASSAEMIA TRAIT

Also known as β thalassaemia minor, this is where the patient has one abnormal copy of the β globin gene and one normal copy (β⁻/β). It is usually asymptomatic, although a microcytic and hypochromic appearance is seen on blood film, hence often mistaken for IDA; it is usually mild due to a higher than normal red cell count – so consider thalassaemia when you see a disproportionately low MCV for the level of Hb. It is diagnosed when an increased proportion of HbA2 is demonstrated by electrophoresis. Recognition of this syndrome is important as it has implications for genetic counselling and may otherwise be misdiagnosed as iron-deficiency anaemia, leading to inappropriate iron therapy.

Reduction or lack of β chains leads to unpaired α chains precipitating.

- Developing erythroblasts (→ ineffective erythropoiesis and reduced red cell synthesis).
- Mature red cells (→ premature haemolysis and shortened red cell lifespan).

The ineffective erythropoiesis and haemolysis are proportionate to the relative excess of α globins. Severe anaemia manifests at 3 to 6 months when the developmental switch from γ globin to β globins occurs. Extramedullary haemopoiesis causes hepatosplenomegaly and expansion of marrow cavities into cortical bone. This impairs structural integrity, predisposing to fractures and causing a characteristic appearance of the skull X-ray (Fig. 3.8).

A severe microcytic (low MCV), hypochromic (low MCH) anaemia is present, with elevated reticulocytes and the presence of normoblasts, target cells and red cell basophilic stippling on the peripheral blood film. DNA analysis will define the responsible genetic mutation. Haemoglobin electrophoresis is also diagnostic and reveals partial (β thalassaemia trait) or complete (β thalassaemia major) absence of HbA (HbF is present instead).

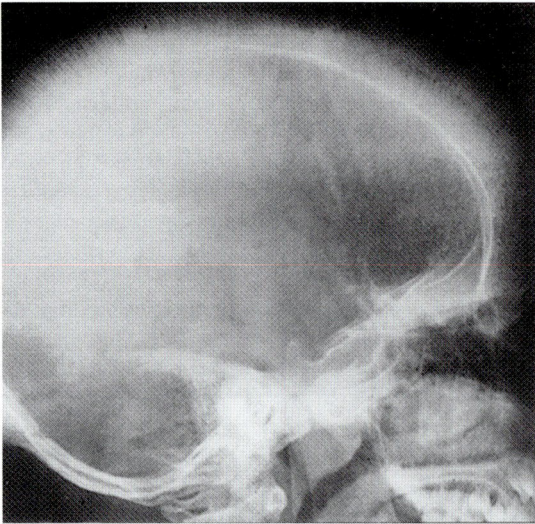

Fig. 3.8 Skull radiograph demonstrating the hair-on-end appearance due to expansion of marrow cavity into cortical bone.

Table 3.6 Features of alpha thalassaemia

Condition	Alpha genes deleted	Functional alpha genes	Electrophoresis
Normal	0	4	HbA (minimal HbF)
Alpha thalassaemia trait	1	3	HbA (minimal HbF) Clinically normal Electrophoresis normal Microcytosis MCV 70–80 fL
Alpha thalassaemia minor	2	2	HbA 90% + Mild anaemia Hb 90–120 g/L Microcytosis MCV 70–80 fL
Haemoglobin H disease	3	1	Haemoglobin H (β tetramer) 5–30% HbA 70% + Marked anaemia Hb 60–100 g/L Marked microcytosis MCV 60–70 fL
Alpha thalassaemia major	4	0	Incompatible with life; death in utero from hydrops fetalis

Hb, Haemoglobin; HbA, adult haemoglobin; HbF, foetal haemoglobin; MCV, mean cell volume.

Regular red cell transfusions are life-sustaining, but these patients are highly vulnerable to iron overload and require chelation therapy and vigilant monitoring of iron status. This susceptibility is exacerbated by enhanced absorption of dietary iron, probably in response to anaemia-induced tissue hypoxia.

Alpha thalassaemia

α Thalassaemia is most common in people of Southeast Asian and West African origin. There are four (rather than two) copies of the α globin gene and α thalassaemia typically results from deletion of one or more of these genes. Clinical severity is proportional to the number of lost (deleted) genes. Deletion of all four genes sadly results in death in utero (from hydrops fetalis), while the deletion of three genes results in a moderately severe anaemia with microcytic, hypochromic red cells and splenomegaly. The abnormal tetramer of unpaired β globins is called haemoglobin H, hence the name haemoglobin H disease. A reduced amount of (normal) HbA and an increased amount of haemoglobin H is seen on electrophoresis.

One deletion (three functional alpha globin genes) is referred to as α thalassaemia trait (Table 3.6). Two deletions (two functional alpha genes) is referred to as alpha thalassaemia minor. This is typically associated with mild anaemia (Hb is normal), although MCV and MCH are reduced and red cell count proportionally elevated. Haemoglobin electrophoresis in α thalassaemia trait is normal.

As with sickle cell anaemia, α and β thalassaemia can only be cured if a patient undergoes bone marrow (stem cell) transplantation. However, due to the risks involved and extensive matching process, it is only viable in a small proportion of patients.

ELECTROPHORESIS: INVESTIGATION OF HAEMOGLOBINOPATHIES

Electrophoresis is a method used to discriminate biological molecules by molecular weight. Samples of interest are processed to isolate chemically the molecule of interest (haemoglobin, in this context).

A detergent denatures the protein samples so that elements of tertiary/quaternary structure cannot confound the outcome and to confer each protein with a uniform negative charge. Each sample is loaded into a depression (loading well) in a gel-phase matrix (typically sodium dodecyl sulphate). The molecular structure of the gel matrix is a network of crisscrossing polymers forming a uniform mesh. When an electric current is applied across the gel, the denatured proteins migrate through the gel. The larger a protein, the less it can travel in a given time, due to more obstruction by the meshwork. The smallest proteins therefore travel the furthest. Since all molecules being analyzed have been conferring with the same negative charge, electrostatic influence is negligible and the distance travelled is inversely related to molecular size alone.

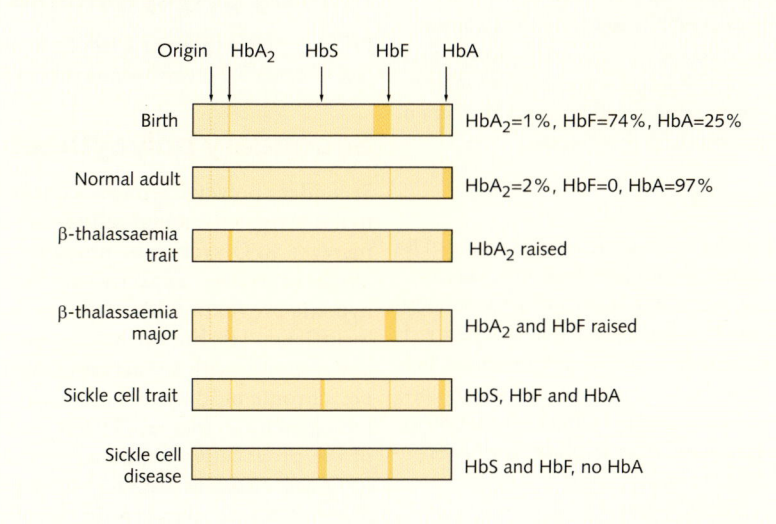

Fig. 3.9 Haemoglobin (Hb) electrophoresis. (From Kapoor R, Barnes KI, Jones V and Horton-Szar D. *Crash Course: Paediatrics*. 4th ed. Mosby, 2013.)

The gel with the migrated proteins is then stained, to allow visualization of each sample's end-position. Every electrophoretic gel also has a control lane that has a mixture of proteins of known molecular size loaded into the corresponding well. This ladder calibrates migration distance of the test protein in terms of molecular size. Then each protein is compared against the control lane to infer its molecular size.

Each type of haemoglobin, for example, HbA, HbF, HbS, will migrate a different difference on gel electrophoresis (Fig. 3.9). The control lane will include examples of each of the abnormal Hb types to allow identification.

MARROW DEFECTS CAUSING ANAEMIA

Aplastic anaemia

Aplastic anaemia is a misleading name because, as it affects haemopoietic stems cells, it reduces all cell counts in all cell lines (pancytopenia), causing leucopoenia and thrombocytopenia as well as anaemia. It is also characterized by aplasia (hypocellularity) of the bone marrow with a reduction in haemopoietic stem cells. Those that are present are defective and unable to repopulate the depleted marrow. ~75% of cases are idiopathic (no cause can be identified); the remaining ~25% cases are due to various factors listed in Table 3.7.

Treatment involves supportive actions: prompt antibiotic treatment in infection, transfusions as needed (red cells or platelets), growth factors and immunosuppression. Most patients are

Table 3.7 Causes of aplastic anaemia with specific examples

Causative mechanism	Examples
Drugs	Antibiotics: chloramphenicol, nitrofurantoin, sulphonamides, ribavirin Antimalarials: quinacrine, chloroquine Rheumatoid arthritis treatment: gold salts, NSAIDs Metal chelators: penicillamine Antiepileptics: phenytoin, carbamazepine
Viral infection	HIV, parvovirus B19, hepatitis B and C, EBV, Varicella-zoster virus
Cytotoxic drugs	Chemotherapeutic agents
Chemical toxins	Benzene, chemical solvents, glue vapour (solvent abuse)
Ionizing radiation	Radiation therapy (cancer treatment) or accidental exposure to ionizing radiation
Pregnancy	—
Autoimmune disease	Any autoimmune disease where immune sensitization develops towards haemopoietic stem cells
Rare genetic conditions	Diamond-Blackfan anaemia Shwachman-Diamond syndrome Fanconi anaemia

EBV, Epstein-Barr virus; HIV, human immunodeficiency virus; NSAIDs, nonsteroidal antiinflammatory drugs.

treated with anti–thymocyte globulin (ATG) as first-line. This product is derived from horses or rabbits and consists of antibodies directed against human T cells. The T cell destruction results in intense immunosuppression. Although some patients achieve lasting remission, others relapse. Stem cell transplant offers a cure for carefully selected patients with this disease.

Pure red-cell aplasia

This is a rare condition. A severe normocytic anaemia with <1% reticulocytes is present, but white cell and platelet counts are normal. It may be triggered by certain drugs, infections and autoantibody formation. Parvovirus B19 infection may cause a transient pure red cell aplasia. Red-cell precursors in the bone marrow are absent, but aside from erythroblast absence, the bone marrow cellularity is normal. Treatment is supportive, focusing on red cell transfusion. Stem cell transplantation may be considered in appropriate candidates.

Other causes

In terms of haematological disease, leukaemia and lymphomas may cause anaemia due to marrow infiltration. Myelodysplasia (see Chapter 5: Myelodysplasia) may present with a macrocytic anaemia.

Any space-occupying lesions that occupy an area of normal bone marrow territory large enough to disrupt the normal architecture may cause anaemia. Metastases or primary neoplasms affecting the bone marrow may have this effect. However, it is more likely that all cell lines would be affected: isolated anaemia in these cases due to bone marrow infiltration would be unusual.

POLYCYTHAEMIA

Polycythaemia (erythrocytosis) is the term used to describe an increase in red cell count above normal levels. It may be primary or secondary.

Primary polycythaemia

Primary polycythaemia arises from an abnormal clone of cells (see Chapter 5: Polycythaemia rubra vera).

Secondary polycythaemia

Secondary polycythaemia is a normal physiological reaction to tissue hypoxia. Renal cells detect hypoxia and in response increase EPO synthesis, upregulating erythropoiesis. The oxygen-carrying capacity of the blood increases. The hypoxia provoking this response may or may not be due to insufficient Hb, but the body is unable to identify the cause and responds with an increase in red cell count. As an example, chronic mild hypoxia seen in heavy smokers is usually indicated by an increased haematocrit. If a reasonable cause of the provocative hypoxia is not clearly apparent, serum EPO can differentiate secondary polycythaemia from primary; EPO is elevated in secondary but not primary polycythaemia.

Secondary polycythaemia is much more common than primary polycythaemia. Since secondary polycythaemia is an appropriate physiological response, treatment is not necessary just to normalize red cell counts. Complications may arise due to increased viscosity; in this instance, venesection to reduce the haematocrit to ≤0.55 may be considered.

Apparent polycythaemia is due to a decrease in intravascular volume unaccompanied by the loss of red cells; this contraction of intravascular volume usually results from dehydration or inappropriate third space redistribution.

Chronic excessive vasoconstriction, as seen in long-term hypertension, results in such a contracted intravascular volume. This specific scenario, known as Gaisbock syndrome, is typically seen in obese males with hypertension and is a favourite in exams as an example of secondary polycythaemia.

● Chapter Summary

- Anaemia (defined as reduced Hb) gives rise to a common set of symptoms but can result from many different underlying causes.
- Symptoms common to anaemia (no matter what underlying cause) include fatigue, exertional breathlessness, palpitations, presyncope/syncope and headache.
- Common causes of anaemia include haematinics deficiency, chronic disease, blood loss or haemolysis.
- Haemolysis may be subclassified by its primary location: intravascular (e.g., all causes of microangiopathic haemolysis) or extravascular (e.g., hereditary enzyme deficiencies).
- Rarer causes of anaemia are hereditary abnormalities of haemoglobin structure such as sickle cell anaemia and thalassaemia or bone marrow disorders such as aplastic anaemia and pure red cell aplasia.
- Enzyme deficiencies affecting glycolysis such as pyruvate kinase or glucose-6-phosphate dehydrogenase lead to shortened red cell survival due to red cell reliance on glycolysis for ATP generation.
- Polycythaemia (an abnormally raised Hb and red cell count) is usually due to various states resulting in chronic tissue hypoxia, but rarely may be due to pathological mutations of red cell precursors (polycythaemia rubra vera, also called primary polycythaemia).

MLA Conditions
Adverse drug effects
Haemochromatosis
Haemoglobinopathies
Malaria
Malnutrition
Pancytopenia
Polycythaemia
Sickle cell disease
Vitamin B12 and/or folate deficiency

MLA Presentations
Fatigue
Jaundice
Pallor

White blood cells | 4

LEUCOCYTE STRUCTURE

'Leucocytes' is the term used to describe *white* blood cells. The structure and characteristics were covered in Chapter 1; please refer back for a refresher if needed. The immunological functions of each type of leucocyte are explained in detail in Chapter 9.

Lymphocytes

Lymphocytes (Fig. 4.1) are the smallest of the white blood cells. The term 'lymphocytes' includes T cells, B cells and natural killer (NK) cells. Lymphocytes usually represent ~20–25% of the blood population of leucocytes. They circulate in blood and the lymphatic system when travelling between bone marrow and lymphoid tissue such as the spleen or lymph nodes. They either produce antibodies (B cells) or kill foreign/infected cells (T cells and NK cells). Some lymphocytes such as memory B or T cells can survive for decades.

Granulocytes

Granulocytes: Neutrophils

Neutrophils (Fig. 4.2) are also known as 'polymorphonuclear' leucocytes. Nuclei are segmented, with 2–5 lobes connected by thin chromatin threads.

Location

Neutrophils circulate in blood for up to 10 hours and represent the majority (~60%) of the leucocyte blood population. They migrate into tissues in response to chemotactic agents, where they survive for a further 1–3 days.

Function

Neutrophils are the first cells to arrive at a zone of inflammation, comprising a prominent aspect of the innate immune system, described further in Chapter 9. Neutrophils destroy microorganisms by:

- Release of hydrolytic enzymes from their granules
- Phagocytosis

Dead neutrophils are the major constituent of pus.

Granulocytes: Eosinophils

Eosinophils (Fig. 4.3) are larger than neutrophils, and the nucleus is bilobed or reniform (kidney shaped). The cytoplasm contains numerous cationic granules with cytotoxic contents including major basic protein and eosinophil-derived neurotoxin, peroxidase and cationic protein.

Location

The vast majority of eosinophils reside mainly at epithelial barriers including lungs, skin and gastrointestinal tract. They circulate in blood for 1–2 days.

Function

Eosinophils play the primary role in attacking multicellular parasitic organisms (see Chapter 11) and are mediators of allergic reaction (see Chapter 12).

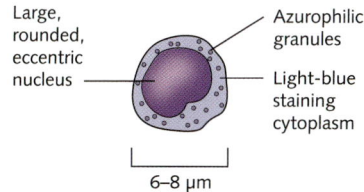
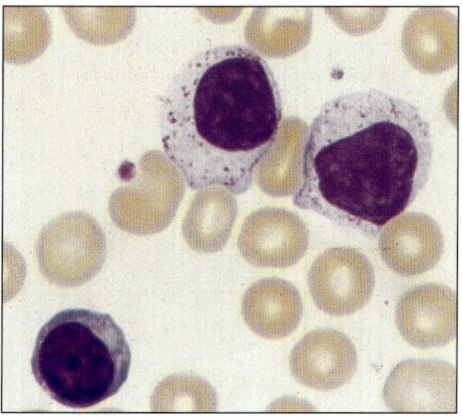

Fig. 4.1 Lymphocyte structure. Line diagram (*left panel*) and film appearance (*right panel*).

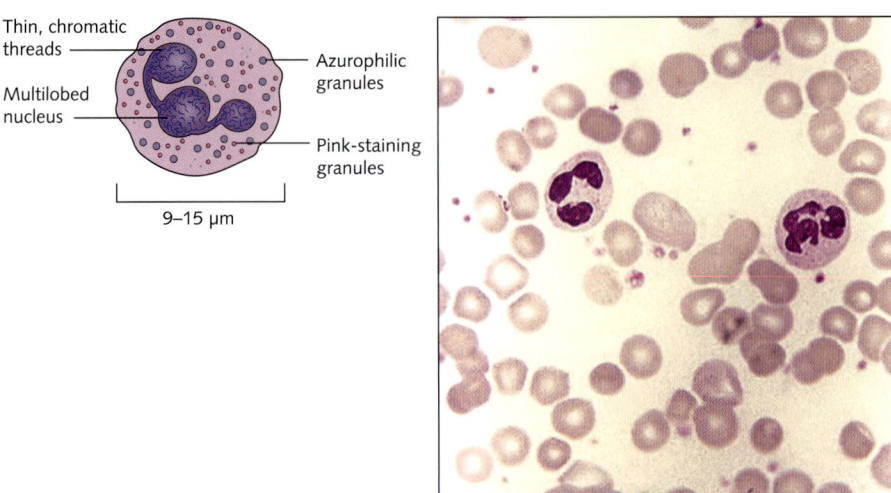

Fig. 4.2 Neutrophil structure. Line diagram (*left panel*) and film appearance (*right panel*). Note that only the azurophilic granules are visible in the film view of the neutrophil (*right panel*). Other granules present (but not visible on the film) include glycogen, tertiary and specific granules.

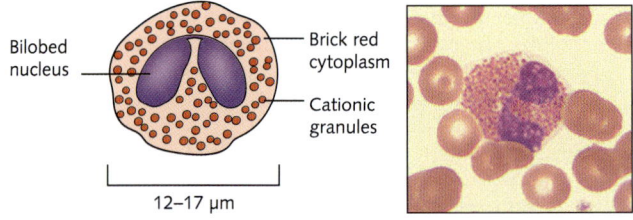

Fig. 4.3 Eosinophil structure. Line diagram (*left panel*) and film appearance (*right panel*).

Basophils

Appearance and structure

Basophils (Fig. 4.4) have a 'S-shaped' nucleus. Cytoplasm is densely packed with large blue-staining (basophilic) granules that may obscure the nucleus and cause bulging outward of the cell membrane, giving a 'roughened' appearance to the perimeter. These granules contain heparin, histamine, chemotactic factors and peroxidase.

Location

Basophils are scarce (<1% of circulating leucocytes), with a lifespan in the circulation of 1–2 days (whilst travelling to lymphoid and nonlymphoid tissues).

Function

Basophils are functionally very similar to mast cells, although their lineages differ, and mast cells are restricted to tissues and thus do not appear in the blood. They both release a similar array of mediators in response to immunoglobulin E (IgE) cross-linking and thus

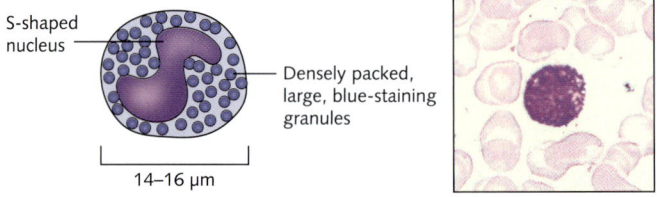

Fig. 4.4 Basophil structure. Line diagram (*left panel*) and film appearance (*right panel*).

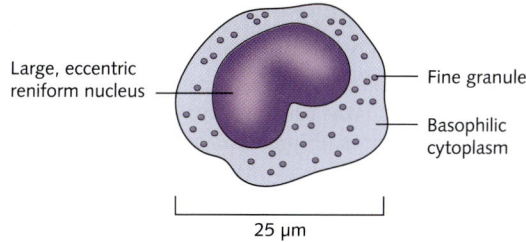
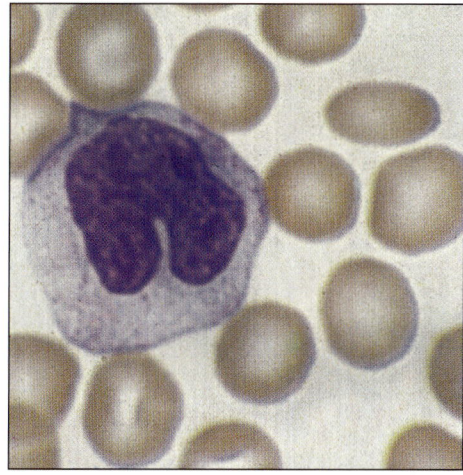

Fig. 4.5 Monocyte structure. Line diagram (*left panel*) and film appearance (*right panel*). The monocyte is surrounded by red cells, giving a good relative indication of the size. Note that the pointed extrusion is due to the 'squashing' between the adjacent cells on the slide rather than a specific feature of monocyte structure.

are thought to participate in type 1 hypersensitivity reactions (see Chapter 12).

Monocytes

Appearance and structure
Monocytes (Fig. 4.5) are the largest leucocytes. Nucleoli are often visible, giving the nucleus a 'moth-eaten' appearance. Basophilic cytoplasm contains numerous lysosomes and vacuole-like spaces, producing a 'ground-glass' appearance. Microtubules, microfilaments, pinocytotic vesicles and filopodia/pseudopodia are present at the cell periphery.

Location
Monocytes spend 1–3 days in blood, where they represent ~2–10% of bloodstream leucocytes. They then enter the tissues, where they differentiate further and become macrophages. Macrophages survive within tissues for months to years.

Function
Macrophages make up the reticuloendothelial system and are found in tissues throughout the body. They phagocytose elderly/damaged red cells, pathogens and cellular debris. They also process and present antigen to lymphocytes as part of the adaptive immune response (see Chapter 10). Macrophages also have a proinflammatory function, releasing a variety of cytokines.

LEUCOCYTE DIFFERENTIATION

Please refer to Fig. 1.2 in Chapter 1 for a detailed overview of white cell differentiation. In brief:

- Lymphocytes (T cells, B cells and NK cells) are lymphoid lineage leucocytes derived from the lymphoid lineage progenitor cell.
- Eosinophils and basophils develop from the myeloid lineage progenitor cells.
- Neutrophils and monocytes develop from the myeloid lineage progenitor cell.

LEFT AND RIGHT SHIFT

'Left shift' describes the phenomenon where an increased proportion of immature neutrophils are released from the bone marrow into peripheral blood (Fig. 4.6). This accelerated release is triggered by inflammatory cytokines produced in response to (usually) inflammation or infection. Left shift can also be seen in certain diseases, including bone marrow disorders. For example, in bacterial infection, the physiological response is a rise in neutrophils. Initially, the demand for mature neutrophils temporarily outstrips the supply available in the bone marrow, so immature neutrophils are also released into blood. Band cells are most common, but earlier versions may also be released in response to increasingly severe inflammatory stimuli.

'Right shift' refers to the converse scenario, where leucocytes persist longer than normal in the circulation and acquire morphological characteristics of 'hypermaturity' (e.g., hypersegmented and enlarged 'giant' neutrophils). This occurs in noninfectious inflammatory processes such as malignancy and bone marrow synthesis disorders such as megaloblastic or iron-deficiency anaemia.

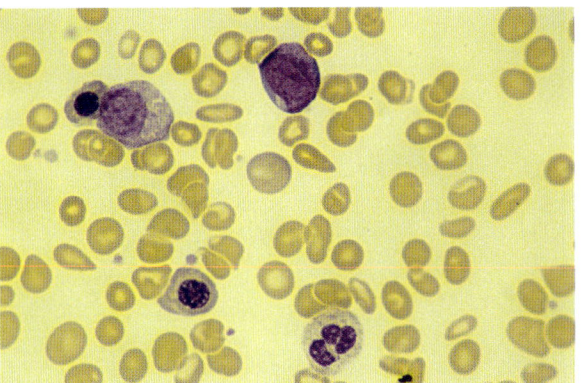

Fig. 4.6 Peripheral blood film showing left shift: a nucleated red blood cell (RBC), dacrocytes (teardrop-shaped RBCs) and immature myeloid cells (promyelocyte and myelocyte). This patient has myelofibrosis. (Source: David Hudnall S. *Hematology: A Pathophysiologic Approach*. 2nd ed. Elsevier; 2023.)

WHITE COUNT DIFFERENTIAL

The white count differential breaks down the leucocyte count into components: neutrophils, lymphocytes, monocytes, eosinophils and basophils. This process is automated and uses stains, cell size and light scatter to differentiate among different cell types. Normal leucocyte parameters and nomenclature of abnormalities are given in Table 4.1. Abnormal leucocyte appearances on blood film may suggest specific disease processes. Table 4.2 details some common morphological abnormalities with corresponding diagnostic inferences.

Table 4.1 White cell count parameters and nomenclature of abnormalities

Parameter	Normal range (×10⁹/L)ᵃ	Abnormality
Total white cell count	4.0–11	↑: 'leucocytosis' ↓: 'leucopoenia'
Lymphocytes	1.3–4.5	↑: 'lymphocytosis' ↓: 'lymphopenia'
Neutrophils	2–7.5	↑: 'neutrophilia' ↓: 'neutropenia' (aka 'granulocytopenia')
Eosinophils	0.04–0.4	↑: 'eosinophilia'
Basophils	0–0.1	↑: 'basophilia'
Monocytes	0.2–0.8	↑: 'monocytosis'

ᵃRanges given represent normal parameters in 95% of the normal population.

LEUCOCYTOSIS

'Leucocytosis' describes an increased total white cell count (i.e., $>11 \times 10^9/L$). One particular type of leucocyte, most commonly neutrophils, usually predominates, with smaller increases in the other types of leucocyte. Many things can lead to a leucocytosis, not all of which are pathological. The nature of the predominant population is mandatory for forming any diagnosis (see Table 4.3 for examples of particular diseases associated with elevation of specific populations of leucocytes).

CLINICAL NOTES

Reactive leucocytosis: An acute rise in total white cell count is usually in response to infection, particularly if it occurs rapidly. This is termed a 'reactive leucocytosis'. If an out-of-proportion rise in lymphocytes, eosinophils and basophils (compared to neutrophils) is noted, consider a nonbacterial infection or haematological malignancy.

CLINICAL NOTES

Benign causes of neutrophilia: These include pregnancy or recent delivery, vigorous exercise, postantibiotic diarrhoea and vaccination. Exogenous factors such as cigarette smoking (possibly the most common cause of mild neutrophilia) or a chronic state of anxiety may also cause a neutrophilia. By far the most common cause you may see in comorbid patients is with concurrent steroid use. Corticosteroids cause neutrophils to migrate more out from the bone marrow into peripheral blood and reduce natural neutrophil apoptosis. For example, a rising neutrophil count in patient with COPD following starting steroids for an acute exacerbation does not mean treatment is not working if they are otherwise clinically improving.

LEUCOPOENIA

'Leucopoenia' describes a *total* white blood count of less than $4 \times 10^9/L$ (see Table 4.1 for definitions).

Causes of neutropenia (<2 × 10⁹/L) and agranulocytosis (<0.5 × 10⁹/L)

Reduced neutrophil count may arise due to inadequate granulopoiesis or an accelerated removal of granulocytes.

Table 4.2 Blood film abnormalities of leucocyte morphology and their diagnostic inferences

Abnormality	Description	Diagnostic inference
Hypersegmentation of neutrophils (right shift)	$\geq$5 lobes per nucleus (hypermature neutrophils)	Megaloblastic anaemia Renal failure Iron-deficiency anaemia
Left shift of neutrophils	Various earlier developmental stages of neutrophil Band cells are the most common, but all stages are possible	Severe infection CML Pregnancy Use of G-CSF
Blast cells	The most immature form of the blood cell lineage (e.g., myeloblast or a lymphoblast could be seen in the peripheral blood in AML and ALL, respectively	Acute leukaemias (AML and ALL: see Chapter 5) Occasional blast seen with leucoerythroblastic reaction (see 'Leucocytosis' section below)
Auer rods	Rod-like accretions of granular material which may appear in the cytoplasm of leukaemic blast cells in AML	AML
Smear cells (also known as 'smudge' cells or 'basket' cells)	Remnants of a cell, lacking a clearly identifiable cell membrane or nucleus These are seen when abnormally fragile cells are abundant in the blood	Reactive lymphocytosis CLL
Leucoerythroblastic change	Presence of immature leucocytes including occasional blast *and* immature (still nucleated) red cells	Severe haemorrhage Severe haemolysis Sepsis Myelofibrosis (either primary or secondary to metastatic disease in bone marrow) DIC

ALL, Acute lymphoblastic leukaemia; AML, acute myeloid leukaemia; CLL, chronic lymphocytic leukaemia; CML, chronic myeloid leukaemia; DIC, Disseminated intravascular coagulation; G-CSF, granulocyte-colony stimulating factor.

Table 4.3 Diseases associated with increases in particular leucocyte population

Leucocyte population	General causative mechanism	Specific examples
Neutrophil (neutrophilia)	Bacterial infection (acute and chronic)	
	Acute inflammation and/or tissue necrosis	Infarction, surgery, rhabdomyolysis, myositis, burns, trauma, vasculitis, RA
	Myeloproliferative disorders	CML, primary myelofibrosis
	Metabolic or endocrine disease	DKA, thyrotoxicosis, gout, eclampsia
	Drugs	G-CSF, steroids, adrenaline
Lymphocytes (lymphocytosis)	Viral infection	EBV, CMV, rubella
	Bacterial infection	TB, brucellosis, syphilis, pertussis
	Parasitic infections	Toxoplasmosis, rickettsial infections
	Neoplastic	CLL, ALL, lymphoma
	Other	Postsplenectomy, postadrenaline
Eosinophils (eosinophilia)	Parasitic infection	Helminth (worm) infections, schistosomiasis, malaria
	Hypersensitivity	Asthma, hay fever
	Drugs	Drug-related eosinophilia, DRESS

Continued

Table 4.3 Diseases associated with increases in particular leucocyte population—cont'd

Leucocyte population	General causative mechanism	Specific examples
	Skin disease	Eczema, psoriasis, urticaria, pemphigus, dermatitis herpetiformis
	Neoplastic	Hodgkin lymphoma, T cell non-Hodgkin lymphoma, CML, hypereosinophilic syndrome, solid tumours
	Postinfectious	Convalescence phase following any infection
Basophils (basophilia)	Myeloproliferative disorders	Classically CML, although basophilia may be seen in PRV, PMF and ET
	IgE-mediated hypersensitivity reactions	Anaphylaxis
	Infection	Viral, helminths, mycobacterial
	Endocrine	Hypothyroidism, diabetes, oestrogen treatment
	Autoimmune	UC, RA
Monocytes (monocytosis)	Neoplastic	Most commonly in CMML, CML and AML May be seen in some lymphoma and myelodysplastic syndromes
	Bacterial infection	TB, bacterial endocarditis, syphilis, typhoid, brucellosis
	Viral infection	Varicella zoster
	Parasitic infection	Malaria, trypanosomiasis, leishmaniasis

ALL, Acute lymphoblastic leukaemia; AML, acute myeloid leukaemia; CLL, chronic lymphocytic leukaemia; CML, chronic myeloid leukaemia; CMML, chronic myelomonocytic leukaemia; CMV, cytomegalovirus; DIC, disseminated intravascular coagulation; DKA, diabetic ketoacidosis; DRESS, drug-related eosinophilia with systemic symptoms; EBV, Epstein-Barr virus; ET, essential thrombocytosis; G-CSF, granulocyte-colony stimulating factor; PMF, primary myelofibrosis; PRV, polycythaemia rubra vera; RA, rheumatoid arthritis; TB, tuberculosis; UC, ulcerative colitis.

Inadequate granulopoiesis

Reduced or ineffective neutrophil production by bone marrow causes neutropenia. Such inadequate granulopoiesis may be secondary to generalized bone marrow failure, which may be primary (myelodysplastic syndrome [MDS], lymphomas, leukaemias [see Chapter 5] or aplastic anaemias [see Chapter 3: Aplastic anaemia]) or secondary (chemotherapy, megaloblastic anaemia, metastatic infiltration or drugs such as methotrexate or azathioprine).

CLINICAL NOTES

Iatrogenic neutropenia: In all instances, drugs are the most common cause of neutropenia. Always review the patient's medications and consider if a known culprit (Table 4.4) could be responsible for a new neutropenia.

Table 4.4 Drugs known to cause neutropenia by therapeutic class (not exhaustive)

Anticonvulsants	Phenytoin, carbamazepine, lamotrigine
Antithyroid	Carbimazole, propylthiouracil
Immunomodulatory	NSAIDs, sulphasalazine, gold, phenylbutazone, penicillamine
Antibiotic	Cephalosporins, co-trimoxazole, chloramphenicol, dapsone, vancomycin
Psychotropic	Clozapine, tricyclic antidepressants, phenothiazines
Gastrointestinal	H2-receptor antagonists (cimetidine, ranitidine)
Antiarrhythmic	Propranolol, digoxin, flecainide, procainamide
Diuretic	Thiazide, furosemide, spironolactone, acetazolamide
Antiplatelet	Dipyridamole, ticlopidine
Oral hypoglycaemics (sulphonylureas)	Tolbutamide, chlorpropamide

NSAIDs, Nonsteroidal antiinflammatory drugs.

Alternatively, inadequate granulopoiesis may be due to a specific failure of neutrophil production. This may be:

- A dose-related drug exposure phenomenon (Table 4.4).
- Rare congenital diseases (e.g., Kostmann syndrome, cyclical neutropenia, Schwachman syndrome).
- Ethnicity—benign ethnic neutropenia (BEN) is seen in some individuals of African, Middle-Eastern and West Indian descent. Usually it is not diagnosed until all other causes have been excluded.

Accelerated removal of granulocytes

Neutropenia due to increased destruction/distribution may be secondary to several mechanisms:

- Drug-induced immune-mediated destruction (Table 4.4): note that drug-induced neutropenia operating via an immune mechanism is *not* dose-dependent
- Immune-mediated destruction (idiopathic or related to coexisting autoimmune disease, e.g., systemic lupus erythematosus)
- Hypersplenism (i.e., splenic neutrophil sequestration, typically accompanied by pancytopenia)
- Severe infection, resulting in rapid exit from the circulation to the site of sepsis

CLINICAL NOTES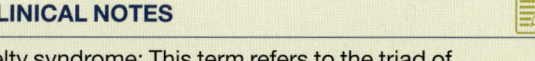

Felty syndrome: This term refers to the triad of rheumatoid arthritis (RA), splenomegaly and neutropenia. It arises as a complication of severe, long-standing RA. With improvements in treatment for RA, this is rarely seen nowadays.

Causes of lymphopenia

Lymphopenia is most commonly secondary to minor, community-acquired viral infections. Other important causes of lymphopenia are shown below.

CLINICAL NOTES

CAUSES OF LYMPHOPENIA

Human immunodeficiency virus (HIV) infection, corticosteroid or other immunosuppressive drugs, chemotherapy, Cushing syndrome, autoimmune disease (e.g., systemic lupus erythematosus, RA, sarcoidosis), Hodgkin lymphoma, MDS, trauma or surgery, liver or renal failure.

Mild lymphopenia has little in the way of clinical consequences. Prolonged severe lymphopenia, however, such as that seen in HIV-positive patients, carries with it the significant clinical consequences of immunodeficiency with primarily recurrent, severe and opportunistic infections.

● Chapter Summary

- Leucocytes are white blood cells. This group encompasses lymphocytes, neutrophils, eosinophils, basophils and monocytes. Each is differentiated by structure and function.
- Increased counts of particular groups of white cells are seen with particular infections, disease states and/or malignancies.
- Decreased counts ('leucopoenia') of white blood cells overall (i.e., $\leq 4 \times 10^9$/L) place the patient at increased rate of infection.
- A decrease in the count of a specific white cell type (e.g., neutrophils: 'neutropenia') allows narrowing of the differential diagnosis because the identity of the cell type with the decreased count will usually be associated with a particular set of conditions.
- Leucopoenia may also suggest disorder of the bone marrow or immune system.
- The blood film, as for red cells, provides extremely useful diagnostic information for various acute and chronic disease states.

MLA Conditions

Pancytopenia
Sepsis

MLA Presentations

Fever

INTRODUCTION

Haematological malignancies can affect the bone marrow, lymph nodes, spleen and blood components. As with all neoplasias, the process begins with an abnormal DNA mutation. The pathological change may occur at any stage in haematopoietic development in any of the cell lineages. The change may occur due to genetic and/or environmental factors, often specific to each malignancy, but always results in:

- Unregulated, increased proliferation producing large numbers of identical daughter cells (clones) and
- Cellular 'immortalization; resistance to normal apoptosis signals

CLINICAL NOTES

CONSTITUTIONAL SYMPTOMS ('B SYMPTOMS')

These include unexplained weight loss, low-grade fever and drenching night sweats. This is clarified early in this chapter, as they are a feature at some point in nearly all haematological malignancies.

Classification of haematological malignancies is complex and has often varied with the categorizing organization, although the World Health Organization (WHO) classification is now considered standard and is widely accepted. Broadly, this is based on the cell of origin, the tissue location and the molecular change(s) resulting from the causative DNA mutation. In this chapter, we will classify them as follows:

- Myeloproliferative disorders: defined by excessive proliferation of one or more specific cell line(s) derived from a myeloid progenitor. These cells retain the ability to mature and differentiate normally. The myeloproliferative disorders typically follow an indolent course.
- Myelodysplastic disorders: a diverse group of bone marrow disorders characterized by clonal proliferation of myeloid cells that mature abnormally and incompletely ('dysplastic' cells). The most immature of these cells are known as 'blasts.'
- Leukaemias (acute and chronic): abnormal clonal proliferation of white blood cells.
- Lymphomas: pathological clonal proliferation of lymphoid cells, usually located in lymph nodes, spleen or extranodal lymphoid tissues.

- Plasma cell dyscrasias: abnormal clonal proliferation of plasma cells, which can secrete detectable levels of paraproteins (monoclonal immunoglobulins or immunoglobulin fragments).

MYELOPROLIFERATIVE NEOPLASMS

Myeloproliferative disorders arise from neoplastic transformation of a cellular precursor of myeloid lineage. The neoplastic cell proliferates, and the cells produced may follow one or more differentiation pathways. Myeloproliferative disorders differ from myelodysplasia and leukaemia in that these neoplastic cells are capable of differentiation and maturing. Myeloproliferative disorders are nonmalignant neoplasms but have the potential to further evolve into acute myeloid leukaemia (AML). Clinically important myeloproliferative disorders are discussed in the following sections.

Janus kinase 2 (JAK2) gene mutation

Janus kinase 2 (JAK2) gene mutations are now seen as one of the defining features of myeloproliferative disorders. This gain-of-function mutation leads to a constitutively active (i.e., active response in absence of cytokine stimulus) proliferation scenario. Testing for the JAK2 mutation (performed on peripheral blood samples) is widely available and has become an integral test in the diagnosis of myeloproliferative disorders.

Polycythaemia rubra vera (primary polycythaemia)

This disorder is characterized by excessively high red cell numbers, resulting from a red cell precursor mutating and acquiring invulnerability to apoptosis. One of the established mechanisms leading to immortalization in polycythaemia rubra vera (PRV) is an increase in sensitivity to antiapoptotic growth factor insulin-like growth factor. The pathologically elevated red cell levels are often accompanied by neutrophilia (in ~66% of cases) and thrombocytosis (in ~50% of cases). Transformation to acute leukaemia (probability of ~5% after 10 years) or myelofibrosis (probability of 20% after 10 years) can occur even if adequately treated. Treated patients have a median survival of at least 10–15 years. Thrombosis is the main cause of death in untreated patients.

Clinical features

Polycythaemia rubra vera often presents insidiously at a median age of 60 years. Symptoms arise secondary to blood hyperviscosity due to increased cell numbers (see 'Clinical Notes: Hyperviscosity Syndrome'). Around 40% of patients also have elevated histamine levels, resulting in gastroduodenal ulcers and pruritus exacerbated by warm baths/showers. On examination patients are plethoric and 30–50% will have palpable splenomegaly or hepatosplenomegaly due to extramedullary haematopoiesis. The most serious complication of PRV is thrombosis, which may be arterial (myocardial infarction, cerebrovascular accident) or venous (deep venous thrombosis, pulmonary embolism).

CLINICAL NOTES

HYPERVISCOSITY SYNDROME

This may be due to increased cell numbers, as in PRV, or paraproteins, as in Waldenstrom macroglobulinaemia. Symptoms include headache, dizziness, tinnitus, vertigo, blurred vision, paraesthesia, oronasal bleeding, stupor and coma. Cerebral, coronary and peripheral vascular insufficiency (resulting from thromboses or flow disturbances) may lead to stroke, myocardial infarction and claudication, respectively.

Diagnostic tests

Full blood count (FBC) demonstrates raised red cell count, red cell mass, haemoglobin and haematocrit (>0.52 in men, >0.48 in women). There may be elevated neutrophil and/or platelet counts. Serum erythropoietin is low while plasma urate and lactate dehydrogenase (LDH) are often elevated. Bone marrow biopsy exhibits trilineage hyperplasia of erythroid, granulocytic and megakaryocytic cells and iron store depletion. Most patients can now be diagnosed on the basis of a raised haematocrit together with the presence of the JAK2 mutation, which is present in >90% of the patients, but there is still value in the above tests, particularly for complicated cases.

COMMON PITFALLS

EXCLUSION OF PHYSIOLOGICAL POLYCYTHAEMIA

Before diagnosing PRV, one must first exclude both *secondary* and *apparent polycythaemia*. Secondary polycythaemia is a predictable and appropriate rise in red cell numbers in response to factors such as chronic hypoxia (e.g., chronic obstructive pulmonary disease, sleep apnoea or cyanotic heart disease) or excessively high erythropoietin (as in some hepatic, endocrine or

renal disease). Red cell mass is increased in this subtype but there is no primary pathology in haematopoiesis. *Apparent polycythaemia* refers to conditions where the red cell mass is not increased but there is a reduced plasma volume. This is often seen in obesity, smoking, diuretics (e.g., thiazides), SGLT-2 inhibitors (e.g., dapagliflozin) and alcohol abuse. Secondary and apparent polycythaemia are vastly more common than myeloproliferative disease and do not share the same risks or complications with the primary form of this disorder.

Treatment

First-line treatment is venesection, lowering the haematocrit to ≤0.45. Aspirin reduces the risk of thrombosis, the major complication of PRV. Cytoreductive drugs such as pegylated interferon (Peg-IFN), hydroxycarbamide and anagrelide can be used. Recently the JAK-inhibitor, Ruxolitinib, has been approved as second-line treatment for PRV.

Primary (essential) thrombocythaemia

Also known as essential thrombocytosis (ET), this is a rare chronic disorder characterized by excessive production of platelets and thus elevated levels of platelets in the blood.

Clinical features

Nearly 50% of individuals with primary thrombocythaemia are asymptomatic at diagnosis, the elevated platelets being identified incidentally on a routine FBC performed for other reasons. Primary thrombocythaemia usually presents in patients older than 50 years but may occur at any age. In symptomatic individuals, the clinical presentation usually relates to complications of thrombus formation in blood vessels. Like PRV, ET can manifest with thrombosis in arteries, veins or the microvasculature. Microvascular thromboses may cause erythromelalgia (red, painful fingers and toes), gangrene and transient ischaemic attacks. Abnormal bleeding may also occur, particularly with platelet counts >1500 × 10⁹/L, which can cause acquired von Willebrand disease (see Chapter 6: von Willebrand disease) but is rarely severe. Around 5% of patients will have palpable splenomegaly. The risk of transformation to acute leukaemia (~1–2% at 10 years) or myelofibrosis (~10% at 10 years) is less than that observed in PRV.

Diagnostic tests

A sustained, unexplained elevated platelet count (>450 × 10⁹/L) suggests the diagnosis. This prompts bone marrow biopsy, which in ET exhibits a large number of abnormal megakaryocytes and hypercellularity. Cytogenetic studies may also identify chromosomal abnormalities associated with the diagnosis. Nearly 90% of patients will have an identifiable mutation. In 60% of patients with an identifiable mutation, it is the JAK2 mutation. CALR and MPL mutations are the next most common.

COMMON PITFALLS

EXCLUSION OF REACTIVE THROMBOCYTOSIS

Before diagnosing ET, one must first exclude *reactive thrombocytosis* as a cause of the raised platelet count which is much more common. Factors such as bleeding, infection, inflammation and iron deficiency anaemia must be first ruled out before considering myeloproliferative disease as the cause. Of particular note, elevated platelet counts are commonly seen postoperatively, especially following splenectomy. Importantly, all types of cancer may lead to thrombocytosis, which is thought to be mediated by increased interleukin-6 (IL-6).

Treatment

Initial management should address common vascular risk factors (i.e., hypertension, hypercholesterolaemia, smoking, diabetes, etc.). As ET has a generally favourable survival, only patients with a high risk of complications undergo treatment. A high risk of complications is conferred by:

- age older than 60 years
- platelet count $>1500 \times 10^9$/L
- history of thrombosis.

Cytoreductive drugs are used to reduce platelet numbers to normal limits. These include hydroxycarbamide, anagrelide, busulphan and interferon alpha. Daily low-dose aspirin is also given to reduce the risk of thrombosis, although caution if the platelet count is $>1000 \times 10^9$/L.

Primary myelofibrosis

Primary myelofibrosis (PMF) is caused by clonal proliferation of a pluripotent stem cell. Fibrous tissue invades and replaces bone marrow territory. This occurs secondary to fibroblast proliferation and extracellular matrix formation, resulting from an abnormally high cytokine secretion (platelet-derived growth factor, transforming growth factor β) from abnormal megakaryocytes. Extramedullary haematopoiesis is a prominent feature, leading to massive splenomegaly and sometimes also hepatomegaly. Myelofibrosis may present de novo or evolve from other myeloproliferative conditions (e.g., PRV or ET). PMF has the worst prognosis of the myeloproliferative disorders. Median survival is just 5 years, and ~25% of cases transform further into AML.

Clinical features

Patients, usually aged between 50 and 60 years, present with constitutional symptoms secondary to a hypermetabolic state. They may also complain of anaemic symptoms (fatigue, shortness of breath, palpitations) or abdominal pain (due to massive splenomegaly).

Diagnostic tests

Elevated white cell and platelet counts and reduced red cell counts are features of the FBC (Fig. 5.1). The film is often diagnostic, revealing poikilocytosis (see Table 2.4), nucleated red cell precursors and granulocyte precursors (i.e., 'Leucoerythroblastic features'). Bone marrow aspirate often results in a 'dry tap' where no aspirate is obtained due to fibrosis of the usual bone marrow territory. Trephine biopsy reveals patchily hypercellular marrow with prominent reticulin fibrosis: this finding is mandatory for diagnosis (Fig. 5.2).

Cytogenetic analysis reveals karyotypic abnormalities in ~50% of patients. These are associated with a poorer prognosis. Approximately 50% exhibit the same JAK2 mutation that is seen in PRV and ET.

Treatment

Supportive transfusion of red cells, androgens, erythropoietin, thalidomide, lenalidomide or splenectomy are all options to control the anaemia. Ruxolitinib is the first approved JAK inhibitor

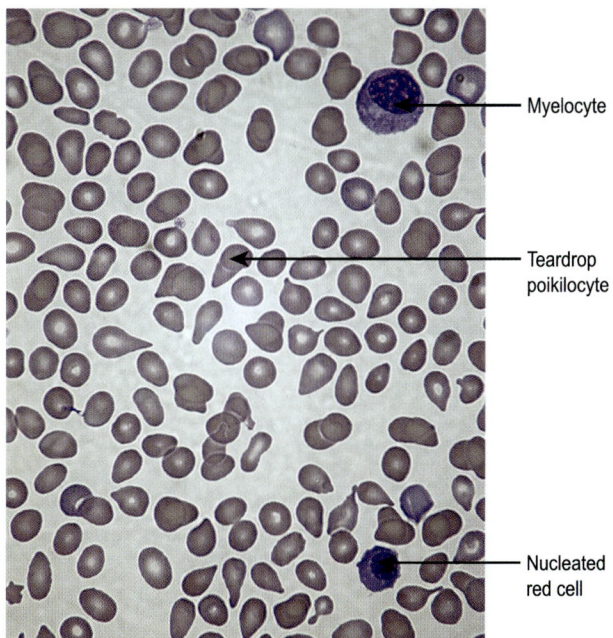

Fig. 5.1 Blood film showing teardrops, nucleated red blood cells and early myeloid progenitor cells. These are 'Leucoerythroblastic changes' and typically seen in myelofibrosis. (From Feather A, Randall D, Waterhouse M. *Kumar and Clark's Clinical Medicine*. 10th ed. Elsevier; 2021).

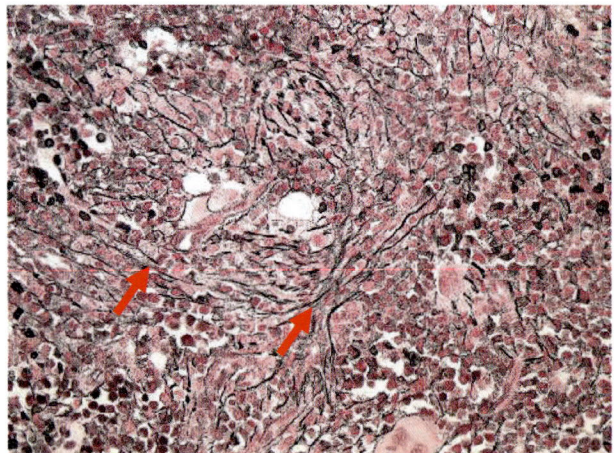

Fig. 5.2 Bone marrow histology showing increased reticulin (*red arrow*) which is typically seen in myelofibrosis. (From Fletcher CDM. *Diagnostic Histopathology of Tumors, 2 Volume Set,* 5th ed. Elsevier; 2021.)

and is the treatment of choice for severe constitutional symptoms or symptomatic splenomegaly. The only curative treatment for PMF is bone marrow transplantation, but this is only appropriate for a small proportion of young patients and represents a very high-risk treatment strategy.

MYELODYSPLASTIC SYNDROMES

A heterogeneous array of disorders; myelodysplastic syndromes (MDS) are defined as a clonal disorder of haematopoietic stem cells where there is replacement of normal marrow by dysplastic, abnormal and immature ('blast') cells. Although the stem cells otherwise retain the capacity to differentiate into mature cells, they fail to mature normally and are functionally suboptimal. The cell counts of any cell line may be reduced. Often more than one cell line is affected. MDS may further develop into AML.

Clinical features

Usually a disease of the elderly, the symptoms depend on the affected cell lines (e.g., neutropenia→recurrent infections, thrombocytopenia→easy bruising). Isolated anaemia is the most common presentation. However, MDS often presents nonspecifically or is discovered incidentally when unexplained cytopenias are further investigated in asymptomatic patients. MDS can develop in patients who have received chemotherapy and/or radiotherapy for another condition.

Diagnostic tests

Full blood count usually reveals cytopenia(s), and blood film demonstrates characteristic morphological abnormalities in the affected cell lines. Red cell macrocytosis is a common finding in MDS, and in one of the subtypes, peripheral monocytosis is an additional common feature. Bone marrow examination, together with cytogenetic analysis, is diagnostic and facilitates classification (Table 5.1), prognostication and treatment decision-making.

Treatment

Treatment (and prognosis) is guided by a prognostic scoring system. In elderly or less fit patients, treatment is essentially supportive. Anaemia can sometimes be managed with erythropoietin injections or lenalidomide but more commonly regular red cell transfusions are required. Thrombocytopenia (if

Table 5.1 The 2022 World Health Organization (WHO) myelodysplastic syndrome subtypes (simplified)	
Name	**BM and PB blasts**
MDS with low blasts (MDS-LB)	BM < 5%, PB < 2%, no Auer rods
MDS with hypoplastic marrow (MDS-h)	BM < 5%, PB < 2%, <25% BM cellularity (adjusted for age)
MDS with increased blasts: - MDS-IB1 - MDS-IB2 - MDS with fibrosis (MDS-f)	 BM 5–9% BM or PB 2–4% BM 10–19% or PB 5–19% or Auer rods BM 5–19% or PM 2–19%
MDS with isolated del(5q) and low blasts	BM < 5%, PB < 2%, no Auer rods with del (5q) mutation alone *or* with 1 additional abnormality (excluding -7 or del (7q))
MDS with SF3B1 mutation and low blasts	BM < 5% or PB < 2%, no Auer rods, >15% ring sideroblasts. Absence of 5q deletion, monosomy 7 or complex karyotype
MDS with biallelic TP53 inactivation (MDS-biTP53)	BM <20% or PB <20%; 2+ TP53 mutations or one mutation with TP53 copy number loss

BM, Bone marrow; MDS, myelodysplastic syndrome; PB, peripheral blood.

associated with abnormal bleeding) is managed with regular platelet transfusions. Some patients can be offered eltrombopag, a thrombopoietin-receptor agonist, to reduce the number of platelet transfusions (see Chapter 6: Haemostasis). Neutropenic patients require appropriate antimicrobial prophylaxis and may benefit from G-CSF. Regular clinical supervision is essential to monitor for development of AML.

In fitter patients, more intensive treatment can be used. Azacytidine, a hypomethylating agent, may induce remissions but is not curative. Chemotherapy (as for AML) followed by stem cell transplant is the only curative option.

LEUKAEMIAS

Leukaemias are characterized by an accumulation of leukaemic cells in bone marrow and often also peripheral blood. Leukaemic cells are 'clonal' (i.e., identical to the original neoplastic cell) and nonfunctional. However, they occupy marrow territory, impairing normal haematopoiesis. This leads to cytopenia in all cell lines. Leukaemias are classified according to:

- Cell lineage – lymphoid or myeloid.
- Maturity of the abnormal cell population: this defines whether the leukaemia is classified as 'acute' or 'chronic,' rather than purely by the clinical course and presentation as one might expect from the name.

Acute leukaemias are defined by proliferation of an immature 'blast' cell and, if untreated, are rapidly fatal. Chronic leukaemias are defined by proliferation of a more mature cell, and the clinical course is more prolonged. Treatment for leukaemias, particularly acute leukaemias, can lead to tumour lysis syndrome.

ACUTE LEUKAEMIAS

Clinical features

Patients are usually very unwell at presentation. Immediate admission and acute resuscitation including intravenous antibiotics, appropriate transfusion and correction of any metabolic abnormalities (these are particularly associated with a high tumour burden) comprise acute management. Intensive chemotherapy is urgently required, or death occurs rapidly from sepsis or bleeding. Constitutional and leucostatic symptoms are common. Symptoms may also relate to the cytopenias and include:

- severe fatigue, pallor and breathlessness (anaemia)
- easy bruising or abnormal bleeding (thrombocytopenia, disseminated intravascular coagulation [DIC])
- fever and recurrent infections (neutropenia)

RED FLAG

NEUTROPENIC SEPSIS

This is the term used to describe invasive bacterial infection occurring in the context of neutropenia ($<1.0 \times 10^9$/L). This is a common and dangerous complication of both the haematological malignancy itself and the treatment-induced suppression of myelopoiesis. Often fever is the only sign of infection; however, patients may be unwell even in the absence of fever. High suspicion in patients likely to be neutropenic is vital, and immediate admission and treatment with empirical intravenous antibiotics must be implemented early to prevent death from septic shock.

RED FLAG

LEUCOSTATIC SYMPTOMS

These arise from blood hyperviscosity due to excessively high levels of abnormal white cells. This 'sludging' of white cells results in impaired tissue perfusion, leading to symptoms of tissue hypoxia, particularly in the brain (blurred vision, headaches, confusion, coma) and lungs (dyspnoea, hypoxia, infiltrates on chest X-ray [CXR]). This hypoxia is exacerbated by the high metabolic demands of rapid blast division. Urgent leucopheresis and commencing concomitant chemotherapy are required.

Other symptoms include:

- Deposition of leukaemic cells in tissue (e.g., gum hypertrophy in AML)
- Lymphadenopathy and hepatosplenomegaly in acute lymphoblastic leukaemia (ALL)
- Infiltration of leukaemic cells in the cerebrospinal fluid (CSF) and (central nervous system [CNS]; most commonly seen in ALL)

There is usually no particular cause identified, but AML and ALL may be associated with radiation, toxins or drug exposure and certain chromosomal disorders (e.g., trisomy 21).

Diagnostic tests

Full blood count exhibits anaemia and thrombocytopenia. The white cell count may be very high or very low. Blood film demonstrates the abnormal morphology of blast cells (Fig. 5.3). Bone marrow biopsy exhibiting blasts is diagnostic, and cytogenetics is mandatory, as the leukaemic cell karyotype is the strongest

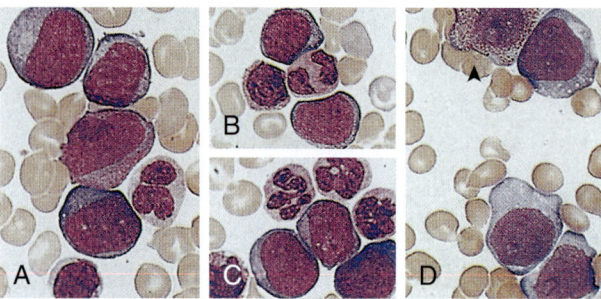

Fig. 5.3 Blood film showing blasts typically associated with acute myeloid leukaemia. (From Skarin AT. *Atlas of Diagnostic Oncology*. 4th ed. Elsevier; 2010).

prognostic factor regarding survival and response to treatment. Molecular genetics are also important, as particular mutations carry prognostic significance. Levels of LDH and uric acid may offer an indication of the tumour burden.

Acute myeloid leukaemia

Acute myeloid leukaemia is the most common adult acute leukaemia. The original neoplastic blast cell is a myeloid precursor cell. Particular chromosomal rearrangements, such as t(15:17), t(8:21) and inversion of 16, have better prognoses than others (e.g., monosomy 7). Importantly, AML can evolve from existing myeloproliferative or myelodysplastic disorders or chronic myeloid leukaemia (CML). As well as accumulation of blasts in marrow and peripheral blood, skin, gum and organ infiltration may occur. The current WHO classification of AML is complex and based on cytogenetic rearrangements and molecular mutations present in the neoplastic clone. The old FAB classification was based on degree of maturation and differentiation of the myeloid lineage (M1 to M7). These subtypes impact on prognosis and crucially whether a patient requires a stem cell transplant. Overall cure rates vary from 30% to 80% depending on the subtype.

HINTS AND TIPS

REMISSION

The term 'remission' describes an absence of disease signs and symptoms. It may be permanent or temporary, ending with reappearance of signs and symptoms ('relapse'). 'Complete remission' describes clinical absence as well as normalized histology and function.

Acute promyelocytic leukaemia

Acute promyelocytic leukaemia (APML) is a particular subtype of AML (M3 in the previous FAB classification). It is characterized by the t(15:17) translocation and (in addition to the findings listed above) often shows features of DIC (see Chapter 6: Haemostasis). It carries a high risk of fatal haemorrhage during the early phase of treatment. However, after the initial phase, it has the best prognosis of all subtypes with cure rates of >80%.

Treatment of AML

This comprises two phases: induction and consolidation. In AML, induction treatment usually comprises cytarabine plus an anthracycline such as daunorubicin. Postinduction treatment usually comprises further chemotherapy, allogeneic stem cell transplantation (SCT) or a combination of the two. Certain specific mutations respond to specific treatments; for example, t(15:17), associated with APML responds to all-trans retinoic acid as well as arsenic trioxide.

CLINICAL NOTES

INDUCTION TREATMENT

'Induction treatment' aims to reduce or eradicate the leukaemic cell population and restore normal bone marrow haemopoiesis (i.e., 'induce' remission). 'Consolidation' treatment aims to destroy lingering but undetectable leukaemic cells.

CLINICAL NOTES

ALLOGENEIC STEM CELL TRANSPLANTATION

Stem cell transplantation aims to replace cancerous marrow cells with disease-free haematopoietic stem cells from donor marrow ('bone marrow transplant') or donor peripheral blood ('peripheral blood stem cell transplant'). Prior to donation, chemotherapy and/or radiotherapy is employed to destroy the native cancerous cells before replacing with the healthy donor cells. Ideally the donor is HLA-matched to reduce the probability of graft-versus-host disease (GVHD), which is when the donor (graft) cells recognize patient (host) cells as foreign, thereby initiating an immune reaction in the transplant recipient. This is primarily a T-cell-mediated disease and a major cause of morbidity and mortality. Immunosuppressive therapy is also used to reduce the chances of GVHD. In addition to GVHD, graft failure (immune rejection of donor cells by the recipient) and organ damage may complicate SCT. This is thus a high-risk procedure with treatment-related mortality of 20–30% (death due to the procedure rather that the underlying condition). For further details, please refer to Chapter 13: Medical intervention.

RED FLAG

HYPERURICAEMIA

This results in painful urate crystal deposition in joints, renal stones and renal failure. To avoid hyperuricaemia, xanthine oxidase inhibitors such as allopurinol or recombinant urate oxidase (e.g., rasburicase) are coadministered prophylactically during chemotherapy (see 'Tumour lysis syndrome').

Acute lymphoblastic leukaemia

The most common childhood cancer, ALL accounts for 80% of all childhood leukaemias. The leukaemic blast cells may be of B-cell (~80%) or T-cell origin. Of note, the Philadelphia chromosome (see subsequent CML section), when seen in ALL (up to 20% of ALL cases), carries a poorer prognosis. As well as the clinical features of acute leukaemias described earlier, hepatosplenomegaly is often present at diagnosis.

Treatment

Fortunately, childhood ALL is more responsive to treatment than AML, with cure rates of >80%. However, adult cure rates are only ~40%. Unlike AML, treatment comprises four phases: induction, consolidation, CNS prophylaxis and continuing then on with maintenance treatment which lasts 2–3 years. In high-risk ALL, SCT is used in place of maintenance treatment.

Induction treatment usually comprises daunorubicin, vincristine, corticosteroids and asparaginase, and if the Philadelphia chromosome is present, tyrosine kinase inhibitors (TKIs) are added (see CML). Allopurinol or rasburicase is used as prophylaxis against tumour lysis syndrome. Consolidation treatment, followed by maintenance treatment, may include cytarabine, methotrexate, mercaptopurine, anthracyclines (e.g., daunorubicin), alkylating agents (e.g., cyclophosphamide), vincristine and epipodophyllotoxins (e.g., etoposide).

Acute lymphoblastic leukaemia has a very high propensity to spread to the CNS, and thus a specific treatment phase for CNS prophylaxis is included. This is further boosted by intrathecal chemotherapy, that is, chemotherapy injected directly into the CSF.

In relapsed disease, monoclonal antibody therapy targeting specific cell surface markers on the blasts can be used (e.g., inotuzumab, anti-CD22) as well as bispecific antibodies (e.g., blinatumomab, anti-CD19 and CD3). Chimeric antigen receptor (CAR) T cells can also be considered in this setting, although allogeneic SCT is preferable. You can read more information about CAR-T cell therapy in Chapter 13: Medical interventions.

RED FLAG

TUMOUR LYSIS SYNDROME

This complication can arise from the breakdown of malignant cells and typically occurs at the start of chemotherapy when the disease is most active. There is an excessive release of proteins and intracellular metabolites (i.e., uric acid) from tumour cells which overwhelm normal homeostatic control. Risk factors for developing this complication include:

- High tumour burden (e.g., high white cell count in acute leukaemias)
- High-grade tumour (e.g., Burkitt lymphoma)
- Increased age
- Preexisting renal impairment
- Concomitant use of drugs that increase uric acid levels (e.g., thiazides, aspirin)

Patients can develop acute kidney injury with hyperkalaemia and hypocalcaemia. If left untreated, they can lead to the development of cardiac arrhythmias, seizures or even result in sudden death.

To prevent this complication, prophylactic medications are prescribed to reduce the production of uric acid. These include allopurinol (a xanthine oxidase inhibitor) or rasburicase (recombinant urate oxidase). It is important not to administer both drugs together, as they will end up blocking each other! Patients are also aggressively hydrated (3 litres of fluids daily) and electrolyte abnormalities are corrected.

CHRONIC LEUKAEMIAS

Chronic leukaemias are often detected incidentally in asymptomatic patients when an elevated white count is noted on FBC. Large numbers of leukaemic cells exist, due to both proliferation and decreased apoptosis. Symptoms develop insidiously and are often secondary to cytopenias (as with the acute leukaemias), which arise due to marrow displacement by leukaemic cells.

Similarly, constitutional or leucostatic symptoms often occur. They differ from acute leukaemias in that:

- the marrow is not infiltrated with immature blasts
- near-normal maturation and differentiation of nonclonal 'normal' cell lines continue in parallel with the neoplastic clone.

Chronic myeloid leukaemia

The original neoplastic cell is a myeloid cell precursor that undergoes uncontrolled proliferation as well reduced apoptosis. This proliferation causes an increase in all cells of myeloid lineage (i.e., granulocytes and their precursors [neutrophils, myelocytes, metamyelocytes, eosinophils, basophils, etc.]). Granulocyte hyperplasia is apparent in the blood, bone marrow and spleen. These cells all display the original neoplastic abnormality, a translocation known as the Philadelphia chromosome. CML cells all possess the potential to transform to AML.

However, unlike the acute leukaemias, the actual leukaemic cell ('blast') population is not dramatically increased in peripheral blood. If the blast population does increase, this may represent the 'accelerated' phase in the disease progression, or above a certain level the transition to AML.

The Philadelphia chromosome

The chromosomal translocation t(9:22) results in movement of the proto-oncogene ABL (normally located on chromosome 9) adjacent to the BCR gene on chromosome 22. This leads to a shortened chromosome 22, which is termed the 'Philadelphia chromosome' and is a hallmark of CML, diagnostic when present in a patient with clinical manifestations of CML. The BCR/ABL fusion gene encodes a constitutively active tyrosine kinase. Expression of this protein leads to development of CML.

Clinical features

Chronic myeloid leukaemia evolves following a predictable course, consisting of three stages: chronic, accelerated and blast crisis. Ninety percent of CML is diagnosed in the earliest chronic stage, when asymptomatic patients are further investigated after markedly elevated granulocytic counts are noted on an FBC. When CML is symptomatic, the symptoms result from splenomegaly, leucostasis or they may be constitutional in nature. Dramatic splenomegaly is present in >50% of patients at diagnosis.

Diagnostic tests

White cell count, attributable to leukaemic granulocytes, is significantly ($>20 \times 10^9$/L) and often dramatically elevated. Basophil, eosinophils and myeloid precursor cells are elevated, and anaemia may be present (Fig. 5.4). Appearance of blasts on film and thrombocytopenia signals progression to the accelerated disease stage. Serum PCR identifies and quantifies the amount of the BCR-ABL fusion gene transcript, thus allowing diagnosis with a simple blood sample. Bone marrow biopsy

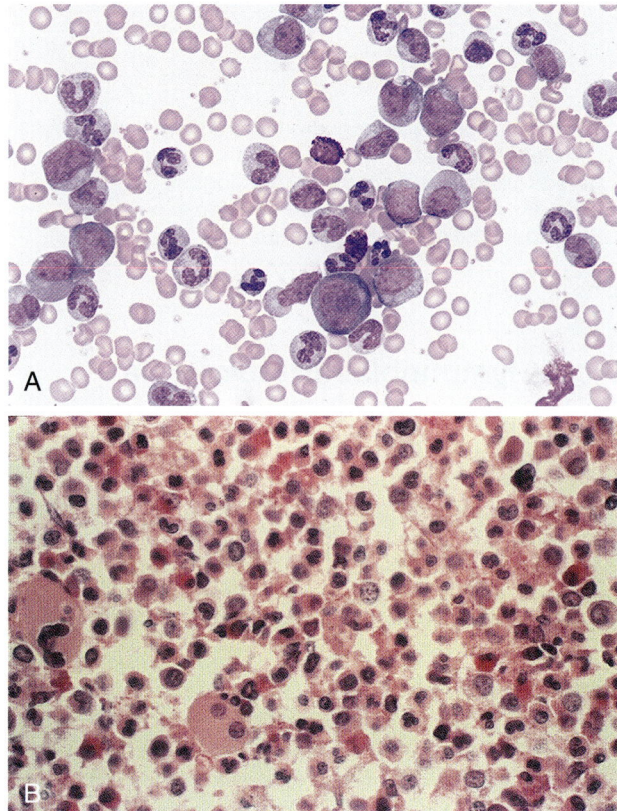

Fig. 5.4 Blood film showing early myeloid precursors, including myelocytes and band cells, typical for chronic myeloid leukaemia. (From Keohane EM, Smith LJ, Walenga JM. *Rodak's Hematology*. 5th ed. St. Louis: Saunders; 2016).

assists with staging and confirmation of the disease, and cytogenetics confirms presence of the Philadelphia chromosome.

Treatment

Because the chromosomal hallmark of CML results in abnormal tyrosine kinase activity, CML treatments centre around TKI. Imatinib was the first of the TKI inhibitors and has become a paradigm for targeted therapies; this has completely changed the landscape of first-line treatment for CML. While in the past, without an SCT, most patients would transform to acute leukaemia, today imatinib and other TKIs can induce complete haematological, cytogenetic and molecular remission. Since its initial development, several other TKIs have been developed which appear to be even more effective than imatinib (see Table 5.6).

If diagnosed in the blast crisis stage, treatment resembles that of the acute leukaemias. Severe leucostatic symptoms may be managed with leucopheresis. However, even at this stage, one of the TKI drugs is added to the treatment.

Chronic lymphocytic leukaemia

The original neoplastic cell is usually a lymphoid B-cell precursor, arrested in development. The resulting leukaemic cell population resemble mature (but nonfunctional) B cells. They infiltrate bone marrow, lymph nodes, spleen and liver. Those in peripheral blood may appear normal or as 'smear cells.' As with other haematological malignancies, chromosomal mutations are common and have an important bearing on the prognosis and response to treatment. Clinical progression is widely variable depending on the stage of the disease at diagnosis. Staging is determined according to number of lymphadenopathy sites, anaemia and thrombocytopenia and presence of various biomarkers. Significantly, up to 5% of cases of chronic lymphocytic leukaemia (CLL) can evolve further into high-grade lymphomas. This evolution is termed 'Richter's transformation'.

Clinical features

Chronic lymphocytic leukaemia is the most common adult leukaemia, is nearly twice as common in males and usually occurs in the elderly (median age at presentation, 72 years). In addition to the features common to the chronic leukaemias listed above, painless generalized lymphadenopathy is the most common presenting symptom. Cytopenias are the other common finding. Patients with CLL are particularly prone to infections even in the absence of cytopenias as they often have hypogammaglobulinaemia with poor antibody response to infections. Patients with CLL also have a high incidence of autoimmune cytopenias, in particular immune thrombocytopenia and autoimmune haemolytic anaemia.

Diagnostic tests

The initial finding is usually a mild to marked elevation in total white cell count due to the leukemic cell population. Unusually, bone marrow examination is not mandatory for CLL diagnosis: diagnosis is instead based on characteristic morphology of leukaemic cells ('smear cells') on blood film, a sustained count $>5 \times 10^9$/L clonal B cells and presence of a diagnostic immunophenotype (Fig. 5.5). Lymphocyte doubling time (LDT) as an index of disease progression can be established with serial measurements.

Treatment

'Early' CLL is simply monitored with regular review because the risk:benefit ratio favours this approach in inactive disease. Treatment is commenced when the disease is deemed 'active.' This is defined by:

- progressive failure of bone marrow haematopoiesis (indicated by worsening cytopenias)
- massive, progressive or symptomatic splenomegaly or lymphadenopathy
- an LDT <6 months
- presence of constitutional symptoms

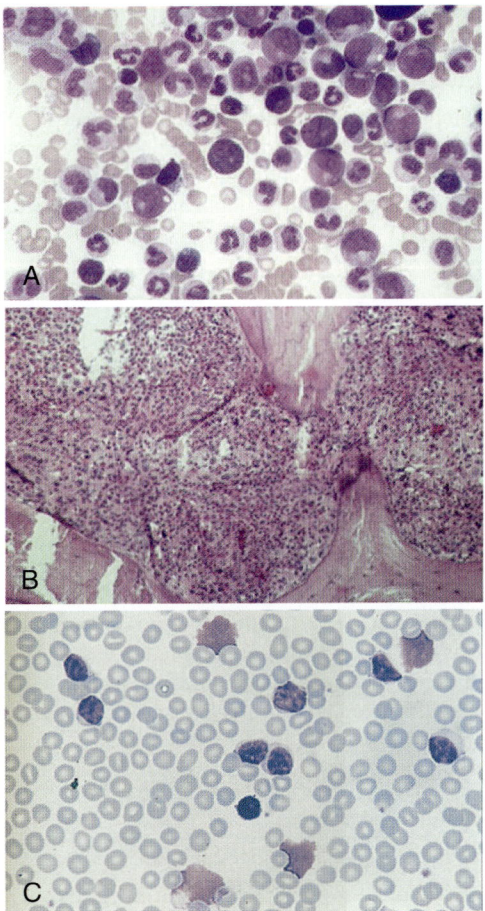

Fig. 5.5 Blood film showing raised lymphocytes as well as smear cells, a typical feature of chronic lymphocytic leukaemia. (From Naish J, Court DS. *Medical Sciences*, 3rd ed. Elsevier; 2018).

Treatment is not to cure but to achieve remission, which can last years. The disease tends to recur, requiring additional treatment strategies. The treatment usually involves various combinations of chemotherapy and immunotherapy drugs. Common chemotherapy drugs used include fludarabine (F), cyclophosphamide (C), bendamustine (B) and chlorambucil (Chl). Commonly used monoclonal antibodies used include rituximab (R), obinutuzumab (O) and ofatumumab (Of). Depending on the fitness of the patient, various combinations are used (e.g., FCR, BR and OChl).

Treatment of CLL has undergone a revolution in the last few years with 'chemotherapy-free' treatments becoming available. These targeted drugs act on the cellular pathways in the B lymphocytes, are orally active and used as continuous daily treatment as long as the disease remains responsive. Ibrutinib, acalabrutinib and venetoclax are three such drugs, all available as both first- and second-line options.

MALIGNANT LYMPHOMAS

Lymphomas are characterized by accumulation of clonal neoplastic cells in lymph nodes and extranodal lymphoid tissue (e.g., lungs). The original mutated cell is a primitive lymphoid cell. They are non-functional and occupy lymph node territory, impairing normal development of immune cells. Lymphomas are categorized as:

- Non-Hodgkin lymphoma (NHL; ~90%)
- Hodgkin lymphoma (HL; ~10%)

Clinical features of lymphomas

Presentation varies enormously among individuals. Common clinical features shared by most lymphomas include:

- Painless, nontender lymphadenopathy (most common sites cervical, then axillary)
- Constitutional, aka B symptoms (fever, night sweats, weight loss)
- Pruritus
- Mild/moderate splenomegaly
- Superior vena cava obstruction or respiratory symptoms in cases with mediastinal lymphadenopathy
- Human immunodeficiency virus infection significantly increases the risk of developing many high-grade B-cell NHL and HL.

COMMON PITFALLS

DIFFERENTIATING LEUKAEMIAS AND LYMPHOMAS

Avoid the common pitfall of oversimplifying leukaemias as being bone marrow diseases and lymphomas being lymph node diseases. Both leukaemic and lymphoma cells are also present in the blood and lymphoma cells may invade marrow too.

Differentiating clinical and aetiological features differentiating HL and NHL are shown in Table 5.2

Lymphoma staging is predominantly clinical, traditionally via the Ann Arbor staging system, shown in Table 5.3. Stages I and II are described as 'limited stage' and III and IV as 'advanced stage.'

Diagnostic tests in lymphomas

Serum uric acid and LDH are often elevated. FBC may show cytopenias. An enlarged lymph node is surgically resected and examined by a histopathologist for histology, immunophenotype and molecular genetics. Bone marrow examination will identify presence and extent of invasion by lymphoma cells. Computed tomography (CT) scanning identifies clinically impalpable or unnoticed areas of lymphadenopathy. A positron emission

Table 5.2 Features differentiating Hodgkin lymphoma from non-Hodgkin lymphoma

Non-Hodgkin lymphoma	Hodgkin lymphoma
Median age of presentation for most NHL tends to be >50 years of age	Presentations peak at ages in both 20s and 60s
Alcohol-induced pain in lymph nodes is not seen in NHL	A small fraction of HL patients may experience alcohol-induced pain of enlarged lymph nodes – a classical pathognomic feature
Cyclical fever not a feature	Patients may experience cyclical fever, known as Pel-Ebstein fever
Tends to involve extranodal lymphoid tissue more than HL Spleen, liver, thymus and mucosally associated lymphoid tissue in the gastrointestinal tract are predilection zones	Less likely to involve extranodal lymphoid tissue
Distant lymph node involvement with the intermediate lymph nodes 'skipped' is common	Lymph node involvement is typically contiguous
May be associated with: • Infection (e.g., EBV or HTLV) • Immunodeficiency (e.g., HIV) • Autoimmune disease • Exposure to radiation therapy or carcinogens • Certain inherited diseases such as ataxia telangiectasia, Fanconi syndrome, etc.	May also associated with: • Infection (e.g., EBV) • Immunodeficiency (e.g., HIV)
Patients more likely to experience cytopenias due to increased likelihood of marrow invasion	Patients less likely to experience marrow invasion and cytopenias
Tumour lysis syndrome occurs more commonly in NHL patients undergoing treatment	Tumour lysis syndrome is very rare in HL patients

EBV, Epstein–Barr virus; HIV, human immunodeficiency virus; HL, Hodgkin lymphoma; HTLV, human T-cell lymphoma virus; NHL, non-Hodgkin lymphoma.

Table 5.3 Cotswold-modified Ann Arbor lymphoma staging system

Stage[a]	Sites of involvement
I	Single lymph node region or one contiguous extranodal lymphatic site (e.g., liver)
II	Two or more lymph node regions on the *same* side of the diaphragm
III	Lymph node regions on *both* sides of the diaphragm, which may involve extralymphatic extension
IV	Diffuse involvement of more than one extranodal lymphatic site (e.g., bone marrow, gut, lung, liver)

[a]*Each stage is further subclassified to indicate absence (A) or presence (B) or one or more of the following three systemic symptoms: unexplained fever (≥38.3°C), night sweats and/or unexplained weight loss ≥10% body weight in the 6 months preceding diagnosis.*

tomography-CT (PET-CT) scan can give further information regarding the extent of the disease and has become mandatory in all high-grade NHL and HL.

Non-Hodgkin lymphomas

These consist of around 60 subtypes with heterogeneous characteristics. Incidence rises with age (median age being 60) and is higher in males. In ~85% the original neoplastic cell is a mature B cell or a B-cell progenitor. The remainder are of T or natural killer (NK) cell origin. They are characterized by grade. Tumour lysis syndrome is a dangerous complication that is not uncommon in NHL patients undergoing treatment.

> **RED FLAG**
>
> **ACUTE PRESENTATIONS OF NON-HODGKIN LYMPHOMA**
>
> Features may include hypercalcemia, tumour lysis syndrome, spinal cord compression, superior or inferior vena cava compression, autoimmune haemolytic anaemia, intestinal or ureteral compression, central nervous system mass lesions or lymphomatous meningitis.

High-grade non-Hodgkin lymphomas

These are aggressive and progress rapidly. The rapid division means they are susceptible to chemotherapy and a significant proportion are curable. They often present acutely. Examples include diffuse large B-cell lymphoma, mantle cell lymphoma and Burkitt lymphoma. T-cell NHL can also manifest cutaneously, which may be localized (Mycosis fungoides) or widespread (Sézary syndrome) (Fig. 5.6).

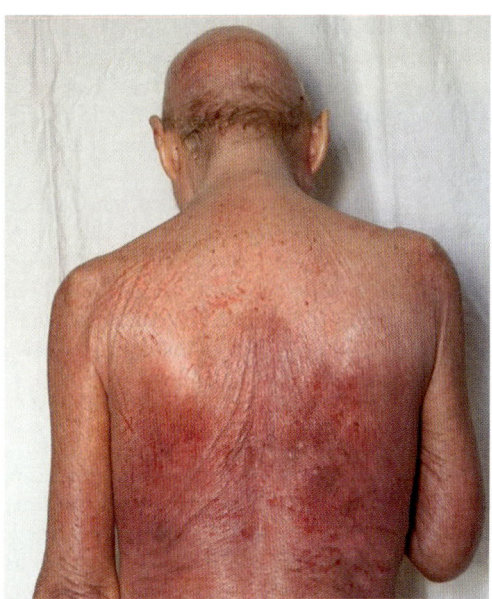

Fig. 5.6 Typical presentation of Sezary syndrome with diffuse erythroderma. (From Shimshak S, Sokumbi O, Isaq N, Goyal A, Comfere N. A practical guide to the diagnosis, evaluation, and treatment of cutaneous T-cell lymphoma. *Dermatol Clin*. 2023 Jan;41(1):209-229. doi: 10.1016/j.det.2022.07.019. PMID: 36410979).

> **RED FLAG**
>
> **SUPERIOR VENA CAVA OBSTRUCTION**
>
> This a dangerous complication of lymphomas where patients can present with facial swelling, chest pain, hoarseness, stridor and headaches. This is usually due to either enlarged lymph nodes or mass causing compression of the superior vena cava obstruction (SVCO). Clinical examination will demonstrate facial and upper extremity oedema with plethora and distended veins along the neck and anterior chest wall. If the patient bends forward, this will exacerbate their symptoms.
>
> If left untreated, SVCO can result in laryngeal oedema and reduced cardiac output, and the outcome can potentially be fatal. Therefore, early recognition of this complication is critical.
>
> Diagnosis is usually confirmed on imaging with CT and management can be both medical and surgical. The former involves using corticosteroids (IV methylprednisolone 1 g daily), although if lymphoma is suspected, a biopsy of the lymph node/mass is usually undertaken first to confirm diagnosis. However, in an emergency, treatment should not be delayed. Surgical intervention usually involves stenting to relieve the pressure.

Low-grade NHL

These are 'indolent,' with clinical signs (e.g., lymphadenopathy/organomegaly) developing slowly. They have a longer median survival but are usually incurable. Examples include follicular lymphoma, small lymphocytic lymphoma and splenic marginal zone lymphoma.

One particular indolent NHL is called mucosa-associated lymphoid tissue (MALT) lymphoma, which usually arises due to persistent chronic inflammation at these sites. Gastric MALT lymphoma is the most common form and is preceded by *Helicobacter pylori* infection. When localized to the gastric mucosa, it often responds to antibiotic therapy aimed at eliminating the bacteria.

Treatment of NHL

The R-CHOP regimen is one of the most commonly employed regimens. This consists of rituximab, cyclophosphamide, doxorubicin, vincristine and prednisolone. Radiation may additionally be utilized. However, there are various regimes used for particular subtypes.

Hodgkin lymphoma

Previously known as Hodgkin disease, HL typically has bimodal age distribution with a first peak in the 20s and the second peak in the 60s, with a slight male preponderance. The original neoplastic cell is a B-cell derivative with a dysfunctional immunoglobulin gene, termed a Reed-Sternberg (RS) cell. Microscopically the RS cell has an 'owl's eye' appearance, with prominent multinucleated nuclei and eosinophilic cytoplasm (Fig. 5.7). The RS cells usually

make up 1–2% of the lymph node cellularity with surrounding reactive macrophages, lymphocytes, plasma cells and eosinophils. Ninety-five percent of HL is 'classical' and classified histologically as follows:

- Nodular sclerosing: the most common subtype. Collagen bands divide affected nodes into nodules.
- Lymphocyte-rich: large numbers of lymphocytes are seen, relative to RS cells. This carries a more favourable prognosis.
- Mixed cellularity: more RS cells are present relative to lymphocytes.
- Lymphocyte-depleted: RS cells are present in the highest proportion relative to lymphocytes. This subtype has the poorest prognosis of all HL subtypes.

The remaining 5% of HL is termed nodular lymphocyte–predominant Hodgkin lymphoma (NLPHL). Clinical staging is the most accurate indicator of long-term prognosis in HL, and as for NHL the revised Ann Arbor system is used. In classical HL, the most common lymph nodes involved are the cervical lymph nodes (~75% of patients) followed by mediastinal, axillary and the para-aortic lymph nodes (see Fig. 1.3).

Treatment

Treatment strategy is chosen according to stage. Many patients require dual treatment with both combination chemotherapy and radiotherapy. With current treatment protocols cure rates vary from ~60 to ≥90%, depending upon the stage at diagnosis.

AGE-SPECIFIC HAEMATOLOGICAL MALIGNANCY RISK

Certain haematological malignancies are more common in different age groups. The *most* common haematological malignancies for each of the following age groups are as follows:

- Childhood: acute lymphoblastic leukaemia
- Adult leukaemia: chronic lymphocyte leukaemia
- Adult lymphoma: diffuse large-cell B-cell lymphoma
- Teenagers/young adults: Hodgkin lymphoma

PLASMA CELL DYSCRASIAS

These are malignant monoclonal proliferations of a neoplastic plasma cell, which synthesize an abnormal immunoglobulin (paraprotein) and/or abnormal light chain. Paraproteins and light chains can be identified in the serum while the light chains can also be found in the urine (Bence-Jones proteins). The most common dyscrasia is monoclonal gammopathy of undetermined significance (MGUS), but multiple myeloma, solitary plasmacytoma and Waldenstrom macroglobulinaemia are also clinically important entities.

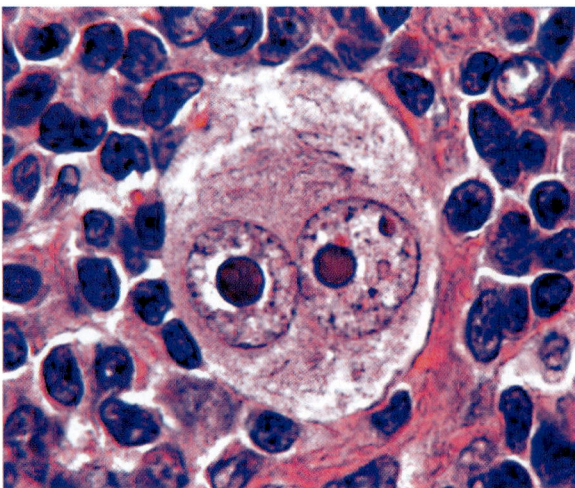

Fig. 5.7 Typical Reed-Sternberg cell with 'owl's eye' appearance seen in Hodgkin lymphoma. (From Harris JP, Roberts DS, Lin HW. *Cummings Review of Otolaryngology.* 2nd ed. Elsevier; 2023. Image courtesy of Dr. Fabio Facchetti, Brescia, Italy).

Multiple myeloma

This is a disease of late middle age onwards with incidence ~5/100,000 annually. Aetiology is unclear, although there is an increased incidence in patients with previous exposure to ionizing radiation. Staging according to International Staging System is from stages I to III according to age, laboratory and cytogenetic findings.

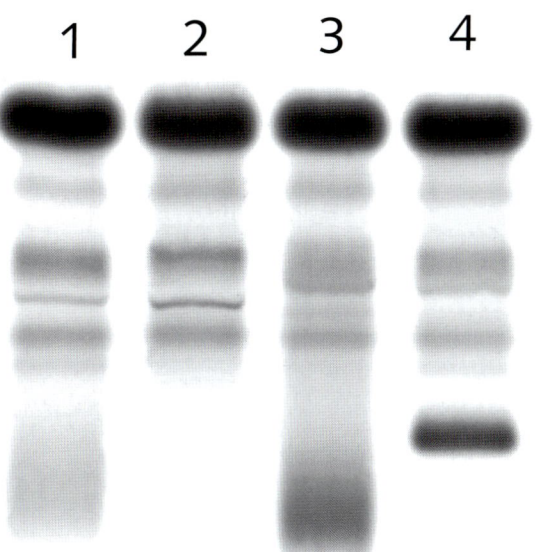

Fig. 5.8 Serum electrophoresis. Electrophoresis uses an electric field to separate proteins across a gel matrix according to various properties including molecular size. Each band, which is visible when stained appropriately, represents a protein of a specific molecular weight. *Lane 1*: normal serum. *Lane 2*: antibody-deficient serum. *Lane 3*: serum from an infected patient, illustrating polyclonal immunoglobulins. *Lane 4*: myeloma patient serum illustrating prominent band representing monoclonal immunoglobulin.

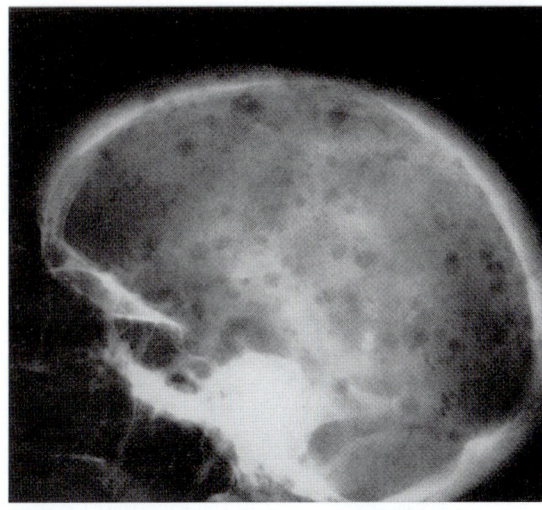

Fig. 5.9 Skull radiograph illustrating a 'pepper-pot skull' in a patient with multiple myeloma. The appearance is of multiple osteolytic bone lesions. (Courtesy Dr M. Makris.)

Clinical features

These are legion, but the four most common are abbreviated as 'CRAB' symptoms.

- Calcium. Hypercalcaemia (due to increased bone resorption).
- Renal. The kidneys are particularly affected, leading to renal impairment in ~25% of patients and severe renal failure in ~5%. This may be secondary to dehydration, nonsteroidal antiinflammatory drug use (for bone pain), recurrent sepsis, hypercalcaemia, renal tubular obstruction from proteinaceous casts and light chain proximal tubular toxicity to proximal tubules.
- Anaemia (normochromic and normocytic) due to plasma cell infiltration of the bone marrow.
- Bone. Lytic lesions (Fig. 5.9) resulting from bone destruction, predominantly affecting the axial skeleton, are a hallmark of the disease, with back pain being a very common symptom. Diffuse osteoporosis results in pathological fractures. Bone pain is the most common symptom of multiple myeloma, present in ~60% of patients.

including confusion, coma, renal impairment, gastrointestinal disturbance, cardiac arrhythmia, bone pain and profound muscle weakness. Symptomatic or marked (>3.5 mmol) hypercalcaemia is therefore treated with aggressive intravenous (IV) hydration with 0.9% saline, IV bisphosphonates and sometimes calcitonin.

Other symptoms include:

- Immune. Neutropenia and lack of functional immunoglobulins results in high susceptibility to persistent and recurrent infections.
- Neurological. Symptoms secondary to spinal cord or nerve root compression by collapse of the vertebrae due to lytic bone lesions (Fig. 5.10).

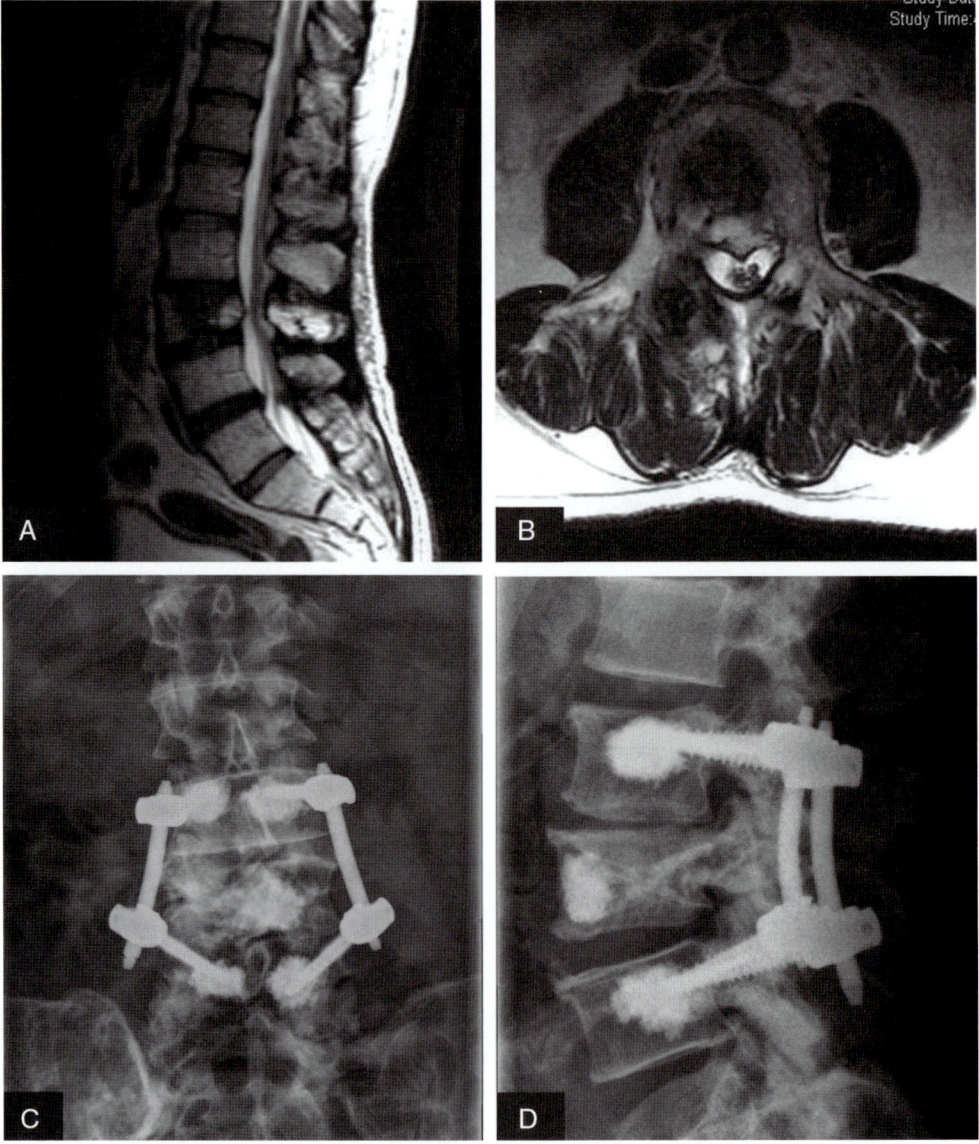

Fig. 5.10 MRI showing lytic lesion causing vertebral collapse and subsequent cord compression in patient diagnosed with multiple myeloma. (From WNEU, 1878-8750, 2018).

- Amyloidosis. Approximately 10% of patients with myeloma will develop amyloid light-chain (AL) amyloidosis.

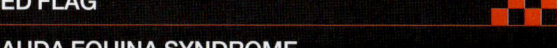

RED FLAG

CAUDA EQUINA SYNDROME

This is an oncological emergency and requires rapid intervention. In patients with multiple myeloma, vertebral collapse from lytic lesions or large extramedullary lesions can result in spinal cord compression and subsequent cauda equina syndrome. Patients typically present with acute lower back pain radiating down both legs as well as paraesthesia and lower body weakness. Classically they will report saddle anaesthesia, due to loss of sensation in the perineum and anal area. As a result, patients will report loss of bowel and/or bladder control with incontinence.

Diagnosis is usually clinical and then confirmed on magnetic resonance imaging (MRI). Intervention usually depends on the underlying cause but can be medical (corticosteroids), surgical (neurosurgical intervention) or radiotherapy.

Diagnostic tests

Blood tests typically show normochromic, normocytic anaemia while rouleaux changes can be seen on the blood film (Fig. 5.11). The erythrocyte sedimentation rate (ESR) is usually raised and there may be renal impairment with high calcium levels.

Serum electrophoresis reveals a prominent discrete band (Fig. 5.8, *lane 4*) representing the paraprotein (immunoglobulin) in 80% of patients. (IgG > IgA > IgD: IgM paraproteins are typically associated with Waldenstrom rather than multiple myeloma.)

In the remaining 20% only *free* light chains are produced; since the clonal plasma cells produce only *one* type of light chain (kappa or lambda), it leads to a very abnormal κ:λ ratio. This is called light chain myeloma. Bence-Jones proteins (which are essentially light chains) are often present in the urine.

In a very small percentage the malignant plasma cell *does not* secrete a paraprotein *or* light chains – this rare variant is referred to as 'nonsecretory myeloma'.

Another marker for multiple myeloma is β2-microglobulin (β2M) which is a component of the major histocompatibility complex (MHC) class I molecules and expressed on all nucleated cells. It is typically increased in multiple myeloma, and high levels are associated with poor prognosis.

Bone marrow examination in multiple myeloma shows >10% occupation by clonal plasma cells (Fig. 5.12). Lytic lesions are typically seen on X-rays although the gold standard imaging modality in current practice is either MRI or PET scans.

Treatment

Without effective treatment, median survival is 6 months. Patients are risk stratified according to presence/absence of specific genetic abnormalities as well as using the Revised International Staging System (R-ISS). The latter incorporates albumin, β2M, LDH and cytogenetics.

Induction therapy is commenced in all patients regardless of suitability for SCT. This usually consists of various combinations of traditional chemotherapy drugs (cyclophosphamide, melphalan), immunomodulatory drugs (thalidomide, lenalidomide), proteasome inhibitors (bortezomib, carfilzomib), monoclonal

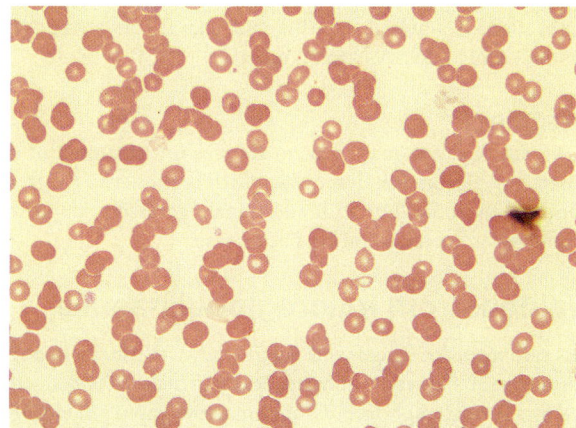

Fig. 5.11 Blood film showing red cell rouleaux (stacked, overlapping cells). These arise due to excessive levels of high-molecular-weight proteins in blood. This is seen in multiple myeloma, but also in other nonhaematological inflammatory conditions.

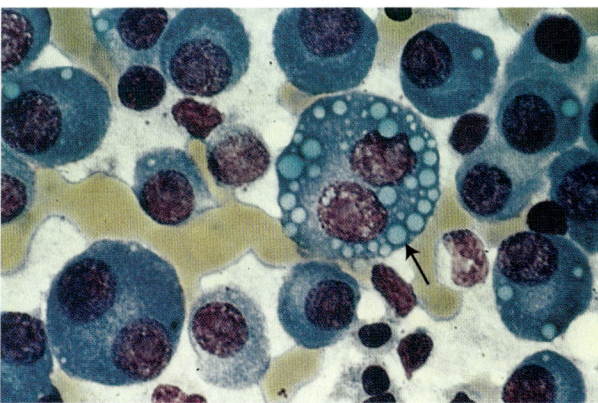

Fig. 5.12 Bone marrow aspirate showing increased infiltrate of abnormal plasma cells typically seen in multiple myeloma. (From Kumar V, Abbas AK, Aster JC, eds. *Robbins and Cotran Pathologic Basis of Disease*. 10th ed. Philadelphia: Elsevier; 2021).

antibodies (daratumumab [anti-CD38]) and a steroid. Fitter patients then receive consolidation treatment with autologous SCT, while others may remain on a single agent as maintenance therapy. Although such treatments can achieve complete remissions, relapse is inevitable and further lines of treatments are necessary. Therapies typically used in the relapsed setting can include a combination of the above as well as more novel options (CAR-T therapy, bispecific antibodies, anti-BCMA therapy). Supportive management includes adequate analgesia, sufficient hydration and bisphosphonates.

Solitary plasmacytoma

A solitary plasmacytoma is a solid tumour consisting of a neoplastic proliferation of plasma cells. They may be osseous (develop in bone) or extraosseous (develop in soft tissue). The former usually progresses to multiple myeloma, but the latter responds well to surgical resection and radiotherapy, thus it has an excellent prognosis.

Monoclonal gammopathy of uncertain significance

When a paraprotein is present but the neoplastic plasma cells occupy <10% of the marrow and clinical features of myeloma are absent, the condition is termed MGUS. This is present in ~3% of people older than 50 years, and the incidence rises to >7% by age 80 years. Only ~1% of patients with MGUS will progress to symptomatic myeloma (if IgG or IgA) or NHL/Waldenstrom (if IgM) annually. There are various prognostic factors and scoring systems that more accurately quantify this risk.

Differentiation between MGUS and MM

Both are plasma cell dyscrasias, but MGUS is benign and asymptomatic, in particular lacking any of the CRAB signs (hypercalcaemia, renal impairment, anaemia and bone lesions) and does not warrant treatment.

Amyloidosis

Amyloidosis refers to the extracellular deposition of abnormal protein variants. These variants restructure into fibrils with a beta-pleated sheet secondary structure. Various soluble serum proteins have the potential to restructure abnormally and deposit in this manner (e.g., immunoglobulin light chains). This subtype is referred to as AL amyloidosis and may occur in association with plasma cell dyscrasias. Amyloidosis is also a feature of other unrelated disorders such as chronic inflammatory illnesses (amyloid A protein [AA] amyloidosis). The hereditary form is referred to as amyloid transthyretin (ATTR) amyloidosis. It may be multisystem, or rarely, localized.

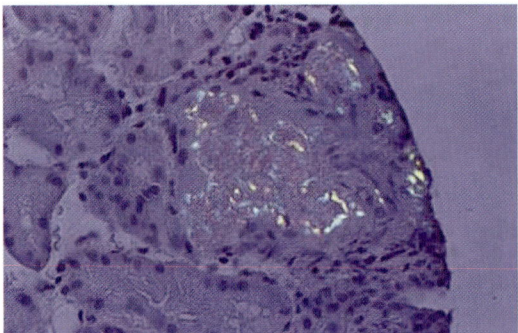

Fig. 5.13 Amyloid: Congo red with Congo red stain, amyloid deposits produce characteristic apple-green birefringence under polarized light. (From YAJKD, 2002).

Clinical features

An enormous range of clinical manifestations may occur, determined by the location, precursor protein type and the extent of deposits. Marked proteinuria in the nephrotic range (renal disease), peripheral and autonomic neuropathies and restrictive cardiomyopathy form the classic triad of symptoms. Other symptoms include organomegaly, CNS disease, skin manifestations and musculoskeletal and pulmonary disease.

Diagnosis

Diagnosis is made when biopsied subcutaneous fat stained with Congo red shows green birefringence on exposure to polarized light (Fig. 5.13). In AL amyloidosis, an abnormal light chain ratio can often be demonstrated in the blood, and bone marrow examination may show evidence of clonal plasma cells. A serum amyloid P component scan (SAP scan) allows detection and localization of amyloid deposits and is available at the NHS National Amyloidosis Centre, London.

Treatment

In AL amyloidosis, management focuses on treatment of the underlying plasma cell dyscrasia, which is similar to the treatment for myeloma, but with additional aggressive supportive treatment for the renal and cardiac disease.

Waldenstrom macroglobulinaemia

This rare disorder (incidence: 3/million/year) usually presents around age 50–70 years, more frequently in males. It is characterized by a B-cell lymphoproliferative marrow-based process, IgM paraprotein and elevated blood viscosity. If hyperviscosity occurs, plasmapheresis may be necessary. Constitutional symptoms, cytopenias and paraneoplastic neuropathy may also occur. Treatment aims to control symptoms and minimize end-organ damage.

INVESTIGATIONS IN HAEMATOLOGICAL MALIGNANCY

Erythrocyte sedimentation rate and plasma viscosity

Erythrocyte sedimentation rate is the rate at which red cells sediment in 1 hour. The 'normal' rate varies with age, gender and pregnancy. The major variable affecting ESR is the concentration of plasma proteins; the higher the concentration, the higher the ESR. ESR corresponds with plasma viscosity, an automated test. It is raised in inflammation (infectious and noninfectious) and, importantly, in malignancy.

Serum lactate dehydrogenase

In malignancy, normal tissues damaged by the neoplastic process experience increased cell death, releasing their intracellular LDH. In addition, the increased metabolic rate of rapidly dividing neoplastic cells enforces increased reliance on glycolysis, resulting in very high intracellular LDH. When these cells die, this LDH is released. Elevated levels are thus used as a serum marker of cellular damage. Malignancies with a particularly large malignant cell load (i.e., many haematological malignancies) can exhibit dramatically elevated LDH. Likewise, haemolysis results in raised LDH. It is useful in approximating disease load in lymphomas and leukaemias, particularly in quantifying response to treatment and prognosis.

Bone marrow biopsies

Biopsies of bone marrow are used to diagnose and/or stage haematological diseases, including malignancies. It is an ambulatory procedure with low morbidity performed under local anaesthesia. Two techniques are employed: bone marrow aspiration and trephine biopsy.

Trephine biopsy

A trephine biopsy is obtained via a large-bore needle, inserted into the iliac crest. This yields a core of bone and marrow, which is examined as a histological specimen. These are useful for assessing marrow cellularity and architecture. Table 5.4 describes the appearance of bone marrow in particular haematological diseases.

Bone marrow aspiration

A fine-bore needle is inserted into the iliac crest. The material aspirated makes individual cells available for microscopy and analysis. A 'smear' is performed, allowing for examination of the stages of haemopoiesis using specialist stains (e.g., MGG dye). The aspirate is also subjected to immunophenotyping and cytogenetic analysis.

Table 5.4 Bone marrow appearance in specific conditions

Disease/disorder	Bone marrow appearance
Iron-deficiency anaemia	Macrophage iron stores absent
Megaloblastic anaemia	Hypercellular marrow with megaloblasts ± giant metamyelocytes
Haemolytic anaemia	Hypercellular marrow with erythroid hyperplasia and reduced ratio of myeloid to erythroid precursors
Aplastic anaemia	Hypocellular marrow
PRV	Hypercellular marrow with hyperplasia of all cell lineages ('panmyelosis')
Essential thrombocythaemia	Hypercellular marrow with a marked increase in megakaryocytes, distributed in loose clusters
Myelofibrosis	Reduced haemopoiesis Hypercellularity in early disease (megakaryocytes form tight clusters) or reactive fibrosis in late disease
Acute leukaemias	Hypercellular marrow with blast infiltration
CLL	Hypercellular marrow with lymphocytic infiltration
CML	Hypercellular marrow with granulocyte and megakaryocyte hyperplasia
Multiple myeloma	Increased presence of clonal plasma cells

CLL, Chronic lymphocytic leukaemia; CML, chronic myeloid leukaemia; PRV, Polycythaemia rubra vera.

A 'Dry tap'

When bone marrow aspiration fails to produce marrow cells, this is a 'dry tap'. Rather than due to technical failure, this is indicative of certain marrow pathologies such as CML, PMF and metastases.

Cytogenetic analysis

Conventional cytogenetic analysis includes visual assessment of chromosomal size and structure on microscopy of metaphase chromosome preparation. Expert analysis may detect abnormalities of ~4–6 MB size or greater using this approach. Molecular cytogenetic analysis, also known as fluorescence in situ hybridization (FISH), can identify particular deletions or duplications associated with particular diseases. This approach identifies if a particular clinical suspicion is correct, since appropriate DNA probes must be used to detect if the particular suspected abnormality is present. Important translocation examples relevant to haematological malignancies are shown in Table 5.5.

Table 5.5 Translocations associated with specific malignancy

Translocation	Malignancy
t(9:22)	Pathognomonic of CML but also may occur in small percentage of ALL The altered chromosome 22 is known as the Philadelphia chromosome
t(14:18)	Follicular lymphoma (NHL)
t(8:14)	Burkitt lymphoma (NHL)
t(15:17)	Acute promyelocytic leukaemia (APML M3)

ALL, Acute lymphoblastic leukaemia; AML, acute myeloid leukaemia; CML, chronic myeloid leukaemia; NHL, non-Hodgkin lymphoma.

Lymph node biopsy

A suspicious enlarged lymph node is biopsied under local or general anaesthesia. Ideally, a superficial site is chosen to limit surgical/anaesthetic morbidity. This investigation is particularly important in lymphomas. Although 'core' biopsies can provide diagnostic material, wherever possible excision biopsy must be performed.

Lymphadenopathy 'red flags'

Painless, nontender lymphadenopathy that is generalized (i.e., involves several noncontiguous areas and feels hard or matted on palpation) suggests a noninfectious cause (i.e., a pathological manifestation of a disease rather than normal physiological reactive lymphadenopathy in response to infection in the drainage territory (see Chapter 1: Lymphadenopathy). Further red flags are raised by features such as hepatic/splenic enlargement and a history of constitutional symptoms accompanying the lymphadenopathy.

Immunophenotyping

This technique detects if particular antigenic protein structures are present on analyzed leucocytes. Normal leucocytes possess a standard array of individual antigens, while characteristically different arrays are present on the abnormal leucocytes seen in leukaemias and lymphomas. This allows diagnosis and classification of the malignancy. Immunophenotyping may be performed on any cell sample (e.g., marrow, blood, tissue). Flow cytometry is the technique most often employed with liquid samples, and immunocytochemistry is used with solid samples.

CHEMOTHERAPY AND TARGETED TREATMENTS

Treatment of haematological malignancies is immensely complex and must always be managed by appropriate specialists. In the past, chemotherapy was the only pharmacological strategy available to treat haematological cancers; however, new 'targeted' agents continue to be developed, allowing the haematologist's therapeutic arsenal to evolve and improve. Examples of targeted agents are shown in Table 5.6.

CLINICAL NOTES

CHEMOTHERAPY

Traditional chemotherapeutic agents arrest cell division and thus nonselectively damage/destroy *all* dividing cells, not just the cancerous cells. Neoplastic cells are more likely to be undergoing division due to their abnormally rapid proliferation than normal cells, so they are more likely to be damaged by the chemotherapy drug. However, 'innocent bystanders' that appropriately undergo rapid division, such as cells regenerating the constantly shedding gastrointestinal tract lining and mucosal surfaces, and hair too, are similarly affected. This accounts for symptoms commonly seen in patients undergoing chemotherapy (i.e., oral mucositis, bowel disturbance, alopecia).

Table 5.6 Examples of new targeted agents

Agent(s)	Target	Condition treated
Imatinib, dasatinib, nilotinib, ponatinib	BCR-ABL fusion protein	CML
Rituximab, ofatumumab, obinutuzumab	CD20	CD20-positive B-cell non-Hodgkin lymphomas
Brentuximab	CD30	CD30-positive lymphomas (e.g., Hodgkin lymphoma)
Ruxolitinib, pacritinib, momelotinib, fedratinib	JAK1/2	PMF
Ibrutinib, idelalisib, acalabrutinib, venetoclax	B-cell receptor pathways	CLL
Nivolumab, pembrolizumab	PD-1 pathway	Hodgkin lymphoma

CLL, Chronic lymphocytic leukaemia; CML, chronic myeloid leukaemia; PMF, primary myelofibrosis.

CLINICAL NOTES

TARGETED TREATMENTS

In contrast, targeted treatments damage *only* the specific cell type associated with the neoplastic disease. For example, rituximab is a monoclonal antibody that binds CD20-positive B cells; thus it selectively recruits the immune system to destroy only B cells, which makes it effective at malignancies of B-cell origin.

● Chapter Summary

- Myeloproliferative syndromes include PRV, ET and PMF. These result in overproduction of specific cell lines, and often evolve further into other types of haematological malignancy.
- Myelodysplastic syndromes usually lead to reduction in counts and functionality of one or more cell lines. They arise from a clonal disorder of the haematopoietic stem cell and may progress to AML.
- Leukaemias are subclassified by the cell progenitor affected (myeloid or lymphocytic) and are termed 'acute' or 'chronic' according to a combination of acuity of presentations, marrow blast infiltration and persistence of normal cell manufacture alongside the neoplastic clone proliferation. Important leukaemias to be aware of include acute and chronic myeloid leukaemias and acute and chronic lymphocytic leukaemias.
- Lymphomas (non-Hodgkin or Hodgkin) present heterogeneously, but symptoms may include painless lymphadenopathy, pruritus, splenomegaly and constitutional symptoms. They arise due to occupation of lymph node territory by abnormal primitive lymphoid cells, which impair normal immune cell maturation.
- Neutropenic sepsis may arise due to haematological malignancy or chemotherapy treatment. It is a medical emergency, presenting with low neutrophil count and typically septic shock. Sepsis must be treated urgently as neutropenic sepsis carries a high mortality.
- Tumour lysis syndrome, a complication of chemotherapy where the neoplastic cell load is very high. Release of intracellular components from the dying cells causes electrolyte derangement, the most acute consequence being hyperkalaemic cardiac arrhythmias.
- Multiple myeloma is most commonly characterized by multifactorial renal impairment, hypercalcaemia, anaemia and lytic lesions of bone. Immune impairment, neurological issues and secondary amyloidosis are also often problematic.
- Important investigations in suspected haematological malignancy include serum ESR, LDH and urate, the FBC, bone marrow or lymph node biopsy, cytogenetics and immunophenotyping.
- Stem cell transplantation involves therapeutic obliteration of diseased bone marrow and recolonization with disease-free donor haematopoietic stem cells. Along with chemotherapy and 'targeted treatments,' SCT represents a key weapon in the haematologist's antimalignancy arsenal.

MLA Conditions

Arterial thrombosis
Hypercalcaemia of malignancy
Leukaemia
Lymphoma
Multiple myeloma
Myeloproliferative disorders
Pancytopenia
Pathological fracture
Spinal cord compression
Spinal fracture

MLA Presentations

Bone pain
Fatigue
Fever
Limb weakness
Lump in groin
Lymphadenopathy
Neck lump
Night sweats
Organomegaly
Petechial rash
Stridor
Weight loss

INTRODUCTION

Haemostasis, defined as the processes occurring to arrest bleeding, is necessary to limit blood loss from damaged blood vessels. Unchecked, blood loss reduces circulating volume, which compromises tissue perfusion. A complex myriad of cellular and biochemical interactions underpins the process of haemostasis. However, it is based on simple principles as follows:

- Vasoconstriction: an increase in vascular tone reduces the diameter of proximal vessels, reducing blood flow to the damaged area. This minimizes blood loss and maximizes interaction between the platelets, coagulation factors and the endothelium. Vasoconstriction occurs in response to factors released by endothelial cells local to the injured area.
- Formation of a primary platelet plug: this initial structure forms a framework for the developing clot and temporarily seals the vessel wall, stopping blood loss. Platelets adhere to underlying tissue exposed by the vessel wall injury and each other with the help of von Willebrand factor (vWF). This step is termed 'primary haemostasis'.
- Reinforcement of the primary plug: circulating coagulation factors undergo a cascade of reactions, ultimately generating fibrin. Fibrin forms a mesh, stabilizing platelets in the developing clot and recruiting passing platelets. This allows the clot to remain until the underlying damage is repaired. This step is termed 'secondary haemostasis'.

CLINICAL NOTES

Bleeding time: This is the time taken for a small cut to stop bleeding, correlating approximately to the time taken for a platelet plug to form (primary haemostasis). It assesses platelet function and is increased in the context of platelet disorders. It is rarely used these days, as it is affected by too many variables, and there is controversy regarding its clinical utility.

PLATELETS

Platelets are nonnucleated, granular cells. The usual lifespan is 7–10 days. At any time, up to one-third of circulating platelets are sequestered within the spleen.

Structure

Platelets exhibit a biconvex discoid shape, which is maintained by a circumferential bundle of microtubules. The cytoplasm contains numerous granules (α, δ and lysosomal) which contain an array of bioactive molecules.

Platelet synthesis ('thrombopoiesis')

Platelets are synthesized from megakaryocytes in the bone marrow. These are large (50–100 μm) precursor cells that originate from pluripotent stem cells under the influence of thrombopoietin (TPO), a hormone produced mainly by the liver. Megakaryocytes develop lobulated, polyploid nuclei and an expanded cytoplasm volume via endomitosis (DNA replication without cellular division). They mature by distributing their cytoplasm into 10–20 processes ('proplatelets') that first radiate outwards, then elongate, narrow and branch. Platelets develop at the tips of proplatelets and disperse into the circulation. Each megakaryocyte may spawn up to 7000 platelets.

Platelet functions

The main functions fulfilled by platelets are primary haemostasis and tissue repair.

Sequence of primary haemostasis

Vessel injury

Endothelial damage exposes underlying subendothelium, causing release of endothelin. Endothelin induces vasoconstriction, reducing blood flow to the damage zone. Circulating vWF binds to exposed collagen myofibrils in the subendothelium.

Transient tethering

Transient tethering of platelets to the damage zone is mediated by a binding interaction between platelet glycoprotein (GP) Ib receptors and collagen-bound vWF in exposed subendothelium. This bond is short-lived but allows an initial monolayer of platelets to cover the damage zone (Fig. 6.1).

Adhesion

Adhesion describes permanent adherence of platelets to the damage zone following transient tethering. In this step, platelet receptors (GP Ia, GP IIa and GP VI) bind directly to the subendothelial collagen. This also leads to cytoskeletal alterations making the platelets flatter and leading to the formation of podia, thus increasing the available surface area for interactions with other platelets.

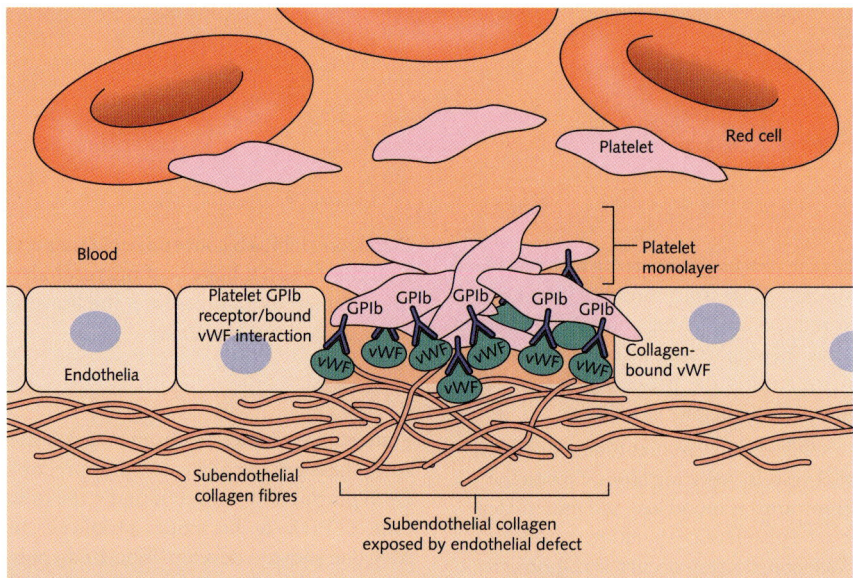

Fig. 6.1 Transient tethering. Circulating von Willebrand factor (vWF) binds exposed subendothelial collagen and is immobilized in an endothelial defect. Platelet GPIb receptors then bind the immobilized vWF. This allows a monolayer of platelets to form over endothelial defects. The tethered platelets are then able to interact with the damage zone in a more permanent way (via platelet receptors GP Ia, GP IIa and GP VI) by binding directly to subendothelial collagen.

Platelet activation and release reaction

The 'release reaction' occurs within 2 seconds of adhesion. This describes the release of bioactive contents from platelet storage granules into the local environment via the surface-opening canalicular system. The release reaction is triggered by calcium ion (Ca^{++}) influx and consequent intracellular (Ca^{++}) elevation.

Bioactive granule contents 'activate' additional platelets for incorporation in the platelet plug. 'Activation' in this context refers to a concert of intracellular signalling cascades that impose multiple changes promoting platelet aggregation, including conformational change of the platelet itself (lens-shape → spiny sphere) and the GP IIb/IIIa receptor. The GP IIb/IIIa receptor activation allows it to bind vWF and fibrinogen.

> **HINTS AND TIPS**
>
> Platelet-synthesized bioactive molecules: Delta ('dense') granules contain calcium adenosine triphosphate, adenosine diphosphate (ADP), serotonin, histamine and adrenaline. Alpha granules contain fibrinogen, vWF, factors V, XI and XIII. Platelets also synthesize thromboxane A2 (TXA2) from arachidonic acid. As well as potentiating platelet aggregation, TXA2 is a potent vasoconstrictor, contributing towards flow reduction to the zone of damage.

Aggregation

Aggregation describes the process of cross-linking between platelets, which stabilizes the developing clot and allows additional recruitment of passing platelets to expand the volume of the clot. Aggregation can only occur following activation, since the GP IIb/IIIA receptor conformation must be competent to bind vWF and fibrinogen. Aggregation is promoted by raised intraplatelet (Ca^{++}) concentration.

Permanent aggregation

Aggregation is rendered irreversible by insoluble fibrin formation. Recruited fibrinogen (bound to activated GP IIb/IIIA receptors) is cleaved to fibrin by thrombin. Thrombin may be:

- Derived from platelets
- Generated by activation of the coagulation cascade (see later in this chapter Coagulation cascade)

Fibrin creates a reinforcing network between platelets in the primary platelet plug, as well as polymerizing to form a mesh-like network which traps additional platelets and blood cells for integration into the clot. Factor XIIIa, activated in the coagulation pathway, further stabilizes the clot by covalently cross-linking fibrin polymers.

Prevention of inappropriate primary haemostasis

In the absence of vessel injury, endothelial cells exert an anti-platelet influence to prevent unnecessary thrombus formation in healthy vessels. Important mechanisms include:

- Endothelial synthesis and release of prostacyclin (PGI2); and nitric oxide, both of which inhibit platelet aggregation.
- Electrostatic repulsion between the negative electrostatic charges of endothelial and platelet surface membranes limits physical interaction.

CLINICAL NOTES

Inappropriate haemostasis: Undue activation of haemostasis compromises the ability of the blood to perform the vital functions of nutrient delivery and waste removal, which rely on its fluid state. Inappropriate thrombosis and thromboembolism impair distal perfusion, resulting in tissue ischaemia.

Tissue repair

Platelets stimulate wound healing by secretion of platelet-derived growth factor, which stimulates mitogenesis of vascular smooth muscle cells and fibroblasts.

ANTIPLATELET DRUGS

Given the pivotal role of platelets in thrombosis, platelets are pharmacologically targeted to reduce disease risk arising from inappropriate thrombosis, for example myocardial infarction (MI) and ischaemic stroke. The following sections discuss anti-platelet drug mechanisms, which are illustrated in Fig. 6.2.

COX inhibition

Cyclooxygenase (COX) is responsible for TXA2 synthesis. Inhibition of COX reduces TXA2 availability and thus impairs platelet aggregation and clot formation. COX inhibitors may be selective for particular subtypes or nonselective (inhibiting all subtypes). They can be reversible or irreversible. Aspirin is the most well-known example of a COX inhibitor. It is nonselective and irreversible, permanently acetylating the enzyme.

Adenosine diphosphate receptor antagonism

These drugs exert their antiplatelet effect by occupying the ADP receptor, preventing ADP binding. Platelet aggregation is thus impaired. Important drugs in this class include clopidogrel, prasugrel, and ticlopidine (irreversible) and ticagrelor (reversible).

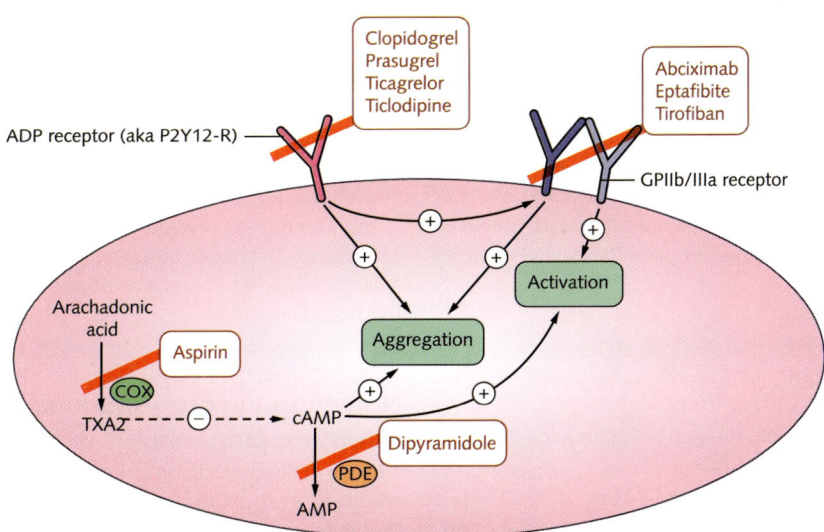

Fig. 6.2 Mechanism of action of antiplatelet drugs. *ADP*, Adenosine diphosphate; *cAMP*, cyclic adenosine monophosphate; *COX*, cyclooxygenase; *PDE*, phosphodiesterases; *TXA2*, thromboxane A2. For detailed explanation of mechanism, see Antiplatelet drugs section.

The ADP receptor is also known as the 'P2Y12' receptor.

GPIIb/IIIa-R antagonism

Antagonism of the GPIIb/IIIa receptor impairs clot formation by impairing:

- Platelet binding to collagen-bound vWF
- Fibrinogen recruitment and subsequent cross-linking between platelets

Abciximab, eptifibatide and tirofiban are examples of this class of drugs.

Phosphodiesterase inhibition

Inhibition of platelet phosphodiesterase prevents intracellular cyclic adenosine monophosphate (cAMP) degradation, resulting in a high cAMP. This disrupts virtually all the changes necessary for platelet activation including degranulation (release reaction), cytoskeletal rearrangement and conformational change of the GPIIb/IIIa receptor. The platelet is unable to undergo adhesion and aggregation, preventing effective primary haemostasis. Dipyridamole is the most commonly encountered antiplatelet drug of this class.

PLATELET DISORDERS

The normal concentration of platelets in blood is $150-400 \times 10^9$/L. A reduced platelet count (thrombocytopenia) or defects of platelet function may increase the risk of bleeding. Thrombocytopenia may present with easy bruising, petechiae, purpura and mucocutaneous bleeding; if very severe, it increases the risk of intracranial haemorrhage. Impaired synthesis, reduced lifespan or excessive consumption of platelets may all result in thrombocytopenia.

Thrombocytopenia: decreased platelet production

The most common explanation for thrombocytopenia is a decrease in platelet production (Table 6.1).

Haematinic deficiency

Vitamin B12 and folate are essential for DNA synthesis; their deficiency impairs megakaryopoiesis and erythropoiesis (see Chapter 3: Megaloblastic anaemia).

Table 6.1 Reduced platelet production: specific causes and their mechanisms

Mechanism of decreased production	Specific causes
Non–immune drug-induced thrombocytopenia	Chemotherapy Antibiotics (linezolid, cotrimoxazole) Antivirals (ganciclovir)
Bone marrow infiltration	Metastatic malignancy Haematological malignancies (leukaemia, myeloma, lymphoma) Fibrosis (e.g., myelofibrosis) Granulomas
Bone marrow failure/ineffective haematopoiesis	Myelodysplastic syndrome Bone marrow failure syndromes (e.g., aplastic anaemia)
Others	Megaloblastic anaemias Chronic liver disease (reduced TPO)

Chronic liver disease

Reduced TPO levels causing impaired megakaryopoiesis is a major contribution to the thrombocytopenia associated with chronic liver disease.

Chronic liver disease is also frequently associated with splenomegaly (secondary to portal hypertension), which can contribute to thrombocytopenia by splenic sequestration (see 'Splenic Platelet Sequestration' below).

Bone marrow disorders

Displacement of normal haematopoietic tissue from the bone marrow, and replacement with other cells may compromise haematopoiesis, resulting in cytopenias. The pathological states that can cause bone marrow infiltration include haematological malignancies (e.g., leukaemia, myeloma, myeloproliferative disorders including myelofibrosis), metastatic tumour cells and granulomas.

Acquired (e.g., myelodysplastic syndrome) and, much less commonly, inherited bone marrow failure syndromes (e.g., aplastic anaemia) may cause thrombocytopenia due to ineffective haematopoiesis.

Non–immune drug-induced thrombocytopenia

Certain drugs have direct cytotoxic effects on megakaryocytes, resulting in impaired megakaryopoiesis. Cytotoxic chemotherapy is an example of par excellence. However, other drugs, such as the antibiotics linezolid and cotrimoxazole, and the antiviral ganciclovir, are also recognized to be associated with myelosuppression.

Thrombocytopenia: shortened platelet lifespan

Reduction in platelet lifespan leads to a reduction in circulating numbers. The following sections discuss the various mechanisms that can lead to shortened platelet survival.

Immune destruction

Platelet destruction by immune mechanisms is discussed in the following sections.

Immune thrombocytopenic

Immune thrombocytopenia (ITP) is an autoimmune disorder resulting in otherwise unexplained thrombocytopenia. The immunological basis for thrombocytopenia is usually the formation of antiplatelet antibodies, resulting in clearance of platelets by the reticuloendothelial system. The presentation and natural history of ITP varies between children and adults. Symptoms include easy bruising and mucocutaneous bleeding.

Children. In children, ITP is usually an acute, self-limiting process, occurring after a viral illness. ITP resolves spontaneously in the majority of patients within 6 months. Failure of spontaneous resolution should prompt further investigation to exclude alternative causes. Treatment is only required if associated with bleeding; options include steroids and intravenous immunoglobulin (IVIg) (see Chapter 7).

Adults. ITP is typically chronic in adults, and may be associated with autoimmune diseases. Incidence is higher in women. ITP is a diagnosis of exclusion; bone marrow assessment is not mandatory, but should be strongly considered in the context of an atypical history, late-onset (i.e., presentation >60 years of age) or poor treatment response.

CLINICAL NOTES

Management of immune thrombocytopenic purpura in adults

Treatment should be initiated if the platelet count is <30. First-line treatment options include steroids (e.g., dexamethasone 40 mg od for 4 days), IVIg (if a rapid response is essential), and anti-D immunoglobulin for RhD+ patients (to saturate Fc receptors). Patients are often steroid responsive, but the treatment response may be transient. Failure to respond to steroids and/or IVIg should prompt reevaluation of the diagnosis of ITP, and other possible causes of thrombocytopenia be reconsidered.

Second-line treatment options include TPO receptor agonists (e.g., romiplostim, eltrombopag, avatrombopag) that stimulate thrombopoiesis, rituximab, steroid-sparing immunosuppression (e.g., mycophenolate mofetil) and splenectomy.

Drug-induced immune thrombocytopenia

In drug-induced ITP, drug-dependent antibodies cause immune-mediated platelet destruction. Thrombocytopenia typically occurs 5-10 days after initial drug exposure, with a platelet nadir of $<20 \times 10^9$/L. Many drugs have been associated with drug-induced ITP, but more common causes include heparin (see below), penicillins, cephalosporins, sulphonamide antibiotics and quinine.

A high degree of suspicion is required for its diagnosis. Management primarily involves discontinuation of the offending drug.

Heparin-induced thrombocytopenia

An important potential complication is heparin-induced thrombocytopenia (HIT), which classically presents with a falling platelet count 5–14 days after starting heparin (especially unfractionated heparin [UFH]) treatment. HIT occurs due to heparin-dependent anti-PF4 antibodies binding heparin/PF4 complexes, causing platelet activation and a potentially lethal prothrombotic state. This may result in venous and arterial thrombosis. Management depends on discontinuing heparin and initiating alternative anticoagulation (e.g., fondaparinux, argatroban) in spite of the thrombocytopenia. Subsequent lifelong heparin avoidance is essential.

Posttransfusion purpura

Posttransfusion purpura occurs when individuals lacking a common platelet antigen (e.g., Human Platelet Antigen-1a [HPA-1a]) are reexposed to the platelet antigen by blood transfusion (e.g., packed red cells or platelets) following a prior sensitization event. Through incompletely understood mechanisms, antibody-dependent destruction of the recipient's own platelets (i.e., 'bystander destruction') causes thrombocytopenia. The treatment is IVIg, and future blood transfusions should be of antigen-negative blood products.

Neonatal alloimmune thrombocytopenia

Neonatal alloimmune thrombocytopenia (NAIT) arises from the transfer of maternal antiplatelet antibodies across the placenta, resulting in foetal and neonatal thrombocytopenia associated with a high (10%) risk of intracranial haemorrhage. It most commonly occurs when a mother negative for a common platelet antigen (e.g., HPA-1a) is sensitized to that antigen by the foetus, resulting in antiplatelet antibody formation. Affects neonates should be transfused with antigen-negative platelets.

Thrombocytopenia: excessive platelet consumption

Three important conditions hallmarked by excessive platelet consumption are discussed here.

Platelet consumption by microthrombi formation (with associated microangiopathic haemolytic anaemia)

Conditions that result in widespread microthrombi formation can cause a consumptive thrombocytopenia, in addition to microangiopathic haemolytic anaemia (MAHA; see Chapter 3: MAHA). Important causes of MAHA include thrombotic thrombocytopenic purpura (TTP), haemolytic uraemic syndrome (HUS) and disseminated intravascular coagulation (DIC).

Thrombotic thrombocytopenic purpura

Although TTP is a rare disorder, its potential diagnosis must always be considered as it is a medical emergency and if untreated, is associated with a mortality rate ~90%. TTP is classically associated with a pentad of MAHA, thrombocytopenia (platelet count typically $10–30 \times 10^9$/L), fever, fluctuating neurological signs and acute kidney injury (AKI) (Fig. 6.3).

Thrombotic thrombocytopenic purpura occurs due to a deficiency of the ADAMTS13 protease, whose normal function is to cleave vWF multimers activated by shear stress. In the absence of ADAMTS13, exposure of vWF multimers to shear stress causes platelet aggregation and microvascular thrombus formation. The majority of cases are acquired (rather than congenital), and are associated with auto-antibodies against ADAMTS13. Some cases may be associated with human immunodeficiency virus (HIV) or pregnancy.

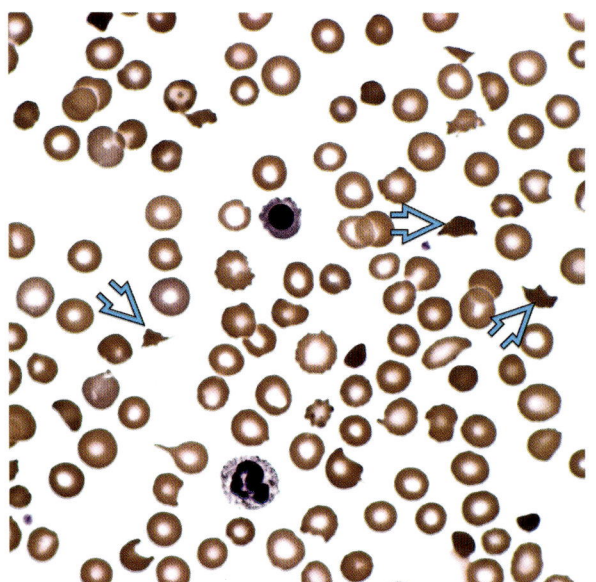

Fig. 6.3 Thrombotic thrombocytopenic purpura blood film. Red cells are fragmented as they pass through microthrombi, and nucleated red blood cells are released from the bone marrow. (From Foucar K. *Diagnostic Pathology: Blood and Bone Marrow*. 3rd ed. Elsevier Health Sciences; 2023).

Thrombotic thrombocytopenic purpura is a medical emergency and plasma exchange should be commenced within 4-8 hours of the diagnosis being suspected; this helps remove antibodies against ADAMTS13 whilst replacing with functional ADAMTS13 that is present in donor plasma. Treatment options also include steroids, caplacizumab (a nanobody directed against vWF) and rituximab. All patients with acute TTP should be transferred for treatment at one of nine specialist centres across the UK.

Haemolytic-uraemic syndrome

Haemolytic uraemic syndrome (HUS) manifests with thrombocytopenia secondary to microthrombi formation and MAHA, similar to TTP. In contrast to TTP, AKI is the dominant feature of HUS. Classical HUS occurs after infection with Shiga toxin-producing *Escherichia coli* (most commonly, the O157:H7 strain) or *Shigella dysenteriae*. Shiga toxin has a predilection for the kidneys and causes cell death that triggers an inflammatory response; ultimately, this results in a prothrombotic state and microvascular thrombus formation. HUS is a common cause of AKI in children. The triad of AKI, low platelets and blood film suggestive of MAHA is diagnostic. Management is generally supportive, but sequelae may be chronic renal impairment.

In contrast, atypical HUS is not associated with infection, but is instead associated with inappropriate complement activation, complement-mediated endothelial damage and resultant microvascular thrombus formation. Treatment involves inhibition of terminal complement activation by an anti-C5 monoclonal antibody (e.g., eculizumab, ravulizumab).

Disseminated intravascular coagulation

Disseminated intravascular coagulation is a life-threatening condition, discussed in detail later in the chapter, associated with a consumptive thrombocytopenia.

Dilutional thrombocytopenia

Rather than a reduction in the absolute numbers of platelets present, significant expansion of intravascular volume results in a dilutional thrombocytopenia. This adverse effect is most commonly encountered secondary to massive transfusion (see Chapter 7: Massive transfusion).

Splenic platelet sequestration

A third of circulating platelets are normally sequestered in the spleen. Splenomegaly increases the proportion of circulating platelets that are sequestered. Thrombocytopenia resulting from functional hypersplenism rarely results in bleeding as the sequestered platelets are released in times of stress.

Defects of platelet function

Impairment of platelet function (i.e., qualitative defect) may be associated with an increased bleeding risk despite a normal platelet count. Causes include:

- Antiplatelet drugs
- Uraemia
- Congenital platelet disorders
- Cardiopulmonary bypass

THE COAGULATION CASCADE

Once a platelet plug (primary haemostasis) has arrested bleeding, the plug is reinforced with by-products of the coagulation pathway (secondary haemostasis). Coagulation involves a cascade of protein activations, culminating with the conversion of prothrombin to thrombin. Thrombin is the end-product of the complex sequence of interaction. Thrombin converts fibrinogen to fibrin and thus mediates reinforcement and stabilization of the clot.

The proteins involved are known as clotting or coagulation factors. They exist in the circulation as inactive proenzymes. The activated enzymes are serine proteases (except FXIII) which cleave other inactive proenzymes to their active versions. All coagulation factors are synthesized in the liver.

> **HINTS AND TIPS**
>
> Clotting factors (coagulation factors) are usually referred to clinically by Roman numerals. However, some are also referred to by particular names: for example, factor II is usually referred to by name as prothrombin. Activated factors have the suffix 'a' (e.g., activated factor VIII = FVIIIa).

The surface of activated platelets within the primary platelet plug functions as a catalytic membrane for complexes of coagulation factors. Platelet presence therefore is mandatory for an intact secondary coagulation response in terms of magnitude and rapidity.

TRADITIONAL PATHWAYS

The traditional pathways represent the historic interpretation of the coagulation process. They are discussed here, as they are still examination topics, plus two commonly used clotting parameters (the activated partial thromboplastin time [APTT] and prothrombin time [PT]), each broadly related to the activity of factors that are differentiated by the concept of each pathway model (Fig. 6.4). They are named according to whether coagulation initiation arises from within (intrinsic) or outside (extrinsic) the circulation.

The extrinsic pathway

The secondary haemostatic response is initiated by tissue factor (TF), a GP expressed within vessel subendothelium and nonvascular cells. Blood passing through normal, nondamaged blood vessels is not exposed to TF. Following vessel wall damage:

- TF is exposed to the circulation
- Circulating factor VII is activated by TF
- TF then forms a complex with FVIIa plus Ca^{++} ions (TF-FVII-Ca^{++})
- This complex then activates factors IX (in the intrinsic pathway) and X (in the common pathway; but note that the extent of factor X activation is small relative to that generated by the intrinsic pathway)

Intrinsic pathway

The intrinsic pathway commences when FXII comes into contact with a negatively charged surface, such as an activated platelet cell membrane.

- This contact activates FXII
- FXIIa then cleaves FXI → FXIa
- FXIa then cleaves FIX → FIXa. In addition, a small amount of FIX is also activated by TF-FVII from the extrinsic pathway
- Circulating thrombin (FIIa) converts a small amount of FVIII to FVIIIa
- FIXa, FVIIIa and Ca^{++} ions together form the 'tenase' complex
- Tenase (FVIIIa-FIXa-Ca^{++}) powerfully activates FX, forming large quantities of FXa
- FXa then enters the common pathway

Common pathway

FXa then combines with FVa and Ca^{++} to form the 'prothrombinase complex,' which cleaves prothrombin (FII) to generate thrombin (FIIa).

Thrombin has many haemostatic functions, including:

- Conversion of fibrinogen to fibrin (most important role).
- Further activation of factors V, VIII and XI. This forms the basis of the amplification process; that is, thrombin further activates proteins of the 'intrinsic' and 'common' pathway to produce even more thrombin.
- Activation of factor XIII.
- Releasing FVIII from its plasma carrier protein (vWF).
- Further platelet activation.
- Binding to thrombomodulin, which then activates protein C. This accounts for the anticoagulant function of thrombin.

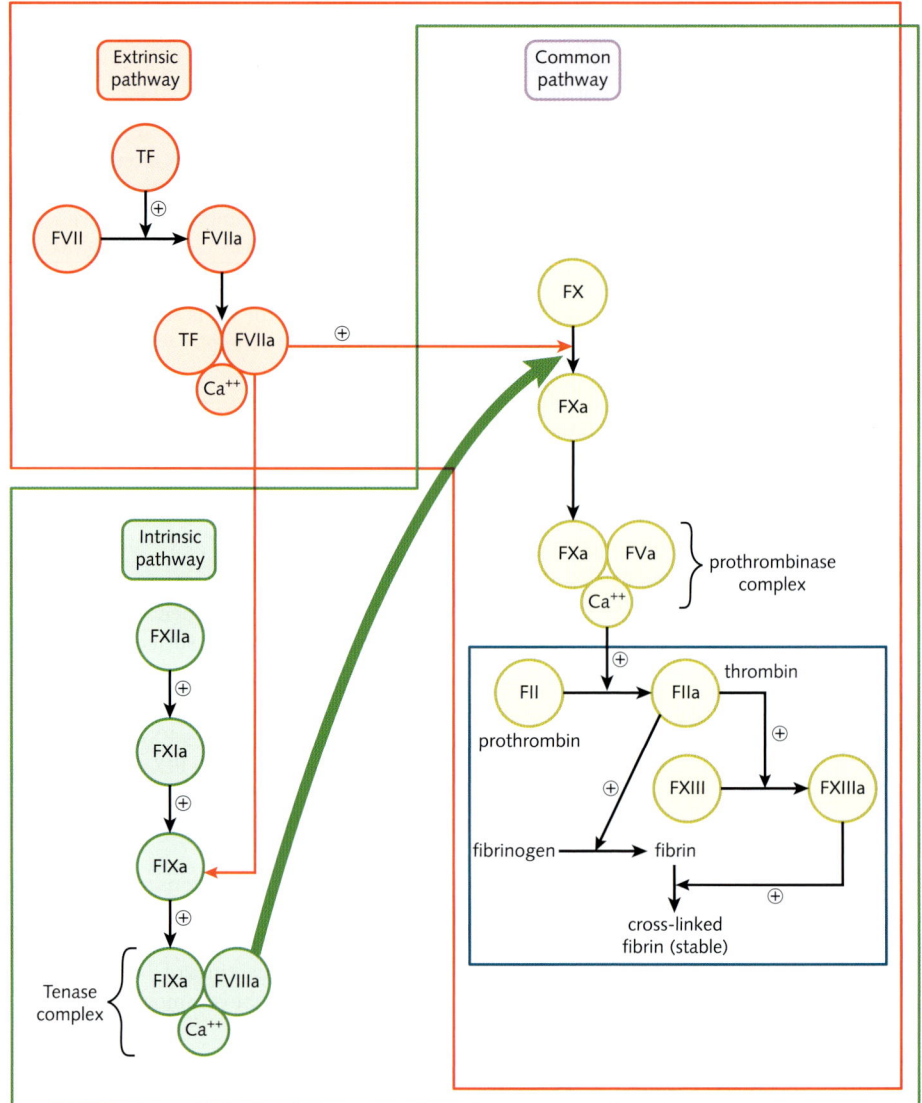

Fig. 6.4 The traditional pathways. See 'Traditional pathways' section for detail of the extrinsic (*shown in red*), intrinsic (*shown in green*) and common (*shown in yellow/mustard*) pathways. *Green outline*: the processes that together are measured by the activated thromboplastin time (i.e., the intrinsic and common pathways). *Red outline*: the processes that together are measured by the PT (i.e., the extrinsic and the common pathways together). *Blue outline*: Processes contributing to the TT.

Fibrinogen → Fibrin

The ultimate outcome of the common pathway is the thrombin-mediated cleavage of soluble plasma fibrinogen to insoluble fibrin (Fig. 6.5). Fibrin monomers spontaneously polymerize (via hydrogen bonds) into long fibres. These create complex networks within the platelet plug. Thrombin-activated FXIIIa further stabilizes the fibrin reinforcement of the clot, mediating covalent cross-linking between fibrin polymers.

CURRENTLY ACCEPTED PATHWAY

The cascades, as explained earlier, have been the accepted interpretations of the clotting system for decades. However, certain clotting factors are important for their own production, the most obvious one being thrombin (FIIa). Thrombin participates in reactions that occur before its own activation, making the cascade approach seem nonsensical. The more recent interpretation

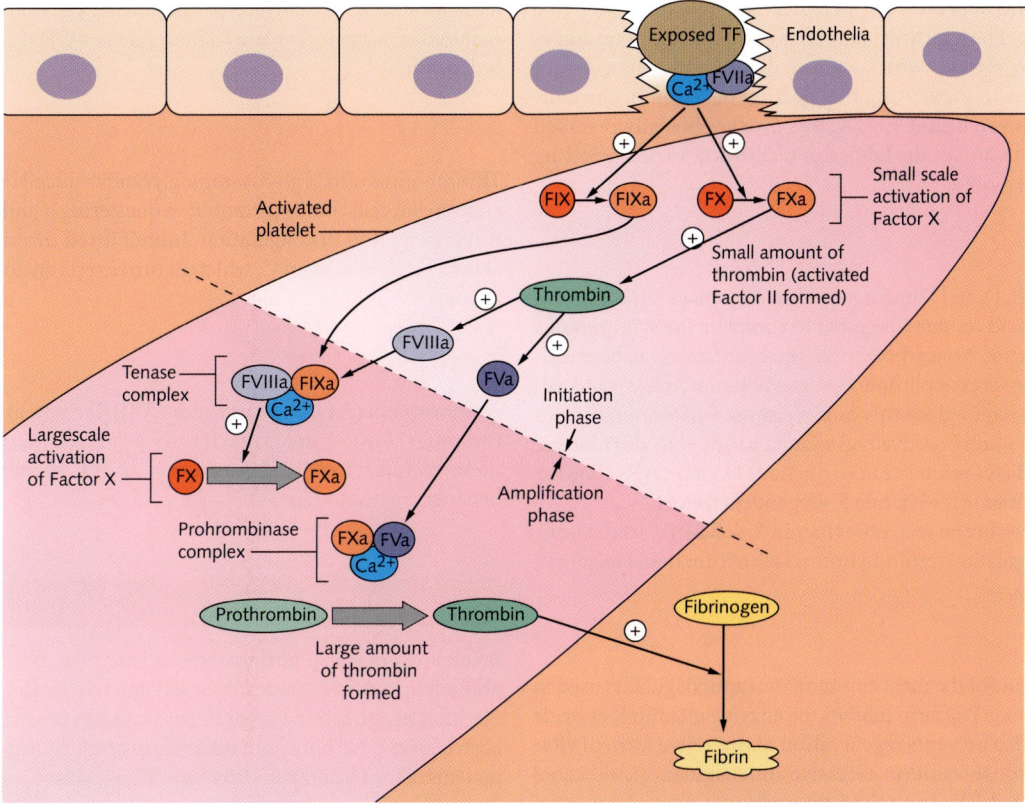

Fig. 6.5 Currently accepted pathways: initiation and amplification phases. Note that the reactions occur at the external surface of activated platelets, an important feature of the clotting cascade incorporated into this more recently accepted version of events.

of coagulation sees the two 'separate' cascades integrated and delineated by two phases: initiation and amplification.

Initiation phase

Initiation commences with TF binding to activated FVIIa. The resultant FVIIa-TF-Ca^{++} complex then activates factors IX and X. The surface membrane of activated platelets then functions as a catalyst for the conversion of a relatively small amount of prothrombin to thrombin by Fxa. Thrombin is then able to activate factors V, VIII and XI.

Amplification phase

The reactions of the amplification phase occur on the external surfaces of activated platelets. FIXa associates with FVIIIa, forming the tenase complex (FVIIIa-FIXa-Ca^{2+}). This complex activates FX much more powerfully than the FVIIa-TF-Ca^{2+} complex. These larger amounts of FXathen form large amounts of prothrombinase complex (FXa-FVa-Ca^{2+}), which is 300,000 times more powerful than lone FXa at converting prothrombin

to thrombin. Far greater amounts of thrombin are thus generated by the amplification phase (see Fig. 6.4).

Calcium

Calcium is vital for coagulation, since it is a component of the TF-FVIIa-Ca^{2+} complex, the tenase complex (FVIIIa-FIXa-Ca^{2+}) and the prothrombinase complex (Fxa-Fva-Ca^{2+}). Furthermore, individual factors II, VII, IX and X (vitamin K–dependent factors) require calcium ions as cofactors for their activation. Coagulation is therefore facilitated by platelet granule release of calcium on activation and markedly impaired in hypocalcaemia.

Calcium chelation for samples

This calcium dependency of clotting is exploited to prevent blood clotting when it would be undesirable, for example storage of donated blood or transfer of samples to the laboratory. Chelation (e.g., with ethylenediaminetetraacetic acid [EDTA]) or deionization (e.g., with citrate) of calcium ions is used in these instances. Thus the 'full blood count' sample is collected in vacutainers that contain EDTA so it remains in the fluid state necessary for performing cell counts and also blood films. The 'clotting sample' is collected in vacutainers that contain citrate, which causes deionization of calcium ions, thus again preventing the clotting of blood in the container. However, unlike EDTA, this process is easily reversed by adding calcium in the laboratory, allowing various clotting times to be studied.

Vitamin K

Factors II, VII, IX and X undergo posttranslational γ-carboxylation at glutamic acid residues, required to complete the synthesis of a functional factor. Noncarboxylated factors are unable to bind activating calcium ions or phospholipid membranes. Active (reduced) vitamin K is required for this carboxylation. Performing the carboxylation oxidizes (inactivating) vitamin K. The epoxide reductase enzyme mediates reactivation (reduction) of vitamin K, allowing further synthesis of the vitamin K–dependent factors.

It can therefore be seen how vitamin K deficiency leads to disordered coagulation resulting from a lack of functional factors II, VII, IX and X.

Warfarin

Warfarin is one of the most common oral anticoagulants used in clinical practice. Warfarin inhibits the enzyme vitamin K epoxide reductase. This prevents regeneration of the active form of vitamin K. Overdose results in excessive anticoagulation, indicated by a prolonged PT (and raised international normalized ratio [INR], see coagulation tests). In massive overdose, it also prolongs the APTT. Treatment of this scenario is covered further in this chapter and in Chapter 7.

REGULATION OF COAGULATION

A number of anticoagulant factors exist to prevent spontaneous activation of coagulation (in the absence of injury) and to limit the activation of coagulation to within the local area in the context of vessel injury.

Tissue-factor pathway inhibitor

Tissue-factor pathway inhibitor (TFPI) is linked via GPI to endothelial cell surfaces. It exerts a background anticoagulant influence by binding the TF-FVIIa-Ca^{2+} complex, thus preventing TF-mediated initiation of coagulation.

Proteins C and S

Protein C is a serine protease that destroys the activated cofactors Va and VIIIa (both factors form part of the amplification process). Protein C is activated when thrombin binds to thrombomodulin,

itself located at the surface of endothelial cells. Protein S is a required cofactor for protein C. Both proteins C and S are vitamin K dependent.

Thrombomodulin

Thrombomodulin, a glycosaminoglycan produced by uninjured endothelial cells, binds thrombin, sequestering it and preventing its participation in coagulation. Immobilized thrombin is then able to activate protein C, which in turn exerts an anticoagulant action.

Antithrombin

Antithrombin (AT), also known as AT III, is a potent inhibitor of thrombin, FIXa, Fxa and FXIIa. AT binds to the active site of these factors. The inhibitory effect of AT is potentiated by heparin.

FIBRINOLYSIS

Breakdown of stable fibrin polymers is termed 'fibrinolysis.' The fibrinolytic system degrades fibrin and thus enables clot breakdown. Fibrinolysis also acts to dismantle any inappropriate fibrin networks obstructing vessel lumens in the absence of injury. Important components of the fibrinolytic system are discussed here.

Plasmin

Plasmin (cleaved from plasminogen) is a serine protease that cleaves peptide bonds within fibrin polymers, degrading fibrin networks and destroying the architecture and stability of a clot. Conversion of plasminogen to plasmin is achieved by tissue plasminogen activator (tPA) or by urokinase.

CLINICAL NOTES

Thrombolysis for ST-elevation MI treatment: In the past, ST-elevation MI was treated with thrombolytic drugs that converted plasminogen to plasmin relying on its action to break clots. These drugs (alteplase, streptokinase and tenecteplase) have been superseded by emergency percutaneous coronary intervention. Alteplase is still the drug of choice in patients with life-threatening pulmonary embolism.

Tissue plasminogen activator

Tissue plasminogen activator is released from activated endothelial cells and is the most important activator of fibrinolysis. It binds to plasminogen, cleaving it to form plasmin, but will only interact with plasminogen bound to fibrin, that is, will only release plasmin in the area of a thrombus.

Antifibrinolytic factors

Thrombin-activated fibrinolysis inhibitor, plasminogen activator inhibitor and α_2-antiplasmin, act to oppose fibrinolysis. The extent of fibrinolysis thus depends on the balance between fibrinolytic promotors (such as tPA) and these antifibrinolytic factors.

OVERVIEW OF HAEMOSTASIS

The role of platelets, the clotting cascade and fibrinolysis in haemostasis are outlined in Fig. 6.6.

COAGULATION ASSAYS

The PT, APTT and thrombin time (TT) are screening tests of haemostasis. However, it is important to emphasize that these are in vitro assays and may not be entirely reflective of haemostatic function in the individual. For example, a patient with Glanzmann's thrombasthenia, a rare platelet function defect, would be expected to have a normal PT and APTT, despite having a severe bleeding phenotype. Conversely, factor XII deficiency (Hageman disease) is not associated with a bleeding disorder, yet may cause a significant APTT prolongation. A thorough bleeding history (which may incorporate the use of a standardized system such as the ISTH Bleeding Assessment Tool) is more informative than screening coagulation assays in the assessment of a patient suspected to have a bleeding disorder.

Whilst a model of coagulation based on intrinsic, extrinsic and common pathways is overly simplistic, it remains

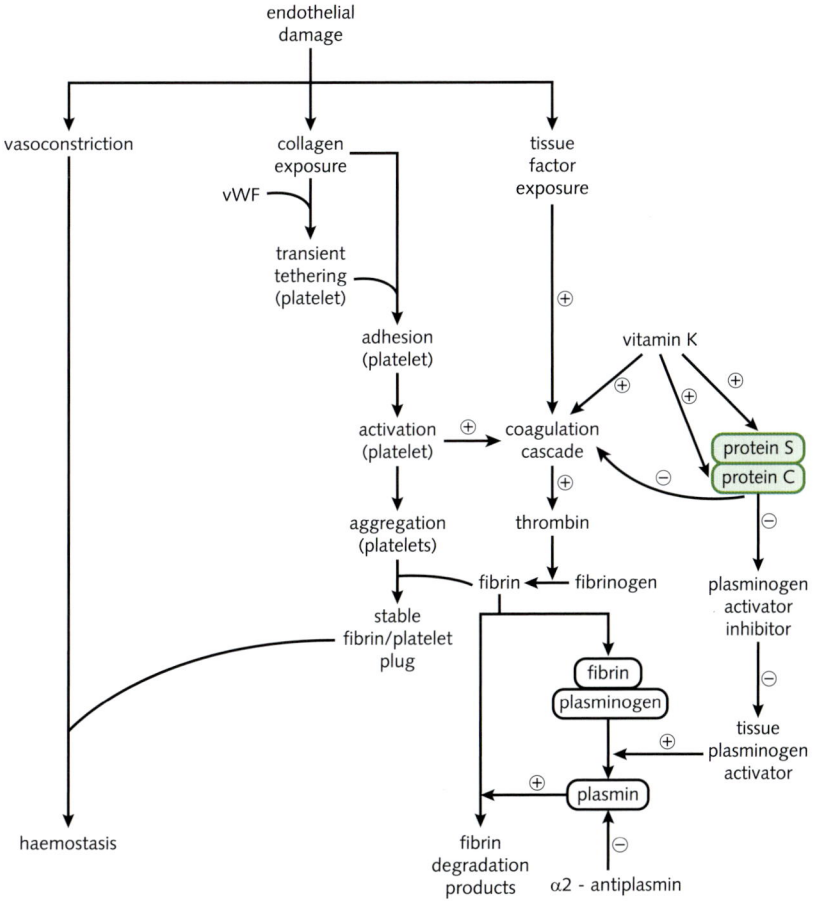

Fig. 6.6 Overview of haemostasis. *vWF*, von Willebrand factor.

Table 6.2 Coagulation assays

Test	Possible causes
Isolated PT prolongation	Factor VII deficiency Warfarin (may also cause slight APTT prolongation)
Isolated APTT prolongation	Factor VIII (e.g., haemophilia A), IX (e.g., haemophilia B), XI, XII deficiency Von Willebrand disease Lupus anticoagulant
PT and APTT prolongation	Factor X, V, II deficiency or combined factor deficiencies DIC Massive transfusion Vitamin K deficiency UFH Direct FXa inhibitor Direct thrombin inhibitor
Fibrinogen low	DIC Massive transfusion Severe liver disease Postthrombolysis Hypofibrinogenaemia, dysfibrinogenaemia

APTT, Activated partial thromboplastin time; DIC, disseminated intravascular coagulation; LMWH, low-molecular-weight heparin; PT, prothrombin time; TT, thrombin time; UFH, Unfractionated heparin.

useful in interpreting coagulation assays since the PT reflects the extrinsic (factor VII) and common (factors X, V, II and fibrinogen) pathways, and the APTT reflects the intrinsic (factors XII, XI, IX and VIII) and common pathways. The pattern of abnormal coagulation assays may be helpful in suggesting potential causes for defective haemostasis; some clinically relevant patterns and possible causes are shown in Table 6.2.

Factor assays can be used to identify deficiencies of specific coagulation factors.

CLINICAL NOTES

Prothrombin time: The PT reflects the activity of the extrinsic (factor VII) and common (factors X, V, II and fibrinogen) pathways.

CLINICAL NOTES

Activated partial thromboplastin time: The APTT reflects the activity of the intrinsic (factors XII, XI, IX and VII) and common pathways.

D-dimers

D-dimers are degradation products formed by the breakdown of cross-linked fibrin. D-dimers are frequently elevated in the context of a significant thrombosis, as well as inflammatory states (e.g., infection, malignancy, surgery, trauma) and DIC. A normal level of D-dimers offers negative predictive value for a thrombosis (i.e., deep vein thrombosis or pulmonary embolism), though it cannot exclude the diagnosis if thrombosis is felt to have high clinical probability.

CLOTTING FACTOR DISORDERS

Acquired factor deficiencies

Vitamin K deficiency

Vitamin K is a fat-soluble vitamin dependent on biliary absorption. Consequently, vitamin K deficiency is associated with biliary obstruction (cholestasis), cirrhosis and malabsorption states. The vitamin K–dependent clotting factors are factors II, VII, IX and X. Deficiency is associated with PT, and to a lesser extent APTT, prolongation.

Liver disease

The liver synthesizes clotting factors and natural anticoagulants (e.g., protein C and S). Impaired synthetic function of the liver is frequently associated with deficiencies in clotting factors, which may manifest in prolongation of the PT and APTT. Cirrhosis may be further associated with thrombocytopenia, which may in part be due to splenomegaly (from portal hypertension) causing splenic sequestration. Beyond indicating impaired synthetic function of the liver, a prolonged PT and/or APTT in the context of liver disease poorly predicts whether an individual patient will have a bleeding tendency. Patients with liver cirrhosis may be prothrombotic, since synthesis of natural anticoagulants may also be impaired, and their activities are not reflected in coagulation screening tests.

Disseminated intravascular coagulation

Disseminated intravascular coagulation occurs due to pathologic and widespread systemic activation of coagulation, resulting in formation of platelet microthrombi and fibrin deposition in small-medium blood vessels, which in turn may cause ischaemic necrosis and organ dysfunction. Furthermore, the widespread activation of coagulation may consume clotting factors, fibrinogen and platelets (i.e., consumptive coagulopathy), paradoxically leading to haemorrhage.

Disseminated intravascular coagulation occurs in response to an underlying cause that results in activation of the coagulation cascade. Causes of DIC include severe infection, trauma, burns, malignancy (notably acute promyelocytic leukaemia), severe transfusion reactions and vascular malformations. Patients with DIC are frequently critically unwell.

The PT, APTT and TT are all prolonged, and fibrinogen and platelet count are significantly lowered. The presence of microthrombi can cause shearing of red blood cells, leading to formation of red cell fragments (schistocytes) and a MAHA.

CLINICAL NOTE

ISTH DIC Score:

Platelet count: >100 × 10⁹/L – 0, <100 × 10⁹/L – 1, <50 × 10⁹/L – 2

PT: <3 s prolonged – 0, between 3 s and 6 s prolonged – 1, >6 s prolonged – 2

Fibrinogen: >1.0 g/L – 0, <1.0 g/L – 2

D-dimer: No increase – 0, moderate between 250 and 5000 – 1, strong increase >5000 – 3

Interpretation: A total score ≥5 means DIC

Management of disseminated intravascular coagulation

Patients with DIC are frequently critically ill, and the acute management should be resuscitation according to an ABCDE approach, with critical care input (e.g., ventilatory or haemodynamic support) as indicated. Ultimately, management of DIC requires identification and treatment of the underlying cause.

Haematologic management is supportive and aimed at the consumptive coagulopathy by transfusion of fresh-frozen plasma (to replace clotting factors), cryoprecipitate (to replace fibrinogen) and platelets (see Chapter 7). Correction of hypothermia and acidosis will facilitate regaining functional haemostasis.

HEREDITARY FACTOR DEFICIENCIES

Von Willebrand disease

Von Willebrand disease (vWD) is the most common hereditary bleeding disorder, arising from reduced vWF activity. vWF is a carrier protein for FVIII, prolonging its circulating half-life, and contributes to primary haemostasis by facilitating the interaction between platelets and endothelium. vWD occurs either due to a quantitative reduction in vWF levels (types 1 and 3) or a qualitative defect in vWF activity (type 2).

Clinical manifestations resemble those of platelet disorders: that is, easy bruising, mucocutaneous bleeding, menorrhagia, epistaxis, or prolonged bleeding following dental extractions, minor wounds, and surgical procedures. See Table 6.3 for clinical

Table 6.3 Differentiation between the three most common hereditary clotting factor deficiencies

Feature	Haemophilia A and B	Von Willebrand disease
Deficient factor	Factor VIII (haemophilia A) Factor IX (haemophilia B)	vWF
Inheritance pattern (excluding de novo cases)	X-linked	Variable, usually autosomal dominant
Gender affected	Males	Males and females
Most likely sites of bleeding	Joints, muscles	Mucocutaneous
Platelet count	Normal	Normal
PT	Normal	Normal
APTT	Prolonged	Normal/ prolonged

APTT, Activated partial thromboplastin time; PT, prothrombin time; vWF, von Willebrand factor.

differentiation between the three most common hereditary clotting factor deficiencies.

The management of vWD depends on the specific type, but may include tranexamic acid (to inhibit fibrinolysis), desmopressin (to stimulate release of vWF from endothelial stores) and factor concentrates. Patients with vWD undergoing invasive procedures should be managed according to individualized perioperative haemostatic management plans.

Haemophilia A: factor VIII deficiency

Haemophilia A is caused by a deficiency of FVIII. As an X-linked recessive condition, it overwhelmingly affects males. Male prevalence of haemophilia A is 1 in 5000. A third arise in absence of family history, due to spontaneous or 'de novo' mutations of the FVIII gene. Bleeding frequency and severity correlate with the plasma level of FVIII. FVIII activity of <1% is associated with severe haemophilia A, 1–5% moderate and 5–40% mild (Table 6.4).

Untreated haemophilia can be associated with significant mortality (e.g., life-threatening bleeding such as intracranial haemorrhage) and morbidity – joint bleeds are painful in the acute setting, with recurrent bleeds resulting in a chronic arthropathy associated with pain and reduced joint function. Patients with haemophilia should be registered with and have their condition managed by a Haemophilia Comprehensive Care Centre.

Children with an FVIII level of <3% (i.e., all patients with severe and some with moderate haemophilia) should be

Table 6.4 Classification of haemophilia severity

FVIII or FIX level (% of normal)[a]	Clinical implications
40%–100%	None
5%–40% (Mild)	Spontaneous bleeding uncommon; bleeding typically provoked by trauma or surgery
1%–5% (Moderate)	Presentation may be variable, resembling either severe or mild haemophilia
< 1% (Severe)	Spontaneous bleeding, predominantly into joints or muscle tissue

[a]FVIII in haemophilia A, FIX in haemophilia B

started on lifelong primary prophylaxis, that is, factor replacement therapy before or immediately after the first bleed, or before the age of two. Alternatively, factor replacement may also be commenced after two or more joint bleeds (i.e., secondary prophylaxis), with the aim of preventing acute bleeds and reducing joint damage. The treatment landscape for haemophilia has evolved considerably and now includes extended half-life factor products, bispecific antibodies (e.g., emicizumab) and gene therapy. Patients with haemophilia (even those who do not receive regular factor prophylaxis) undergoing invasive procedures should be managed according to individualized perioperative haemostatic management plans at specialist centres.

CLINICAL NOTES

X-linked inheritance: As for all X-linked diseases, daughters of an affected male will be obligate carriers, and sons will be unaffected. Daughters of carriers will have a 50% chance of being carriers themselves, but their sons will always be affected. Carriers considering pregnancy should be referred to specialist centres to discuss their options, which include preimplantation and prenatal genetic diagnosis, and individualized birth plans.

CLINICAL NOTES

Inhibitors: The immune system of haemophilia patients may recognize factor products as 'foreign' and become sensitized, resulting in inhibitor (antibodies directed against the clotting factor) formation. It is essential to detect inhibitors since they render factor products ineffective and require alternative treatment strategies.

ETHICS

Before donor screening programmes and development of recombinant factors, iatrogenic blood-borne infections such as hepatitis B and C and human immunodeficiency virus were a significant cause of comorbidity in haemophilia patients, with significant medical (e.g., cirrhosis), psychological and social (e.g., stigmatization) impacts. The final report from the Infected Blood Inquiry, an independent public statutory inquiry, is anticipated shortly and is expected to report upon the decision-making and balance of responsibilities that resulted in haemophilia patients acquiring blood-borne infections from infected blood products.

Haemophilia B: factor IX (9) deficiency

Haemophilia B (also known as 'Christmas disease') is caused by a deficiency of FIX. Like haemophilia A, it is X-linked, thus patients are almost always men. The two diseases are clinically indistinguishable, laboratory factor assays being required to differentiate them. Haemophilia B is however five times less common. Treatment and management are similar to that of haemophilia A, albeit with FIX replacement (rather than FVIII) – crucially, the aim is to prevent spontaneous bleeds, avoid long-term disability from arthropathy resulting from recurrent bleeds, and to manage the bleeding risk associated with invasive or surgical procedures.

Clinical presentation of haemophilias (A and B)

Haemarthrosis (bleeding into joints) is the most common feature of haemophilia, followed by muscular haematomas; together representing 95% of presentations. Nose bleeds, gastrointestinal (GI) bleeds, haematuria and prolonged bleeding following surgery or dental extraction may also be the presenting complaint in haemophilia. An isolated prolonged APTT in a bleeding patient is suggestive of haemophilia (A or B).

Complications of haemophilias (A and B)

Acute complications reflect the consequences of impaired haemostasis and include, among others, intracranial haemorrhage, haemorrhagic shock and compartment syndrome. Chronic complications arise from chronic organ damage from bleeds; these include, most commonly, arthropathy associated with pain and impaired function from recurrent haemarthroses but may also include neurological deficits from intracranial haemorrhage.

Patients may become sensitized to recombinant factor products, resulting in the formation of inhibitors, or antibodies directed against the factor products that render them ineffectual. It is essential to recognize the development of inhibitors since different treatment strategies are required.

Factor replacement therapy in haemophilia A or B

In haemophilia A, factor VIII is replaced with recombinant FVIII, whilst in haemophilia B, factor IX is replaced with recombinant FIX. Depending on the severity (Table 6.4) of haemophilia, patients may either receive continuous prophylaxis or on-demand treatment with recombinant factor products.

During acute bleeding episodes, patients are advised to administer their own supply of recombinant factor, and attend hospital; specialist advice from the patient's haemophilia centre should be sought. Replacement should be aimed to correct to 100% of normal levels for 'severe' or life-threatening bleeds. Other 'minor' bleeds (e.g., haemarthroses, muscle haematomas or oral mucosal and muscular bleeds) should be corrected to 30% to 50% of normal levels.

Other clotting factor deficiencies

Hereditary deficiencies of the other coagulation factors are rare. The prevalence of certain hereditary deficiencies may be higher amongst specific populations (e.g., FXI deficiency amongst Ashkenazi Jews).

THROMBOSIS

A pathologic thrombus can develop in both the arterial or venous circulation. Arterial thromboembolism is the underlying pathology in MI and ischaemic cerebrovascular accident (and thus the leading cause of death in the developed world). Venous thrombi can form anywhere but are most common in the deep veins deep vein thrombosis (DVT) of the legs. Embolization of such a venous clot to the pulmonary vasculature (PE) can be fatal.

> **HINTS AND TIPS**
>
> Definitions: thrombosis versus thrombus: Formation of a clot is termed 'thrombosis.' A clot remaining at the site of formation is a 'thrombus.' However, if dislodged, the thrombus is referred to as a thromboembolism.

Virchow triad describes three factors which predispose to thrombus formation:

- Venous stasis
- Endothelial injury/dysfunction
- Hypercoagulability

Venous stasis

Blood flow is typically laminar (nonturbulent). If laminar flow is interrupted, venous stasis ensues, increasing the risk of thrombosis. Mechanical (metallic) heart valves are associated with turbulent flow and thrombotic risk, though the extent of risk depends on the site (e.g., mitral vs. aortic) and specific type of valve. Metallic heart valves generally require lifelong anticoagulation.

Other common clinical scenarios that illustrate the association between venous stasis and thrombotic risk include immobility and atrial fibrillation (AF). Calf muscle activity pumps venous blood in the lower limbs back towards the heart (the 'calf-muscle pump'). In immobility, this pumping action is absent and stasis of the venous blood predisposes to thrombosis.

Atrial fibrillation results in ineffectual atrial emptying, stasis and atrial thrombus formation. Dislodged thrombi may get trapped in the cerebral circulation, causing ischaemic stroke. Patients with paroxysmal or permanent AF should be risk assessed (e.g., CHA2DS2-VASc score) for the risk of ischaemic stroke, and anticoagulation offered if the benefits outweigh the risks of anticoagulation.

> **CLINICAL NOTES**
>
> Atrial fibrillation stroke risk: Patients with paroxysmal and permanent AF are generally at increased risk of ischaemic stroke; the risk is influenced by additional factors such as age, previous cerebrovascular accidents, sex, heart failure, hypertension, vascular disease and diabetes. The risk of ischaemic stroke can be estimated by risk scores such as the CHA2DS2-VASc score. Similarly, the risk of major bleeding associated with anticoagulation should also be considered (e.g., by risk scores such as the ORBIT or HAS-BLED scores). Counselling patients on their individual risk of ischaemic stroke and risk of bleeding from anticoagulation is central to patient-centred decision-making in this regard.

Endothelial injury/dysfunction

Endothelial injury/dysfunction may occur in context of a myriad of scenarios, including shear stress, atherosclerosis, infection, inflammation and immune-mediated damage. This results in activation of primary haemostasis and consequently thrombosis.

Hypercoagulability

Disruption to the equilibrium of coagulation factors and natural anticoagulants in favour of the former can result in hypercoagulability and an increased tendency to thrombosis. Hypercoagulability may be associated with antiphospholipid syndrome (APLS), malignancy, inflammatory states, pregnancy and the combined oral contraceptive pill, etc.

SECONDARY (ACQUIRED) THROMBOPHILIAS

Specific conditions associated with an increased incidence of thrombosis are outlined in Table 6.5. Acquired thrombophilias are considerably more common than hereditary thrombophilias.

Antiphospholipid syndrome

The clinical presentation of APLS is that of recurrent venous or arterial thrombosis and/or pregnancy morbidity (e.g., recurrent miscarriage). In addition to clinical criteria, the diagnosis also requires the presence of laboratory criteria – the persistent presence of either a lupus anticoagulant (an antibody directed against phospholipid-binding proteins, resulting in phospholipid-dependent prolongation of phospholipid-dependent coagulation assays) or anticardiolipin or anti-b2-glycoprotein 1 antibody. The disease can be idiopathic or secondary to other autoimmune disorders, notably systemic lupus erythematosus (SLE).

The presence of a lupus anticoagulant typically prolongs the APTT by binding to phospholipid, which is a necessary cofactor for in vitro clot formation in the APTT assay; in this context, the prolonged APTT is a laboratory artefact rather than suggesting a haemostatic defect. On the contrary, it is important to emphasize that APLS is a prothrombotic state.

Patients with an unprovoked venous thromboembolic (VTE) event, VTE associated with only a mild provoking factor, and certainly recurrent VTE should be screened for APLS, since the diagnosis may influence the choice of anticoagulation.

Acquired genetic traits

Myeloproliferative neoplasms (MPN) (see Chapter 5) and paroxysmal nocturnal haemoglobinuria (PNH) are clonal disorders, caused by the acquisition of genetic mutations in haematopoietic progenitors, which are associated with increased risk of venous and arterial thrombosis, particularly thrombosis at unusual sites (e.g., splanchnic, cerebral venous sinus).

A consequence of the genetic mutations causing PNH is chronic complement activation. The clinical presentation may be dominated by thrombosis, intravascular haemolysis or cytopenias (aplastic anaemia).

Given that specific management should be initiated if an underlying MPN or PNH is diagnosed, screening for these conditions may be warranted in patients with thrombosis at unusual sites, particularly if accompanied by cytopenias or a cell count consistent with an MPN (see also Chapter 5).

PRIMARY (HEREDITARY) THROMBOPHILIAS

Several hereditary thrombophilias are described below; however, it is important to emphasize that genetic testing is frequently unhelpful and does not actually influence clinical management. Indeed, testing for hereditary thrombophilias should not be performed routinely, and should be restricted to specific cases such as those with strong family histories, where diagnosis may influence management (e.g., AT deficiency in pregnancy).

Antithrombin deficiency

Antithrombin deficiency is an autosomal dominant condition affecting 1 in 2000 people, conferring approximately a 15-fold

Table 6.5 Factors associated with increased thrombosis

Factor	Mechanism
Immobilization	Venous stasis
Obesity	Chronic inflammation Impaired fibrinolysis
Pregnancy	Lower limb venous stasis (IVC compression) Increased levels of coagulation factors I, II, VII, VIII, IX and X Reduced levels of protein S
Oestrogen therapy	Increased plasma levels of factors II, VII, IX and X Reduced levels of AT and tPA
Cigarette smoking	Abnormal endothelial and platelet function
Certain cancers	Cancer cell expression of procoagulant factors (e.g., tissue factor) Tumour cell interactions with endothelium
Nephrotic syndrome	Renal loss of clotting factors
Myeloproliferative disorders	Hyperviscosity Expression of procoagulant factors and adhesion molecules Inflammatory cytokine release
Sickle cell anaemia	Abnormal platelet activation Abnormal activation of coagulation cascades Vasoocclusion (by sickled cells) and impaired blood flow
Antiphospholipid syndrome	Activation of endothelial cells and platelets by antiphospholipid antibodies

IVC, Inferior vena cava; tPA, tissue plasminogen activator.

increased risk of thrombosis. Deficiency may either be quantitative (type 1) or qualitative (type 2).

Deficiencies of proteins C and S

Protein C and S are natural anticoagulants; hence heterozygous deficiency of either increases the risk of thrombosis by five- to sevenfold. Protein C or S deficiency may be quantitative (type 1) or qualitative (type 2). Severe protein C or S deficiency may manifest as neonatal purpura fulminans, or widespread spontaneous intravascular thrombosis resulting in organ damage.

Factor V (FV) Leiden

FV Leiden (FVL) is a polymorphism of *FV* gene that renders FV less resistant to inactivation by activated protein C. FVL is the most common heritable thrombophilia in the European population, but its effect is modest with an increased relative risk of thrombosis of approximately fivefold. Thus, the majority of individuals with the FVL mutation will never suffer a thromboembolic event.

Prothrombin G20210A

This gene variant, with a prevalence of 1–2% in Europeans, increases prothrombin levels and is associated with a slightly increased relative risk of thrombosis of approximately threefold.

VENOUS THROMBOEMBOLISM

Deep vein thrombosis occurs most commonly in deep veins of the lower limbs. Unilateral swelling, tenderness and erythema (redness) of the overlying skin are suggestive of a DVT. The Well's score may be used to determine if exclusion of a DVT could be achieved with a negative D-dimer test (low pretest probability of DVT) or a Doppler ultrasound scan is warranted (high pretest probability of DVT).

CLINICAL NOTES

Well's score: This is a validated risk stratification tool used to estimate the probability of a DVT, to help guide the choice of subsequent investigations (i.e., D-dimers and ultrasound scanning). 1 point is scored for presence of each of the risk factors (active cancer, paralysis/lower limb immobility, previous confirmed DVT or major surgery in the last 12 weeks) and examination findings (unilateral pitting oedema on suspect limb, collateral superficial venous dilation, calf circumference ≥3 cm than asymptomatic calf, unilateral

swelling of entire leg, tenderness localized to deep venous regions). Where an alternative diagnosis is at least as likely as a DVT to account for the symptoms and signs, –2 points are scored. Scores range from –2 to +9, and a score of 1, 0, –1 or –2 suggest a DVT is unlikely.

The main danger of DVT is embolization to the PE. However, postthrombotic syndrome (chronic changes to skin and tissue overlying the zone of the DVT, associated with the risk of venous ulceration and chronic pain) is an important chronic complication. DVTs are common, particularly in hospital patients with risk factors. Treatment is necessary to reduce the likelihood of PE.

Clinical presentation of pulmonary embolism

Whilst massive PE present with haemodynamic instability or even cardiac arrest, small PE may be subtle and nonspecific in their presentation. A high index of suspicion is essential, particularly in patients with risk factors. The following symptoms may suggest a PE: (pleuritic) chest pain, dyspnoea, haemoptysis. Clinical signs may include hypoxia, tachycardia, tachypnoea and systemic hypotension.

Massive PE – an acute PE with haemodynamic instability – is life-threatening and should be managed by systemic thrombolysis. Submassive PE is an acute PE without haemodynamic instability, but with evidence of right ventricular dysfunction (right heart strain) or myocardial necrosis. Besides anticoagulation, patients with a submassive PE should be considered for thrombolysis, or if systemic thrombolysis contraindicated, be considered for thrombectomy or catheter-directed thrombolysis. Acute PE without severe features is considered low risk.

Diagnosis is with computed tomography pulmonary angiogram (CT-PA) or a ventilation perfusion (VQ) scan. Assessment for Right Ventricular (RV) dysfunction by echocardiogram, and correlation with cardiac biomarkers (troponin, B-type natriuretic peptide [BNP]) for evidence of myocardial necrosis may be helpful. Treatment with anticoagulation should be initiated when the diagnosis is confirmed or empirically if a significant delay in diagnostics is anticipated. In the context of haemodynamic instability, systemic thrombolysis is warranted.

ANTICOAGULATION

The main use of anticoagulants is to prevent inappropriate thrombus formation or extension of an existing thrombus. Anticoagulants do not affect platelet plug formation (primary haemostasis), nor do they destabilize existing thrombi. They act at specific stages in the coagulation cascade to ultimately prevent fibrin formation. The type of anticoagulant and duration of use depends on the indication for treatment. Important indications for anticoagulation therapy include:

- Prophylaxis against thrombosis, for example postoperatively, prolonged immobilization, AF, mechanical heart valves
- Treatment for acute thromboembolic events, for example DVT, PE
- During certain invasive procedures, for example cardiopulmonary bypass or haemofiltration

Some anticoagulants require therapeutic monitoring (e.g., APTT or anti-Xa levels for UFH, INR for warfarin), whereas others (e.g., direct oral anticoagulants [DOACs]) are administered in fixed doses. The main complication of anticoagulant use is haemorrhage, and the potential benefit of anticoagulation should be weighed against the risk of bleeding associated with anticoagulation. Examples of high-risk factors for bleeding include:

- Ongoing active internal bleeding
- History of haemorrhagic stroke
- Recent eye, brain or spinal cord surgery
- Severe liver disease
- Severe thrombocytopenia
- Peptic ulcers
- Oesophageal varices
- Frequent mechanical falls

The choice of a specific DOAC can generally be made on the basis of local policy, but haematology input is warranted for complex cases (e.g., cancer-associated thrombosis, recurrent VTE). Important variables for the commonly used anticoagulants are summarized in Table 6.6.

Warfarin

Warfarin is a functional vitamin K antagonist and thus impairs synthesis of the vitamin K–dependent factors, factors VII, IX, X and II (affected most → least) and the natural anticoagulants, protein C and S. The PT (presented as INR) is used to monitor warfarin's anticoagulatory effect, since the factors affected by warfarin impair the extrinsic pathway more than the intrinsic pathway.

CLINICAL NOTES

International normalized ratio: This is the measured PT normalized to a control to correct for reagent and instrument interlaboratory variability. A high INR equates to a more prolonged PT, that is, increased tendency to bleed, or alternatively less tendency to clot.

Table 6.6 Comparison of unfractionated heparin, low-molecular-weight heparins, warfarin, dabigatran and the anti-Xa inhibitors (rivaroxaban, apixaban and edoxaban)

Drug	Warfarin	UFH	LMWH	Dabigatran	Rivaroxaban, Apixaban and Edoxaban
Mechanism of anticoagulant action	Vitamin K epoxide reductase inhibition (reduced levels of II, VII, IX, X)	Anti-Xa and anti-IIa activity by potentiating AT III activity	AT potentiation, anti-Xa activity > anti-IIa activity	Direct FIIa (thrombin) inhibition	Direct FXa inhibition
Administration route	Oral	IV or SC	SC	Oral	Oral
PT	Prolonged	Prolonged	Normal	Prolonged but variable	Prolonged
APTT	Normal/prolonged	Prolonged	Normal	Prolonged but variable	Prolonged
TT	Normal	Prolonged	Normal/mildly prolonged	Prolonged	Normal
Test used to monitor	INR	APTT or anti-Xa	None required regularly; anti-Xa for select situations	None required regularly; dabigatran level for select situations	None required regularly; DOAC level for select situations
Reversal	Vitamin K, Prothrombin complex concentrate (PCC)	Protamine	Protamine	Idarucizumab ('Praxbind')	Andexanet alfa (licensed for rivaroxaban and apixaban)

APTT, Activated partial thromboplastin time; AT, Antithrombin; INR, international normalized ratio; IV, intravenous; LMWH, low-molecular-weight heparin; PT, prothrombin time; SC, subcutaneous; TT, thrombin time; UFH, unfractionated heparin.

Table 6.7 Target INR ranges

Indication	Target INR range
AF	2–3
Mechanical heart valve (aortic)	2–3 (low thrombogenicity),[a] 2.5–3.5 (medium thrombogenicity),[a] 3–4 (high thrombogenicity)
Mechanical heart valve (mitral)	2.5–3.5 (low thrombogenicity), 3–4 (medium or high thrombogenicity)
DVT/PE treatment dose	2–3

[a]Increase target INR by 0.5 if presence of patient-related risk factors (e.g., previous arterial thromboembolism, AF, LVEF <35%, mitral stenosis, left atrium diameter >50 mm).
AF, Atrial fibrillation; DVT, Deep vein thrombosis; INR, international normalized ratio; PE, pulmonary embolism.

Table 6.8 Drugs interacting with warfarin

Potentiate action (increase INR)	Attenuate action (decrease INR)
Alcohol	Certain antiepileptics (carbamazepine, phenytoin)
SSRIs	Azathioprine
Certain antibiotics (cephalosporins, macrolides, fluoroquinolones, metronidazole)	Rifampicin
Tricyclic antidepressants	
Thyroxine	
Amiodarone	

INR, International normalized ratio; SSRIs, selective serotonin reuptake inhibitors.

Target INR ranges vary with treatment indication and are shown in Table 6.7. As warfarin has a half-life of 40 hours, a dose change usually takes 4–5 days to influence the INR.

Since warfarin crosses the placenta and is teratogenic, it is contraindicated in early pregnancy whilst foetal organogenesis is occurring. Heparin does not cross the placenta and is therefore safer in early pregnancy when anticoagulation is necessary.

Warfarin treatment interferes with numerous other drug actions, and its own action is affected by multiple drugs. Common examples are given in Table 6.8.

Warfarin over-anticoagulation and reversal

In the event of over-anticoagulation with warfarin, or if a need for reversal of anticoagulation arises, warfarin should be withheld, and oral/parenteral vitamin K administered, with the dose and method of administration (i.e., oral vs. intravenous) depending on the INR and the time frame available for anticoagulation

reversal (e.g., prior to an invasive procedure). In the presence of bleeding, or if extremely rapid reversal of anticoagulation is required (e.g., for emergency surgery), prothrombin complex concentrate (PCC), which contains the vitamin K-dependent factors II, VII, IX and X (see Chapter 7 for further details) may be necessary. Local guidelines will be available to direct management, and haematology input may be helpful. Used inappropriately, PCC may result in thrombotic complications.

Unfractionated heparin

Heparin is a glycosaminoglycan that binds to and potentiates AT III, inactivating factors IIa and Xa. UFH contains molecules ranging in weight from 5000 to 30,000 kDa. The different chain lengths affect both activity and clearance; larger molecules are more rapidly cleared from the circulation. UFH generally does not require dose adjustment for renal impairment.

Unfractionated heparin has a short half-life, and its anticoagulation effect wears off after 1–4 hours. Thus, a continuous intravenous infusion is necessary to achieve anticoagulation with UFH, and regular monitoring and titration based on the APTT or anti-Xa level is necessary. Reversal of UFH may be achieved by administration of protamine. UFH infusions may be particularly useful in settings conducive to close monitoring (e.g., ICU/HDU), where the ability to rapidly discontinue anticoagulation is greatly valued; conversely, it is frequently challenging to achieve stable anticoagulation with UFH infusions on a general ward setting.

As discussed above, HIT usually causes thrombocytopenia 5–14 days after starting heparin (especially UFH) treatment and is associated with a potentially lethal prothrombotic state. Heparin must be discontinued immediately, and alternative anticoagulation (e.g., fondaparinux, argatroban) initiated in spite of the thrombocytopenia.

Low-molecular-weight heparin

Low-molecular-weight heparins (LMWHs) have a mean molecular weight of 5000 kDa. In contrast to UFH, the anticoagulant effect of LMWHs is primarily through inhibition of Fxa. Administration is parenteral, typically subcutaneously. Crucially, LMWHs have predictable pharmacokinetic and pharmacodynamic properties, and their use is ubiquitous in the hospital setting (e.g., routine VTE prophylaxis). As LMWHs depend on renal excretion, dose reduction for renal impairment is advised. Dosing for extremes of weight should be according to local policies. Although their anticoagulant effect can be monitored by the anti-Xa level, it is not generally advised except for specific situations (typically guided by haematology advice), for instance, in cases of suspected therapeutic failure. Compared to UFH, the risk of HIT is lower with LMWH. Long-term use of LMWH is not advised as it may result in a loss of bone mineral density and an increased risk of osteoporosis.

Fondaparinux

Fondaparinux is a synthetic heparin pentasaccharide which only inhibits Fxa (i.e., no FIIa inhibition). Administration is parenteral, typically subcutaneously. Fondaparinux depends on renal clearance, and has a long half-life of 17–21 hours, which makes it less attractive than LMWHs as a 'default anticoagulant' in the hospital setting. Specific situations where it may be used include treatment of HIT and acute coronary syndromes.

Direct oral anticoagulants

Direct oral anticoagulants have predictable pharmacokinetic and pharmacodynamic properties, and as such are administered orally as fixed doses without the need for regular therapeutic monitoring; these properties make them particularly attractive anticoagulants. Compared to warfarin, they are associated with fewer drug–drug interactions. The choice of a specific DOAC should be in accordance with local policy.

Some hesitation about their use persists as reversal agents are only licensed in specific settings and are not universally available. Nevertheless, bleeding in the context of DOAC use can be managed, for instance by administration of PCC, though reference to local guidelines is essential.

> **RED FLAG**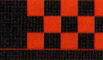
>
> Reversal of dabigatran: A reversal agent, idarucizumab ('Praxbind'), is available for use in acute haemorrhage scenarios.
>
> Reversal of apixaban and rivaroxaban: A reversal agent, andexanet alfa, is available within England for use in acute GI haemorrhage. In Scotland, this agent can also be used for intracerebral haemorrhage.

Direct thrombin inhibitors

Dabigatran is an oral thrombin (FIIa) inhibitor that can be used for VTE prophylaxis (e.g., orthopaedic surgery postoperative prophylaxis) or therapeutic anticoagulation. Idarucizmab (Praxbind®), a monoclonal antibody directed against dabigatran, is licensed as a reversal agent of dabigatran in the context of life-threatening bleeding or emergency surgery.

The parenteral thrombin inhibitors, bivalirudin and argotraban, are infrequently used but have specific applications (e.g., HIT).

Direct Fxa inhibitors

This class of oral anticoagulants includes rivaroxaban, apixaban and edoxaban, and can also be used for VTE prophylaxis or therapeutic anticoagulation. Andexanet alfa (Andexxa®), a recombinant modified version of Fxa lacking coagulant properties, is able to bind and sequester direct Fxa inhibitors. Andexanet alfa is licensed for the reversal of rivaroxaban and apixaban in the context of life-threatening gastrointestinal bleeding.

THROMBOPROPHYLAXIS

Hospital inpatients are at increased risk of VTE for a variety of reasons, including surgery, immobility and their underlying illness. All inpatients must therefore have their individual VTE risk assessed and documented, and appropriate VTE prophylaxis initiated.

Mechanical thromboprophylaxis approaches include regular mobilization, compression stockings and pneumatic intermittent compression devices. Pharmacologic thromboprophylaxis may include any of the anticoagulants, but subcutaneous LMWH are the most commonly used drugs.

THERAPEUTIC THROMBOLYSIS

Whilst anticoagulants prevent extension of existing clots and new clot formation, they do not directly break down existing clots. Thrombolysis, or the dissolving of blood clots, may be achieved by fibrinolytics such as plasminogen activators. Recombinant human tissue-type plasminogen activator (tPA) (e.g., alteplase, reteplase, tenecteplase) are generally used first line. Streptokinase, which is derived from group A β-haemolytic streptococci, has been superseded by recombinant alternatives due to its frequent association with immunological reactions.

As systemic thrombolysis does not discriminate between physiologic and pathologic thrombi, it is associated with a high risk of bleeding complications. Specific indications may include:

- Massive PE (acute PE with haemodynamic instability); consider thrombolysis for submassive PE (acute PE without haemodynamic instability but with evidence of right ventricular dysfunction or myocardial necrosis).
- ST-elevation MI (STEMI) within 12 hours of symptom onset, and where primary percutaneous coronary intervention (PCI) cannot be delivered within 120 minutes.
- Acute ischaemic strokes (following exclusion of intracranial haemorrhage) within 4.5 hours of symptom onset. Patients should also be assessed for suitability for mechanical thrombectomy.

Thrombolysis is contraindicated if there is a high risk of bleeding, including in the context of bleeding disorders, active or previous intracranial haemorrhage, active or recent severe/dangerous bleeding, trauma, surgery and recent stroke (except if thrombolysis being administered for ischaemic stroke within 4.5 hours of symptom onset). Nevertheless, if thrombolysis is considered, local guidelines and the Summary of Product Characteristics of the specific fibrinolytic should be consulted.

Chapter Summary

- Haemostasis consists of the sequence of vasoconstriction, primary haemostasis and finally secondary haemostasis
- Primary haemostasis consists of specific changes to platelets (adhesion, activation and aggregation) which results in formation of a platelet plug at the site of the developing clot
- Secondary haemostasis consists of activation of the coagulation cascades, ultimately converting soluble fibrinogen to insoluble fibrin and stabilizing the clot
- Antiplatelet drugs reduce the probability of thrombus formation by inhibiting key stages in platelet activation and are used where inappropriate thrombus formation is likely, for example, cardiovascular disease
- Thrombocytopenia may result from shortened lifespan or reduced production. Platelets may also be functionally impaired, which may lead to the same set of symptoms as a reduced platelet count, that is, increased tendency to bleed including spontaneously
- The coagulation pathways are cascades of clotting factor activation, which convert a platelet plug to a mature clot (secondary haemostasis). The traditional models were subdivided into extrinsic, intrinsic and common pathways, whilst the currently accepted model consists of an initiation phase followed by an amplification phase
- Haemostatic defects are more commonly acquired (e.g., iatrogenic, DIC), but may be inherited (e.g., haemophilia, vWD)
- A thorough bleeding history is critical for assessing a patient with a suspected bleeding disorder
- If a haemostatic defect is suspected, screening tests may include an FBC, PT, APTT and Clauss fibrinogen
- Risk factors for thrombosis generally relate to Virchow's triad: venous stasis, hypercoagulability and endothelial dysfunction
- Selection of the most appropriate anticoagulant depends on multiple factors, including the reason for anticoagulation/prophylaxis, duration of treatment, preferences regarding mode of administration, renal impairment and availability of reversal agents
- Thrombolysis with fibrinolytic drugs may be used to limit serious/life-threatening complications secondary to acute pathologic thrombus formation (e.g., ischaemic stroke, massive PE, STEMI without primary PCI availability)

MLA Conditions

Adverse drug effects
Arterial thrombosis
Deep vein thrombosis
DIC
Epistaxis
Haemophilia
Pancytopenia
Patient on anticoagulant therapy
Patient on antiplatelet therapy
Pulmonary embolism
VTE in pregnancy and puerperium

MLA Presentations

Bleeding antepartum
Bleeding from lower gastrointestinal (GI) tract
Bleeding from upper GI tract
Bleeding postpartum
Bruising
Epistaxis
Haemoptysis
Painful swollen leg
Petechial rash
Purpura

INTRODUCTION

'Blood transfusion' refers to the therapeutic use of any 'blood product', which includes blood components (e.g., red cells, platelets, fresh frozen plasma [FFP]) and its derivatives (e.g., cryoprecipitate). Nowadays, whole blood transfusion has become extremely uncommon and is only rarely used. Storage temperatures and 'shelf-lives' of the various blood products are given in Table 7.1.

Up-to-date information about donor selection, blood component manufacture and specifications are available is online (https://www.transfusionguidelines.org/red-book).

Patient blood management

Blood components, when used appropriately, save lives. Yet, they may be associated with transfusion reactions and are a scarce resource, so they should be used judiciously. Patient blood management (PBM) is an evidence-based, multidisciplinary

Table 7.1 Storage temperatures and shelf-lives of donated blood components

Blood component	Storage features	Maximum shelf life	Storage solution	Approximate volume per unit/bag/pool/pack	Usage instructions at room (i.e., ward) temperature	Usual duration of intravenous administration
Red cells	4°C (±2°C)	35 days	Saline, adenine, glucose, mannitol (SAGM)	~220–340 mL per unit	Use within 4 hours of removal from blood fridge. May be returned to blood bank within 30 minutes, but no longer	1.5–3 hours per unit
Platelets	Agitated, 22°C (±2°C)	7 days (if bacterial screening performed, otherwise, 5 days)	citrate-phosphate-dextrose (CPD) (pooled); acid citrate dextrose (apheresis)	~340 mL (pool) ~150 mL (apheresis unit)	Use within 2 hours of removal from the agitator. May be returned to blood bank within 30 minutes, but no longer	20–30 min per pool/unit
Granulocytes (BUFFY COAT)	22°C (±2°C), but must *not* be agitated	24 hours	White cell additive solution	~60 mL per pack (10 packs represent a typical adult dose)	Must be infused as soon as possible after collection from donor	The entire dose should be infused over 1–2 hours
FFP	<–25°C	36 months	None	~270 mL per bag	Must use within 4 hours of thawing. Must be thawed at 37°C. Once thawed, FFP cannot be returned to blood bank	20–30 mins per bag

Continued

Table 7.1 Storage temperatures and shelf-lives of donated blood components—cont'd

Blood component	Storage features	Maximum shelf life	Storage solution	Approximate volume per unit/bag/ pool/pack	Usage instructions at room (i.e., ward) temperature	Usual duration of intravenous administration
Cryoprecipitate	<−25°C	36 months	None	190 mL per pool (2 pools represent a typical adult dose)	Must use within 4 hours of thawing. Must be thawed at 4°C. Once thawed, cryoprecipitate cannot be returned to blood bank.	~10 min per pool
Fractionated plasma products						
Immunoglobulins	22°C	Up to 3 years	Saline Glycine	Use immediately after opening		
Clotting factors	<30°C	Up to 3 years	Typically powder for reconstitution	Use immediately after reconstitution		
Albumin	<25°C	Up to 3 years	Saline	Use immediately after opening		

FFP, Fresh frozen plasma.

approach to optimize the care of all patients potentially requiring transfusion by avoiding inappropriate transfusions, thereby ensuring availability of blood components when necessary.

Patient blood management emphasizes that the individual patient should be at the centre of any decision to transfuse blood; that is to say, avenues to avoid transfusion should be explored if clinically appropriate. Thus, haematinic (e.g., iron) deficiency should be aggressively corrected, haemostatic defects corrected (e.g., with vitamin K, FFP; refer to Chapter 6), antifibrinolytics (specifically, tranexamic acid) used in the context of trauma, post-partum haemorrhage and cardiac surgery, and appropriate intra-operative measures (e.g., cell salvage) adopted to reduce the need for blood transfusion. Likewise, evidence-based restrictive trans-fusion thresholds should also be adopted.

Donation process

In the United Kingdom (UK), donated blood comes from healthy, unpaid volunteers. Altruistic donation is associated with lower rates of transfusion-associated infections. Volunteers must be at least 17 years of age; donors older than 65 years are subject to annual health reviews. Regular donors cannot donate more frequently than every 16 weeks (women) or 12 weeks (men).

Donors must have a predonation haemoglobin (Hb) concentration of 125 g/L in females or 135 g/L in males and are screened by a finger-prick Hb measurement.

Donation is either of whole blood or of a single component, for example, platelets, by apheresis. Whole blood is leucode-pleted, then separated into blood components. Blood components may be pooled from several donors to manufacture specific blood products (e.g., manufacture of one unit of pooled platelets from four donations).

The safety of blood components in the UK is strictly regulated by risk mitigation steps; for example, the risk of transfusion-asso-ciated infections is reduced by donor screening, infection screen-ing on blood donations, specific protocols for sample collection (e.g., arm cleansing and diversion of the initial part of the blood donation to reduce bacterial contamination) and strict controls for storage and testing (e.g., screening of platelet components for bacterial contamination) of manufactured blood components.

Donor Health Check

Prior to donation, all donors have to complete a Donor Health Check, a confidential screening questionnaire regarding their general health, travel history (to minimize the risk of transmis-sion of malaria, *Trypanosoma cruzi* and other emerging diseases)

Table 7.2 Mandatory infection screening tests performed on all collected samples

Infection	Parameter used for testing
Hepatitis B	Hepatitis B surface antigen (HBsAg) HBV DNA[a]
Hepatitis C	Anti-HCV antibodies HCV RNA testing
HIV 1 + 2	Anti-HIV 1 + 2 antibodies HIV RNA testing[a]
HTLV	Anti-HTLV I/II antibodies
Syphilis	Syphilis antibodies (antitreponemal Ab)
HEV	HEV RNA

Ab, Antibody; DNA, deoxyribonucleic acid; HBV, hepatitis B virus; HCV, hepatitis C virus; HEV, hepatitis E virus; HIV, human immunodeficiency virus; HTLV, human T-lymphotropic virus; RNA, ribonucleic acid.
[a]Not mandatory, but generally performed in the UK. HIV RNA testing is mandatory in Scotland.

and lifestyle (to reduce the risk of transfusion-associated infections).

Donor deferral evolves with scientific consensus opinions. An example of permanent exclusion criteria includes infection with hepatitis B, C, human immunodeficiency virus (HIV), human T-lymphotropic virus (HTLV) or syphilis. Temporary exclusion includes sexual activity with another man and commercial sex work, where donors have to wait at least 3 months following the last sexual activity before blood donation.

Infection screening

At a minimum, mandatory screening for hepatitis B, C, E, HIV, HTLV and syphilis is required (Table 7.2). Additional screening for *Trypanosoma cruzi*, West Nile virus and malarial antibodies may be performed depending on travel history.

Leucodepletion

All blood products (with a few specific exceptions, e.g., granulocytes) produced in the UK have been universally subjected to leucocyte depletion (leucodepletion). Universal leucodepletion reduces the risk of white-cell–borne infection including variant Creutzfeldt–Jakob disease (vCJD) transmission and cytomegalovirus (CMV), and of immune reactions in the recipient, such as transfusion-associated graft-versus-host disease (GVHD).

RED CELL ANTIGENS

Transfused red cells must be ABO compatible (Box 7.1), and recipients should also not have any clinically significant antibodies that would react with the transfused red cells. To understand

this concept, it is important to have an appreciation of red cell antigens.

RED FLAG

ABO-incompatible transfusion: Naturally occurring IgM antibodies in the recipient's plasma bind to antigens on the donor red cells. This activates the complement pathway leading to intravascular destruction (haemolysis) of red cells and a huge release of inflammatory cytokines. Shock and fatal multiorgan failure may ensue. Accidental transfusion of an ABO-incompatible blood product is a 'never event' that most commonly arises because of human error.

Red cell antigens are molecules capable of provoking an immune response. The surface of the red cell membrane contains various carbohydrate and glycoprotein molecules that can potentially act as antigens. Transfusion of blood product(s) may expose the individual to foreign red cell antigens that trigger an immune response.

There are many different red cell antigen systems; the most clinically significant are the ABO and Rh systems.

THE ABO BLOOD GROUP SYSTEM

The ABO system refers to various forms of the H antigen, which is an oligosaccharide molecule expressed on the red cell membrane. The genes for the ABO blood group system encode transferases that modify the H antigen. This is summarized in (Table 7.3).

'A' antigen

If an individual possesses the gene for the A transferase, the H antigen will be modified by an *N*-acetyl galactosamine moiety, forming the 'A' antigen.

'B' antigen

If an individual possesses the gene for the B transferase, the H antigen will be modified by a galactose moiety, forming the 'B' antigen.

Genetics of the A, B and O antigens

There are three alleles: A, B and O. A and B are codominant. Therefore, although there are six possible genotypes (i.e., O/O, A/O, A/A, B/O, B/B and A/B), there are only four phenotypes:

- group A (A/O or A/A)
- group B (B/O or B/B)

Table 7.3 Blood group, corresponding red cell antigens, genotype, antibodies and ABO compatibilities

Blood group	Genotype	Form of H antigen	Antibodies	ABO compatibility: that is, can receive red cells from donors with blood group(s)	ABO incompatibility: must NOT be transfused with red cells from donors with blood group(s)
O[a]	O/O	H (unmodified)	Anti-A Anti-B	O	A, B or AB
A	A/A, A/O	A	Anti-B	O and A	B or AB
B	B/B, B/O	B	Anti-A	O and B	A or AB
AB	A/B	A and B	None; immune tolerant to A, B and O antigens	A, B, O, AB	Can safely receive transfusion from all ABO types[b]

[a]Group O individuals are termed 'universal donors', since their red cells do not exhibit A or B antigens and thus can be safely transfused to any ABO blood type without causing an ABO incompatibility reaction.
[b]Group AB individuals are termed 'universal recipients', since they can safely accept any ABO type. This is because they have immune tolerance to both A and B antigens, as these are normally expressed on their own red cells.

- group AB (A/B)
- group O (O/O)

Anti-A and anti-B antibodies

ABO antibodies are naturally occurring IgM antibodies and will be made by infants from approximately 3–6 months of age, in the absence of sensitization to any foreign red blood cells (RBCs). This phenomenon arises in response to structurally similar antigens present in intestinal bacteria and/or ingested food molecules.

As the A and B antigens are simply modified versions of the H antigen, group A, B and AB individuals will still have a small amount of the unmodified H antigen and regard it as 'self'. Consequently, groups A, B and AB individuals can receive blood from group O donors, who are 'universal donors' (see Table 7.3).

Group O individuals will have anti-A and anti-B antibodies, and thus can only receive blood from other group O donors. Group A individuals will have anti-B antibodies and can receive blood from either group A or O donors. Group B individuals will have anti-A antibodies and can receive blood from either group B or O donors. Group AB individuals have neither anti-A nor anti-B, can receive blood from donors of any ABO group, and as such are 'universal recipients' (Table 7.3).

Clinical significance

ABO antibodies are naturally occurring and do not require prior sensitization for formation. Thus, an individual can suffer potentially fatal immediate transfusion reactions if transfused ABO-incompatible blood, even if it is their first transfusion episode. Hence, every transfusion has to be ABO compatible.

Rh BLOOD GROUP SYSTEM

There are five main Rh antigens: C, c, D, E and e. These are encoded by two genes: *RHD* and *RHCE*. D is the most immunogenic, but antibodies to any of the Rh antigens are potentially clinically significant. Less than 1% of Africans and Asians are RhD negative, whilst up to 15% of Caucasians are RhD negative.

Antibodies against Rh antigens are usually IgG but are not naturally occurring and require a sensitization event (i.e., exposure to a 'nonself' Rh antigen) for formation. Re-exposure to the antigen, for example, on a subsequent transfusion episode, can trigger an anamnestic (memory) antibody response manifesting as a delayed haemolytic transfusion reaction.

Haemolytic disease of the foetus and newborn

If an RhD–woman becomes pregnant with an RhD+ foetus, the mother will likely become sensitized during pregnancy or delivery and develop anti-D antibodies. The time required for the immune system to respond to the foreign RhD antigen and to develop a high anti-D titre means the first pregnancy is generally unaffected. However, if the woman subsequently becomes pregnant with another RhD+ foetus, the previously developed anti-D antibodies will cross the placenta and can cause haemolysis of foetal RBCs, leading to haemolytic disease of the foetus and newborn (HDFN).

The degree of immune haemolysis and the resultant severity of anaemia is variable. In the most extreme scenario, it can cause hydrops fetalis (prenatal heart failure in utero); a lesser degree of haemolysis may result in anaemia, jaundice and hepatosplenomegaly.

Whilst HDFN is most commonly caused by anti-D, it can also be associated with other red cell antibodies (e.g., anti-c, anti-K).

Sensitizing events

Sensitization can occur through transfusion of blood expressing foreign red cell antigens. To reduce the risk of sensitization, blood should be ABO- and RhD-matched; women of childbearing age should also receive K-matched blood. In the context of major haemorrhage where blood is required before the group of the recipient can be determined, women of childbearing age (i.e., <50 years) should receive group O RhD– K⁻ red cell units to reduce the risk of HDFN.

Foeto–maternal haemorrhage, or the entry of foetal red cells into the maternal circulation, may also result in sensitization. Some possible causes of FMH include:

- Delivery
- Maternal trauma during pregnancy
- Ectopic pregnancy
- Miscarriage, termination of pregnancy, intrauterine death
- In utero procedures including amniocentesis/chorionic villous sampling

Prophylactic anti-D

Anti-D immunoglobulin is manufactured from the plasma of donors with high anti-RhD titres. In addition to transfusing women of childbearing age only with ABO-, RhD- and K-matched red cell units, the risk of HDFN can also be dramatically reduced by routine administration of anti-D immunoglobulin to all RhD– women between 28 and 30 weeks of pregnancy. This protects an RhD– woman against sensitization by foetal RhD+ cells that cross into maternal circulation as part of normal pregnancy or during delivery. The administered anti-D immunoglobulin is believed to coat circulating RhD+ cells; therefore, the immune system of a RhD– woman does not detect the presence of the RhD antigen and forms anti-D antibodies. Further episodes of foetomaternal haemorrhage (see previous section) can also be covered by anti-RhD immunoglobulin.

OTHER RED CELL ANTIGENS

There are many other blood group systems, including Kell, Kidd, Duffy, Lewis, P, I and MNS. Some antibodies against these red cell antigens may also be clinically significant, and are associated with delayed haemolytic transfusion reactions or HDFN.

RED CELL TRANSFUSIONS

Red cell transfusions are indicated for restoring oxygen-carrying capacity in patients with low Hb or blood loss, when alternative treatment strategies are ineffective or inappropriate. Indications include significant acute blood loss (e.g., due to trauma, surgery or obstetric haemorrhage), symptomatic anaemia (see Chapter 3: Anaemia), and temporary (e.g., following chemotherapy) or permanent (e.g., transfusion-dependent thalassaemia, myelodysplastic syndrome) bone marrow failure.

Selection of appropriate donated red cells for transfusion

Group and Screen (G&S)

Prior to transfusion, the ABO and RhD status of the patient is determined by grouping. This is performed by testing a sample of the patient's red cells for a reaction against known antibodies ('forward grouping') – a positive reaction (agglutination) indicates the presence of that red cell antigen on the patient's red cells. ABO status is also confirmed by 'reverse grouping' – the presence of anti-A and anti-B in the patient's serum is determined by its ability to cause agglutination of donor group A or B red cells.

An antibody screen is performed by reacting the patient's serum with a screening panel of donor red cells, specifically selected to express certain red cell antigens, such that collectively, the screen would be expected to detect the vast majority of clinically significant red cell antibodies. If the screen is positive, further tests (e.g., antibody panel) are required to identify the specific red cell antibody, so that its potential clinical significance can be determined.

As any one sample could be mislabelled leading to 'wrong blood in tube', each patient must have at least two G&S samples collected on separate occasions, to minimize the risk of inadvertently transfusing incompatible blood to a patient.

Cross-matching

If a patient requires a red cell transfusion, compatible units are identified by cross-matching. A G&S sample collected within the last 7 days (or within 72 hours if the patient is pregnant, or if they had received a transfusion within the preceding 3 months) is required.

The majority of blood is issued by electronic issue – identifying compatible units based on accurate determination of the ABO and RhD groups of the patient and of donor units, and exclusion of the presence of clinically significant red cell antibodies in the patient by a sensitive antibody screen.

Electronic issue may be inappropriate for various reasons, including a positive antibody screen, the historical presence of red cell alloantibodies, or recent ABO-incompatible bone marrow or solid organ transplant. A serologic cross-match (indirect antiglobulin test) is necessary in these settings – if the patient's serum is able to cause agglutination of donor units, the patient may contain red cell antibodies that would react against that donor unit, indicating possible incompatibility.

Emergency transfusion

The 2022 SHOT report indicates that transfusion delays are the most common cause of transfusion-related mortality in the UK. Patients should not die from not receiving a blood transfusion in a timely fashion.

In emergencies, whilst a G&S is still pending, group O RhD– K– red cell units can be issued to women of childbearing age, and group O RhD+ units to men and women of non–childbearing age (to preserve stocks of group O RhD– units).

Other features important for selecting appropriate donation products

Irradiated units

Gamma irradiation of cellular components ensures that any residual leucocytes following leucodepletion are nonviable, to further reduce the risk of transfusion-associated GVHD (TA-GVHD). All granulocyte concentrates are irradiated. TA-GVHD occurs when residual leucocytes engraft in the recipient and mount an immune response against the recipient, which is typically fatal. Irradiation reduces the shelf-life of red cells to 14 days. Indications for irradiated units (see https://b-s-h.org.uk/guidelines/guidelines/guidelines-on-the-use-of-irradiated-blood-components) include:

- Hodgkin lymphoma (lifelong indication even after completion of treatment)
- Previous exposure to purine analogues (e.g., fludarabine or bendamustine)
- Severely impaired cell-mediated immunity (e.g., severe combined immunodeficiency)

CMV seronegative units

The risk of CMV transmission is significantly reduced by universal leucodepletion. Thus, the indications for CMV seronegative units are limited:

- Neonates up to 12 months of age
- Pregnant women
- Intrauterine transfusions

Washed red cells

Sequential washing of the cells can be performed to remove most traces of residual donor plasma, though this will result in a lower red cell dose. Washing units can be specifically requested from NHS Blood and Transplant (NHSBT) for named recipients with a history of severe allergic reactions to red cell transfusions.

Administration of red cells

Consent

Unless a patient lacks capacity and transfusion is lifesaving, patients must provide informed consent for transfusion.

Confirming correct blood and correct recipient

Around 1 in 13,000 transfusions are administered to the wrong patient. It is vital for rigorous measures to be taken to minimize potential error.

> **CLINICAL NOTES**
>
> Error reduction in transfusion: Appropriate measures to take to reduce errors, as summarized in SHOT's Ten Steps in Transfusion (https://www.shotuk.org/wp-content/uploads/myimages/Ten-steps-in-transfusion.pdf), include:
>
> - Repeated identity and document checking, ideally with two people *and* the patient at all stages from pretransfusion sample collection to commencement of transfusion
> - A final pretransfusion check should be performed at the bedside including the patient
> - If available electronic transfusion management technology with barcode recognition should be used as an additional level of positive patient identification
> - Avoidance of unnecessary transfusions
> - Avoidance of out-of-hours transfusions
> - Adherence to local transfusion guidelines

Procedure

Any indwelling cannula may be used for blood transfusion, via a standard blood-giving set with a mesh filter. Drugs must never be added to the blood bag.

Monitoring

Patients receiving a red cell transfusion should at a minimum have their pulse rate, respiratory rate (RR), blood pressure (BP), and temperature measured before starting the transfusion and then 15 minutes after the start of the transfusion and up to 60 minutes after the transfusion has ended.

ALTERNATIVES TO RED CELL TRANSFUSIONS

Some individuals are averse to receiving blood products. This may be because of concern about the associated risks or religious beliefs.

> **ETHICS**
>
> Jehovah's Witnesses: The brethren are the largest group of individuals in the UK with beliefs advocating refusal of blood products. The majority will not accept major blood

components such as red cells, platelets and fractionated plasma. However, individual beliefs differ, and it is vital to clarify and clearly document what an individual would be prepared to accept in terms of blood products, and under what circumstances. Jehovah's Witnesses who are undergoing elective surgery should be preoperatively optimized for surgery to correct any anaemia (e.g., by correcting any haematinic deficiencies); this may also include the use of recombinant growth factors (i.e., erythropoietin) to stimulate red cell synthesis.

For such individuals, alternatives to blood transfusion are necessary. Unfortunately, these alternatives are only practical when advanced notice of potential blood loss, for example, surgery, is available. They are not therefore useful in cases of emergency haemorrhage.

These alternatives are particularly relevant in the context of valid, informed refusal of transfusion by an adult with capacity. With children under 16 years of age, the law differs.

ETHICS

Medicolegal aspects: In the context of a patient lacking capacity, a lifesaving transfusion can be given as a Best Interests decision. However, if an adult (>16 years of age) patient has capacity to refuse blood products, or if they have clear evidence of prior refusal to receive blood products (e.g., Advanced Decision), clearly acknowledging the potentially fatal consequences of refusal, it is medicolegally and ethically necessary to respect the patient's decision.

ETHICS

Parental refusal of lifesaving transfusions for their children: Where a parent(s)/guardian(s) wish(es) to withhold transfusions on behalf of a child, in a scenario where transfusion would be lifesaving or essential for the child's well-being, a Specific Issue Order can be rapidly obtained from a court. Children (<16 years of age) are not legally entitled to refuse lifesaving treatments, and this includes transfusion.

Emergency alternatives to red cell transfusion

The only practical alternative to transfusion in an emergency haemorrhage scenario is an attempt to restore the depleted circulation volume with crystalloid or colloid. Whilst this may temporarily increase perfusion pressure, it will not compensate for the impairment of oxygen delivery to organs and tissues, and will also cause haemodilution of remaining red cells, clotting factors and platelets. If a cell-saver (see 'Nonemergency alternatives to red cell transfusion' below) is present and practical, this may be benefit, but they are not universally available and even cell-savers are unacceptable to some individuals.

Nonemergency alternatives to red cell transfusion

- Intraoperative cell salvage: red cells lost in the surgical field are collected, washed and returned to the patient, using an automated cell-saver. It can be particularly beneficial in certain 'clean' surgeries, for example, knee and hip replacements but is not applicable in cancer resections or where any infective material may be present.
- Prior autologous donation: an individual can donate their own blood in advance of the situation where a need for red cell transfusion is anticipated. However, this strategy is generally unfeasible since it is inappropriate with predonation anaemia.
- Optimization of haematinics: iron, vitamin B12 and folate are essential for erythropoiesis, so any haematinic deficiency should be identified and corrected.
- Stimulation of erythropoiesis: administration of erythropoietin can be used prior to increase the patient's red cell counts in advance of planned surgery.
- Normovolaemic haemodilution: immediately before surgery, blood is collected from the patient. The volume collected is replaced by crystalloid or colloid, restoring intravascular volume. The intravascular blood is, however, now haemodiluted. For a given volume of surgical blood loss, a smaller number of red cells are lost, reducing the impact on Hb levels. Immediately postoperatively, the collected blood is 'returned' to the patient.

OTHER TRANSFUSION PRODUCTS

Platelets

A dose of platelets is either a unit of pooled platelets (from four pooled whole blood donations), or an adult therapeutic dose (ATD) of platelets obtained from a single donor by apheresis. Platelets must be stored at room temperature ($22 \pm 2°C$) with constant agitation to avoid aggregation. Their shelf-life is 5 days, or 7 days with screening for bacterial contamination.

One dose is administered over 15–30 minutes and typically raises the platelet count by $20–40 \times 10^9$. Though platelets express ABO antigens and ABO-incompatible platelets may exhibit slightly reduced survival, this is rarely clinically significant. As such, platelet transfusions can be ABO-incompatible, if the plasma of the unit does not contain anti-A/B antibodies that are likely to cause significant haemolysis of recipient red cells.

The cause of thrombocytopaenia should be identified as platelet transfusion is contraindicated in some causes of thrombocytopaenia, notably thrombotic thrombocytopaenic purpura (see Chapter 6: Thrombotic thrombocytopaenic purpura) and heparin-induced thrombocytopaenia (see Chapter 6: Heparin-induced thrombocytopaenia). Platelet transfusion in these settings further drives these disease processes. Platelet transfusion thresholds include:

- Bleeding:
  - Intracranial or intraocular haemorrhage: $<100 \times 10^9$/L
  - Severe bleeding: $<50 \times 10^9$/L
  - WHO grade ≥ 2 but not severe: $<30 \times 10^9$/L
  - As part of a major haemorrhage protocol
- Prophylactic
  - Absence of bleeding: $<10 \times 10^9$/L
  - With additional risk factors for bleeding (e.g., sepsis): $<20 \times 10^9$
  - Preoperative: depends on procedure, for example, $<50 \times 10^9$ for major surgery

Certain complications are more common with platelet than with red cell transfusions, reflecting the greater plasma content (e.g., allergic and febrile reactions, transfusion-related lung injury [TRALI]) and the storage conditions (e.g., bacterial contamination).

Granulocyte concentrates

Though evidence for benefit is limited, granulocytes (neutrophils), following discussion with NHSBT, are occasionally transfused to neutropenic patients with life-threatening bacterial or fungal infection. Granulocyte concentrates include red cells and platelets, and must be ABO and Rh D compatible and irradiated to reduce the chance of TA-GVHD.

Plasma derivatives

Due to concern about potential transmission of vCJD, plasma used in the UK since 1999 has been manufactured using donations from countries with a low risk of vCJD.

Fresh frozen plasma

Fresh frozen plasma is frozen soon after collection to preserve the activity of the coagulation factors. The recommended dose is 12–15 mL/kg. FFP may be indicated to treat bleeding associated with coagulopathies caused by deficits of multiple clotting factors (e.g., DIC).

Fresh frozen plasma ABO compatibility depends on preventing the passive transfer of anti-A/B antibodies that can cause haemolysis of recipient red cells, and is summarized in (Table 7.4). Whilst group AB plasma is universally compatible, stocks are very limited so rarely issued.

Immunoglobulins

Normal immunoglobulins

The Igs extracted from several thousand blood donations are pooled and used as replacement therapy for patients with severe Ig deficiency. It can also be used for treatment of some autoimmune diseases, for example, immune thrombocytopoenic purpura (see Chapter 6: 'Immune thrombocytopoenic purpura'), though the precise mechanism for its activity is not fully defined.

Specific immunoglobulins

Anti-D immunoglobulin is the most commonly used specific immunoglobulin as prophylaxis against HDFN. Administration of specific immunoglobulins against certain infectious agents can be used to reduce the risk of serious illness by passive transfer of immunity. Some specific immunoglobulins used in the UK are:

- Tetanus Ig can be given to patients that have *not* recently completed a tetanus toxoid vaccination course if they are injured by a mechanism likely to involve clostridium tetanus exposure (e.g., soil-contaminated cuts, foreign body penetrations, human/animal bites)
- Hepatitis B Ig, which is given to unvaccinated individuals that sustain a high-risk injury such as a needlestick injury
- Rabies virus Ig and varicella zoster virus Ig

Human albumin solution

Albumin solution contains albumin purified from plasma. It contains no antibodies or clotting factors and can be given without regard to the recipient's blood group. It is available in various

Table 7.4 Fresh frozen plasma compatibility

Blood group	Antibodies produced	Can receive FFP safely from blood groups	Can donate FFP safely to blood groups
O	Anti-A, anti-B, anti-A, B	O, A, B or AB	O only
A	Anti-B	A, AB	A, O
B	Anti-A	B, AB	B, O
AB	None	AB	AB, A, B, O

FFP, Fresh frozen plasma.

concentrations. Indications are largely for treatment of complications of liver failure or nephrotic syndrome. Severe hypersensitivity reactions can occur.

Cryoprecipitate

Cryoprecipitate is the insoluble precipitate formed by thawing FFP at 4°C. It contains factors VIII and XIII, vWF, fibronectin and fibrinogen; however, it is typically used as a means of fibrinogen replacement. An adult dose represents two 'pools' (each pool representing five donations). Indications for cryoprecipitate generally relate to treatment of hypofibinogenaemia in the context of bleeding (e.g., DIC, as part of a major haemorrhage protocol).

Single clotting factor concentrates

With the exception of factors V, X and II, all other factors are available as single-factor concentrates. They are used for treatment of specific bleeding disorders. However, recombinant factor VIII and IX products are typically used for the treatment of haemophilia A and B, respectively, which eliminates the risk of transfusion-associated infection.

Combined clotting factor concentrates: prothrombin complex concentrate

Prothrombin complex concentrate (PCC) contains the vitamin K– dependent factors II, VII, IX and X. It rapidly and effectively reverses the effect of warfarin. Compared to FFP, beyond greater efficacy, PCC is associated with reduced risk of serious allergic reactions and transfusion-associated circulatory overload (TACO) due to its smaller volume.

Note that Octaplex® (a brand of PCC) is different from Octaplas® (a brand of solvent detergent-treated FFP).

COMMON PITFALLS

Octaplex versus Octaplas: Octaplex® is a brand of prothrombin complex concentrate, whilst Octaplas® is a brand of solvent detergent treated FFP. Octaplas® is a licensed medicinal product made from a large pool of donors, with more standardized concentrations of clotting factors. Solvent detergent treatment inactivates bacteria and most encapsulated viruses, including hepatitis B and C and HIV.

TRANSFUSION REACTIONS

Although transfusions are generally extremely safe procedures, they can, nevertheless, be associated with transfusion reactions. They can be divided by time of onset – that is, acute (within

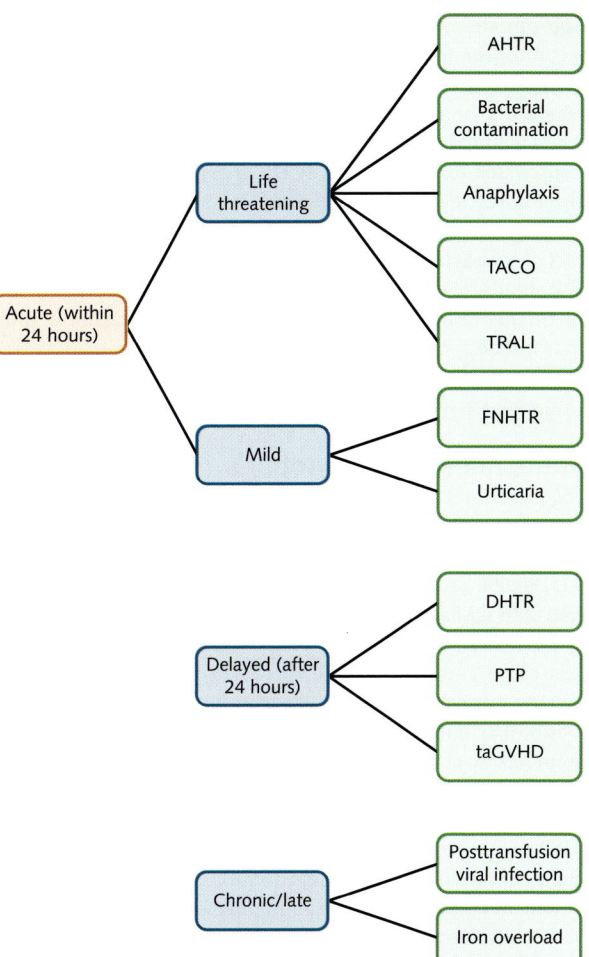

Fig. 7.1 Classification of transfusion reactions according to time of onset following the transfusion. *AHTR,* Acute haemolytic transfusion reaction; *DHTR,* delayed haemolytic transfusion record; *FNHTR,* febrile nonhaemolytic transfusion reaction; *PTP,* posttransfusion purpura; *TACO,* transfusion-associated circulatory overload; *TA-GVHD,* transfusion-associated graft-versus-host disease; *TRALI,* transfusion-associated lung injury.

24 hours) or delayed (>24 hours) – and by underlying mechanism (Fig. 7.1).

Management in suspected acute transfusion reaction

Whenever an acute transfusion reaction is suspected, the transfusion should be paused. The patient should be assessed by a clinician and vital signs measured. If the patient is well and vital signs normal, a nonsevere transfusion reaction is likely, and the transfusion may be resumed, perhaps at a reduced rate.

Appropriate medication may be prescribed, for example, paracetamol for febrile nonhaemolytic transfusion reaction, for symptomatic relief. However, if the patient is unwell, the giving set should be disconnected, and the patency of intravenous access maintained with saline infusion. The patient should be resuscitated following an ABCDE approach, with critical care input if necessary. Specific immediate management relevant to the suspected diagnosis (e.g., intramuscular adrenaline in suspected anaphylaxis) should be urgently undertaken. The suspect unit should be retained and returned urgently to the blood bank for further testing and to allow recall of associated donations if appropriate.

Haemolytic transfusion reactions

Acute haemolytic reactions

The most severe and feared acute haemolytic transfusion reactions are caused by ABO incompatibility, where anti-A/B antibodies react against incompatible donor red cells. This occurs in ~1/180,000 red cell transfusions, usually due to human error. Anti-A/B IgM antibodies fix complement and cause severe intravascular destruction (haemolysis) of donor red cells. C3a and C5a cause vasodilation and increased vascular permeability, causing intravascular fluid redistribution into tissues and profound distributive hypotension and shock. This may be compounded by acute renal failure. A consumptive coagulopathy may result in DIC. Death occurs in 15% of cases of ABO incompatibility and may result from as little as 30 mL of transfused ABO-incompatible blood. Patients are anxious (often experiencing a sensation of impending doom), flushed, feel extremely unwell and may complain of abdominal or loin pain. Symptoms occur soon after the start of the transfusion. Dark urine caused by haemoglobinuria (due to free Hb from the lysed RBCs) is a classical sign pointing to intravascular haemolysis.

Delayed haemolytic transfusion reactions

Delayed (>24 hours after transfusion, but typically 7–10 days after transfusion) haemolytic transfusion reactions occur in previously allo-immunized patients due to an anamnestic (memory) response. Red cell antibodies (e.g., against Rh, Kidd, Kell blood group systems) of the IgG type cause extravascular haemolysis (i.e., reticuloendothelial and splenic removal of antibody-coated donor cells). The clinical presentation may be anaemia, failure to achieve a Hb increment following transfusion, jaundice, fever or haemoglobinuria. Management is typically supportive, though in some settings IVIg and steroids, or even further transfusion may be necessary.

Febrile nonhaemolytic reactions

An isolated pyrexia (≥38°C or ≥1.5°C above baseline, if baseline <37°C) not associated with any other derangement in blood oxygen saturation (SpO$_2$), RR, heart rate (HR) or BP may be managed by temporarily pausing the transfusion and/or administering an antipyretic such as paracetamol. A reduction in the transfusion rate may be helpful. Increased frequency of observations should be implemented. Shivering, myalgia and nausea may accompany the fever. Febrile nonhaemolytic reactions occur in 1–2% of red cell transfusions and represent the most common transfusion reaction.

However, a rise in temperature >2°C above baseline, or any derangement of other observations or symptoms suggestive of a haemolytic or bacterial contamination reaction should warrant immediate cessation of transfusion and be managed as for all suspected acute transfusion reactions.

Hypersensitivity reactions

Severe allergic or anaphylactic reactions

Severe allergic reactions are more common with FFP and plasma-rich transfusion products such as platelets. This is a potentially fatal acute complication of transfusion. Pallor, tachycardia, desaturation and hypotension, urticarial rash, wheeze (bronchospasm), stridor (laryngospasm) and swelling of the lips and tongue may be observed. Increased vascular permeability causes the hypotension which may progress to severe distributive shock, loss of consciousness and death. Anaphylaxis should be treated as per national guidelines, and specific treatment (e.g., 0.5 mL of 1:1000 adrenaline IM in adults) should be administered.

An extremely small proportion of severe allergic reactions to blood components can be attributed to the presence of anti-IgA antibodies in patients with IgA deficiency, though no single allergic trigger can be identified in the majority of cases. Patients experiencing recurrent/severe allergic transfusion may benefit from washed products or solvent detergent FFP.

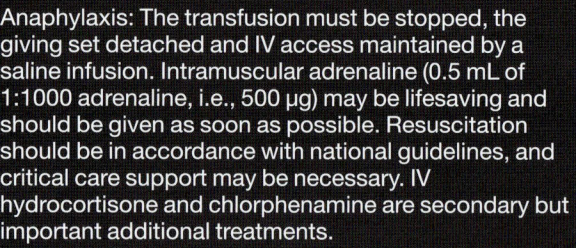

RED FLAG

Anaphylaxis: The transfusion must be stopped, the giving set detached and IV access maintained by a saline infusion. Intramuscular adrenaline (0.5 mL of 1:1000 adrenaline, i.e., 500 µg) may be lifesaving and should be given as soon as possible. Resuscitation should be in accordance with national guidelines, and critical care support may be necessary. IV hydrocortisone and chlorphenamine are secondary but important additional treatments.

Mild allergic reaction

Itching ('pruritus') or an urticarial rash unaccompanied by a change in vital signs or any more worrisome symptoms most likely represents a mild allergic reaction. Mild allergic reactions are relatively common, especially with platelet or FFP transfusions. Antihistamines (e.g., chlorphenamine) may reduce the symptoms.

Transfusion-related lung injury

Severe breathlessness and a productive cough with frothy pink sputum occurring within less than 6 hours (typically within 2 hours) of transfusion may suggest TRALI. Hypotension caused by abnormal redistribution of intravascular fluid into the lung parenchyma is not uncommon. A fever may be present. TRALI results from donor antibodies reacting with the recipient's neutrophils. Inflammatory sequestration in the lungs leads to non-cardiogenic pulmonary oedema (with a clinical picture of acute respiratory distress syndrome). Treatment is supportive, potentially requiring critical care support.

Implicated donors are typically females sensitized by previous pregnancy. The risk of TRALI is mitigated by manufacturing FFP from male donors, resuspending pooled platelets in male plasma, and screening female apheresis donors for leucocyte antibodies.

Transfusion-related circulatory overload

Transfusion-associated circulatory overload describes new onset (or exacerbation of existing) pulmonary oedema within less than 6 hours of a transfusion. This manifests as acute respiratory distress (breathlessness, ↑ RR and desaturation) and is associated with signs of intravascular hypervolaemia, for example, elevated jugular venous pressure, hypertension and tachycardia. Patients with low body weight that receive a large volume transfusion, for example, in massive haemorrhage, and patients with preexisting cardiac or renal insufficiency are at particular risk. TACO and TRALI are occasionally difficult to distinguish; Table 7.5 provides useful distinguishing features.

Infection

Bacterially contaminated transfusion product

This most often occurs with platelets (as they are stored at 22°C), but rarely occurs with red cells. An acute, severe response is seen very soon after the transfusion starts. Symptoms and signs may be very similar to an acute haemolytic or hypersensitivity reaction, with hypotension, shock and reduction in consciousness. Rigors and elevation of temperature >2°C above baseline may distinguish bacterial contamination from these other serious acute transfusion reactions.

Viral infection from infectious donation

Viral infection secondary to transfusion with blood products derived from a virally infected donor is a rare complication of transfusion. The risks are <1 in 1.2 million for hepatitis B, <1 in 7 million for HIV and <1 in 28 million for hepatitis C.

Table 7.5 Differentiating between TACO and TRALI

Clinical features	TRALI	TACO
Onset after transfusion	Usually <2 hours	Within 6 hours
Tachycardia	Yes	Yes
BP	Hypotensive or normotensive	Hypertensive or normotensive
Respiratory distress (↑ RR, ↓ SpO$_2$, dyspnoeic)	Yes	Yes
Pyrexia	Likely	Unlikely
Fluid challenge	Improves, or no change	Worsens
Diuresis	Worsens	Improves
Underlying mechanism	Intravascular hypovolaemia caused by abnormal fluid redistribution	Intravascular hypervolaemia

BP, Blood pressure; RR, respiratory rate; SpO$_2$, blood oxygen saturation; TACO, transfusion-associated circulatory overload; TRALI, transfusion-related lung injury.

Transfusion-associated graft-versus-host disease

This delayed complication of transfusion is fortunately very rare, as it is usually fatal. It arises from leucocytes contaminating a blood product engrafting in the recipient, and the donor lymphocytes mounting a graft-vs-host immune response against the recipient's cells and tissues. Symptoms typically develop within 30 days of transfusion, and include rash, pyrexia, diarrhoea, deranged liver function tests and bone marrow aplasia. Universal leucodepletion minimizes the chance of this occurring. Patients with impaired cell-mediated immunity are at particular risk for transfusion-associated GVHD, hence they should receive irradiated cellular components (see section on Irradiated Units above) to ensure any residual lymphocytes are rendered incapable of proliferation. Granulocytes, which are not leucodepleted, and have a particularly high leucocyte content, must always be irradiated.

Iron overload

This chronic complication arises from recurrent transfusions (see Chapter 2: Iron overload), so it is of most relevance in transfusion-dependent individuals (e.g., transfusion-dependent thalassaemia, sickle cell anaemia) for whom strategies such as iron chelation and exchange blood transfusions may be necessary.

Posttransfusion purpura

This delayed transfusion reaction typically manifests between 5 and 12 days following a transfusion (see Chapter 6: Posttransfusion purpura).

MAJOR HAEMORRHAGE

This encompasses a range of scenarios ranging from acute blood loss with haemodynamic instability to bleeding requiring massive transfusion. A physiological definition based on response to resuscitation is preferred; for instance, HR >110 bpm or systolic BP <90 mmHg, following adequate resuscitation are some proposed thresholds.

In all scenarios, the primary priority is obtaining haemostasis. Transfusion of appropriate blood products should aim to:

- maintain a sufficient intravascular volume to maintain end-organ perfusion pressure
- prevent an excessive fall in Hb impairing the oxygen delivery to perfused tissues
- replacement of blood components (platelets and clotting factors) to enable haemostasis to be achieved

Major haemorrhage should be managed by major haemorrhage protocols, which are site-specific protocols that prespecifies the ratio and order of blood products, and how blood products can be made available to the bleeding patient without need for escalation for approval. A commonly used ratio is 4:4:1 (RBC:FFP:platelets) for the first major haemorrhage pack (MHP) followed by the second MHP which has all the aforementioned in same ratio but added two pools of cryoprecipitate. In the context of major haemorrhage due to trauma, tranexamic acid should be administered as early as possible, up to 3 hours following trauma.

G&S samples should be sent, ideally prior to transfusion. Prior to the G&S results being available, the patient should be issued group O, RhD−, K− red cells if she is a woman of child-bearing age. Depending on local protocol, men and women of non–childbearing age may be issued either group O RhD− or RhD+ red cells. Whilst the major haemorrhage is ongoing, the FBC, coagulation screen and fibrinogen should be checked regularly (e.g., every 30–60 minutes) so that targeted replacement can be initiated. The aim is to maintain Hb >80 g/L, platelet count $>50 \times 10^9$/L, INR <1.5 and fibrinogen >1.5 g/L. Hypocalcaemia (that may arise from chelation by citrate in the blood components) should be corrected to encourage coagulation.

Complications associated with massive transfusions

All the usual complications associated with transfusion are possible, but large-volume transfusions required in major haemorrhage scenarios may also be associated with dilutional coagulopathy, hypothermia (from cold resuscitation fluids and blood products), hypocalcaemia, hyperkalaemia (from lysis of red cells in red cell components) and metabolic acidosis. These factors impair coagulation and should be corrected as part of haemostatic resuscitation.

● Chapter Summary

- Blood donation is a standardized and altruistic process in the UK. A questionnaire assesses the general health, travel history and lifestyle factors to ensure safety of the donor and to minimize the risk of transfusion-associated infections.
- Donated whole blood is used to manufacture various blood products, including cellular components (red cells, platelets) and plasma derivatives (e.g., FFP, cryoprecipitate).
- Different blood products have specific requirements in terms of processing, storage solution and temperature and lifespan.
- Blood is a scarce resource and though transfusion is very safe, it may be associated with complications, so it should only be performed if indicated.
- There are many blood group systems, but the most important is the ABO system. ABO-incompatible transfusions are a never event, and mostly happen due to human error.
- Other blood group systems may also be associated with clinically significant issues, for example, HDFN due to anti-D from an allo-immunized RhD− woman crossing the placenta to affect an RhD+ foetus.
- The 'group and screen' determines the blood group of a patient and screens for the presence of red cell antibodies. Most red cell units can be issued electronically, but some require a serological cross-match.

- Complications of transfusion can be divided into immediate (e.g., ABO incompatibility), early (e.g., transfusion-associated lung injury) or late (e.g., infection).
- Major haemorrhage should be managed according to prespecified major haemorrhage protocols.

MLA Conditions

Postpartum haemorrhage
Transfusion reactions

MLA Presentations

Bleeding antepartum
Bleeding from lower GI tract
Bleeding from upper GI tract
Bleeding postpartum
Massive haemorrhage
Postpartum haemorrhage

Principles of immunology 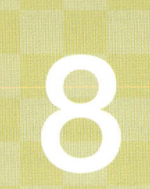 8

AN INTRODUCTION TO IMMUNOLOGY

The immune system is represented throughout the body and plays a role in most pathological processes. It works as a network with many different components; to get your head around immune function and malfunction, it helps to have an idea of the overall picture before diving into the details.

This chapter aims to introduce the bigger picture of immunology while avoiding the detail, which will be covered later. Try to understand the concepts and links that are covered here and revisit them as you progress through the later chapters.

The need for an immune system

The threat of many different types of infection is present for all living things. Methods to defend against these threats are required and have evolved as the nature of pathogens has also evolved. Humans face encounters with a multitude of pathogens, from aerosols of virus particles to multicellular parasites. These threats are diverse in their mechanisms of entry into the body (e.g., broken skin, airway mucosa, contaminated food) as well as their strategies of attack within the body and methods of reproduction. For example, pathogens can replicate within cells or populate the lumen of the gastrointestinal tract. Many of these pathogens can rapidly mutate, meaning that a threat that the body has encountered before may not appear in the same way if encountered again. Therefore, an immune system must be broad in its recognition of pathogens and in its mechanisms of response, yet swift enough to destroy a rapidly reproducing population.

The body also regularly encounters a plethora of harmless organisms that share characteristics with pathogens. In addition, the environment we live in and the tissues of the body itself contain many molecules that are a similar structure to molecules found on the surfaces of pathogens. For this reason, the immune system must be regulated to attack the harmful and tolerate the harmless.

Problems that arise in the immune system can lead to a breakdown in this balance:

- A fault in system function could lead to severe and repeated infection
- A loss of immune regulation could lead to unnecessary tissue damage

These immunologic problems are explored in Chapter 12.

Innate immunity

The innate immune system constitutes the first-line defence against pathogens and potentially harmful microorganisms and is present from birth. It is particularly important, as it provides a rapid immune response against pathogen invasion, protecting the host until the adaptive immune responses take over (days to weeks).

It is made up of cellular, humoral and physical defences, all tasked with the initial prevention of infection. Its functions include:

- Detection of pathogens and initiation of first-line defence mechanisms (through pattern recognition) to prevent invasion and eradicate the pathogens.
- Maintenance of immune homeostasis involves a fine balance between the proinflammatory responses (recruited to eradicate the pathogens) and the antiinflammatory responses (suppressing the inflammation to allow the body's physiology to return to its baseline).
- Activation of the adaptive immune system to take over.

The components of the innate immune system are highly conserved and include:

- Physical barriers
- A variety of cells (such as macrophages, mast cells and natural killer cells)
- Cell receptors (such as the Toll-like receptors)
- Antimicrobial enzymes (such as lysozyme) and peptides
- Cytokines (such as chemokines, interferons, interleukins)
- The microbiome, which involves a variety of bacterial, fungi and viruses that live normally (colonize) in the body

The full details of the innate immune system are covered in Chapter 9.

HINTS AND TIPS

Pathogens are detected by the innate immune system in many ways, including pattern recognition molecules, opsonization (when immune molecules mark a pathogen for destruction) and antibody binding.

Adaptive immunity

The innate immune system's nonspecific nature means that it cannot always eliminate infectious organisms, as there are some pathogens they cannot recognize. The ability to recognize and provide protection against any pathogen is a unique feature of the adaptive immune system. Furthermore, the innate immune system does not lead to immunological memory.

Lymphocytes are the primary cells of the adaptive immune system. A given lymphocyte bears an antigen receptor of a single specificity; however, the specificity of each lymphocyte is different. That means that the millions of lymphocytes carry millions of different receptors with variable specificity, which allows recognition of an endless diversity of antigens.

When a lymphocyte encounters an antigen, it gets activated and differentiates into effector cells. Then the following occur:

- Clonal selection: The activated lymphocyte proliferates to produce many identical copies of itself, known as a clone. These cells now bear receptors of identical specificity to those of the parental cell from which they derived.
- Clonal expansion: This takes about 4 to 5 days, explaining why the adaptive immune responses are delayed.
- Clonal deletion: Lymphocytes bearing potentially self-reactive receptors are removed before they mature.
- Lasting protective immunity: Once the antigen is removed, effector cells undergo apoptosis. However, a small number persist and become memory cells. It is due to these cells that a more rapid immune response is mounted when the same antigen is encountered again.

The innate and adaptive immune systems are compared in Table 8.1, components of each system are summarized in Table 8.2.

HINTS AND TIPS

T cells coordinate the adaptive immune response as well as eradication of certain pathogens. B cells secrete antibody which neutralizes pathogen directly and aids the innate immune system in pathogen recognition.

The link: presentation of antigen

Both the innate and the adaptive immune systems are able to distinguish between foreign and self molecules. The innate immune system relies on the recognition of specific types of molecules found on pathogens but not on the host, called 'pathogen-associated immunostimulants'. Adaptive immunity is driven by the recognition of small molecular units found on pathogens, and these units are called antigen (antibody generator). In infection, innate

Table 8.1 Essential differences between the innate and adaptive immune systems

	Innate immune system	Adaptive immune system
Response to pathogens	Rapid – response does not change with repeated exposure	Slower – requires repeated exposure to develop
Specificity	Each component can defend against various types of pathogen (it is not antigen specific)	Each component can only defend against one type of pathogen (it is antigen specific)
Mechanisms of defence	Broad and are effective against many pathogens (e.g., phagocytosis, complement)	Specific to each pathogen (e.g., antibody)

Table 8.2 Components of the innate and adaptive immune systems

	Innate system	Adaptive system
Cellular components	Monocytes/macrophages Neutrophils Eosinophils Basophils Mast cells Natural killer cells	B cells/plasma cells T cells
Molecular components	Complement Cytokines Acute phase proteins Interferons	Antibody Cytokines

immune cells kill pathogens and process their remains to produce antigen. This is then presented to adaptive immune cells by professional antigen-presenting cells, linking the innate and adaptive immune systems. The adaptive immune system then coordinates the response, as described earlier. This process of antigen presentation is also used by the majority of body cells to flag up any intracellular infection to the immune system. Antigen presentation and recognition is covered in more detail in Chapter 10.

In immunization, a harmless molecule bound to an immunostimulant is injected, leading to the activation of the adaptive immune system, causing long-lasting protection against this molecule.

● Chapter Summary

- Pathogens vary greatly in nature
- A broad and efficient immune system is required to prevent infection while avoiding tissue damage
- The innate immune system is broad in its recognition of pathogens and can activate the adaptive immune system
- The adaptive immune system is more targeted, develops with pathogen exposure and is driven by antigen presentation from the innate immune system
- An ineffective immune system can result in severe infection; an unregulated immune system can result in tissue damage

Innate defences can be classified into three main groups:

1. Barriers to infection
2. Cells
3. Serum proteins and the complement system

BARRIERS TO INFECTION

Physical and mechanical

Skin and mucosal membranes act as physical barriers to the entry of pathogens. Tight junctions between cells prevent the majority of pathogens from entering the body. The flushing actions of tears, saliva and urine protect epithelial surfaces from colonization. High oxygen tension in the lungs, as well as body temperature, can also inhibit microbial growth.

In the respiratory tract, mucus is secreted to trap microorganisms. They are then mechanically expelled by:

- Beating cilia (mucociliary escalator)
- Coughing
- Sneezing

Chemical

The growth of microorganisms is inhibited at acidic pH (e.g., in the stomach and vagina). Lactic acid and fatty acids in sebum (produced by sebaceous glands) maintain the skin pH between 3 and 5. Enzymes such as lysozyme (found in saliva, sweat and tears) and pepsin (present in the gut) destroy microorganisms.

Biological (normal flora—the microbiome)

The microbiome is a dynamic collection of organisms (bacteria, viruses and fungi) that live normally in and on our body (skin, respiratory system, gastrointestinal and urogenital tract). It constitutes an essential element of the innate immune system, as it influences the effectiveness of the immune responses and maintains the balance between proinflammatory and antiinflammatory responses, promoting immune homeostasis. The microbiome may change in response to various factors, such as stress, diet, medications and other environmental factors.

Dysbiosis refers to the loss of the gut homeostasis, resulting in a change in the distribution, composition or diversity of the microbiome. Increasing evidence supports a correlation between the microbiota and disease development, such as cancer, cardiovascular disease, diabetes and neurological disorders.[1,2] For that reason, manipulation of the microbiota, as a potential disease treatment, has attracted a lot of interest. Faecal microbiota transplantation (FMT), which refers to the introduction of faecal matter from a donor to the intestinal tract of a recipient, has emerged as a potential treatment for various conditions, such as the *Clostridium difficile* infection (CDI), cancer and inflammatory bowel disease (IBD), with very promising results (cure rates up to 90% in CDI).[3,4] Other approaches include the use of pro- and prebiotics, administration of antibiotics and engineering of gut bacteria.

CLINICAL NOTES

Clostridium difficile (*C. diff*): Hospitalized patients that are being treated with certain antibiotics (such as clindamycin, cephalosporins and fluoroquinolones) are at greater risk of developing a *C. diff* infection because of the disruption of the patient's normal gut flora. *C. diff* infection causes watery diarrhoea, nausea and abdominal pain; possible complications include toxic megacolon and sepsis. The infection can rapidly spread between patients in a ward, so adequate hand washing and isolation of infected patients are essential.

CELLS OF INNATE IMMUNITY

The cells of the innate immune system consist of:

- Phagocytes
- Natural killer (NK) cells
- Degranulating cells
- Dendritic cells (DCs)

Phagocytes

Phagocytes (macrophages and neutrophils) engulf and then destroy pathogens. Macrophages are long-lived sentinel cells stationed at likely sites of infection; upon infection, they release cytokines that recruit the shorter-lived but more actively phagocytic neutrophils.

Neutrophils (for structure and production, see Chapter 1: Neutrophils)

Neutrophils comprise 50% to 70% of circulating white cells. Neutrophils are the first cells recruited into the site of inflammation and in the act of killing pathogens they die; in fact, dead neutrophils are the major constituent of pus. Neutrophils migrate from the bloodstream in response to tissue damage, complement proteins and chemicals released by macrophages (see Chapter 11). As they are phagocytes, they have an important role in engulfing and killing extracellular pathogens. The process of phagocytosis and the mechanisms of killing are shown in Fig. 9.1. During inflammation, neutrophil production is stimulated by the cytokine granulocyte colony-stimulating factor. A high neutrophil count is part of the acute phase response (see clinical notes section on 'Acute Phase Response). Neutrophils can be activated and recruited either by interleukin (IL)-8 and tumour necrosis factor (TNF) secreted by macrophages, or by IL-17 secreted by T cells of the adaptive immune system.

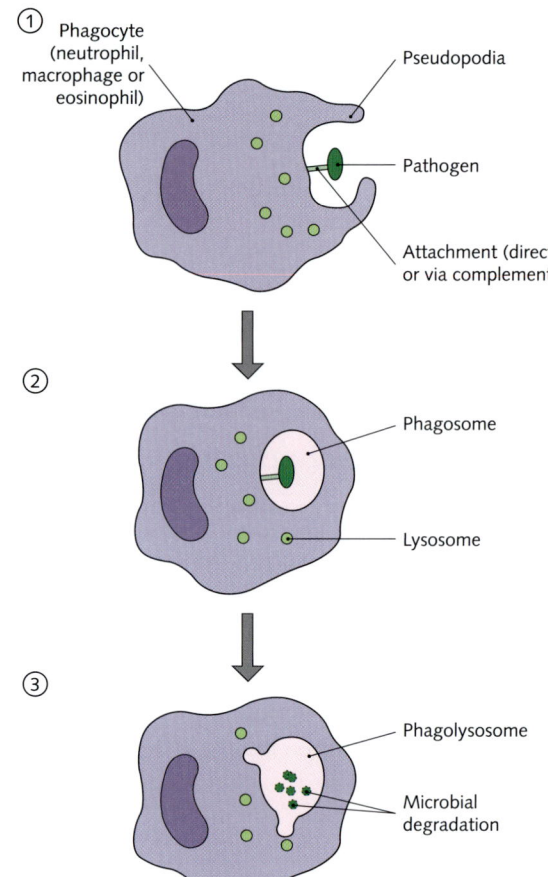

Fig. 9.1 Phagocytosis. Pseudopodia surround the pathogen. (1) They fuse around the organism, producing a vesicle known as a phagosome. (2) Lysosomes fuse with the phagosome to form phagolysosomes. (3) Proteins within the lysosome, and other granules that fuse with the phagolysosome, lead to degradation of the organism. The microbial products are then released.

CLINICAL NOTES

Neutropenic sepsis: Neutropenic individuals are at an increased risk of serious bacterial infections and sepsis. Neutropenic sepsis is often difficult to detect because of the decreased immune response to pathogens; any suspicion of infection should be investigated, and the patient treated accordingly. Treatment of neutropenic sepsis includes fluid resuscitation (in case of hypotension) and broad-spectrum antibiotics, along with antivirals or antifungals, depending on the suspected offending organism. Close monitoring of clinical parameters (blood pressure, oxygen saturation, heart rate and temperature), along with biochemical markers (such as C-reactive protein (CRP) and lactate) is essential for a favourable outcome.

Monocytes and macrophages

Monocytes and macrophages comprise the other major group of phagocytic cells. Monocytes account for 5% to 10% of the circulating white cell count and circulate in the blood for approximately 8 hours before migrating into the tissues, where they differentiate into macrophages; these macrophages can live for decades. Some macrophages become adapted for specific functions in particular tissues, for example Kupffer cells in the liver, glial cells in the brain and osteoclasts in bone.

In comparison to monocytes, macrophages:

- Are larger and longer lived
- Have greater phagocytic ability
- Have a larger repertoire of lytic enzymes and secretory products

Macrophages phagocytose and destroy their targets using similar mechanisms to neutrophils. The rate of phagocytosis can be greatly increased by opsonins, such as immunoglobulin (Ig) G and the complement protein C3b. Neutrophils and macrophages have receptors for these opsonins, which may be bound to the antigenic surface. Intracellular pathogens, for example *Mycobacterium,* can prove difficult for macrophages to kill. They are either resistant to destruction inside the phagosome or can evade by entering the macrophage cytoplasm. For the immune system to act against these pathogens, T-cell help is required (see Chapter 10).

In addition to phagocytosis, macrophages can secrete a number of compounds into the extracellular space, including cytokines (TNF, IL-8 and IL-1) and hydrolytic enzymes.

Macrophages express a wide array of surface molecules including:

- Receptors for complement and the Fc portion of IgG
- Pattern recognition molecules (PRMs)
- Cytokine receptors, for example, TNF-α and interferon-γ (IFN-γ)
- MHC and B7 molecules (to activate the adaptive immune response)

Macrophages can be activated by:

- Cytokines such as IFN-γ
- Contact with complement or products of blood coagulation
- Direct contact with the target through PRM stimulation

Following activation, macrophages become more efficient phagocytes and have increased secretory and microbicidal activity. They are also able to process and present antigen in association with class II major histocompatibility complex (MHC) molecules, stimulating the adaptive immune system (see Chapter 10).

In comparison to neutrophils, macrophages:

- Are longer-lived (they do not die after dealing with pathogens)
- Are larger (diameter 25–50 μm), enabling phagocytosis of larger targets
- Move and phagocytose more slowly
- Retain Golgi apparatus and rough endoplasmic reticulum and can therefore synthesize new proteins, including lysosomal enzymes and secretory products
- Can act as antigen-presenting cells (APCs)

Killing by phagocytes

The process of phagocytosis allows cells to engulf matter that needs to be destroyed. The cell can then digest the material in a controlled fashion before releasing the contents. The process of phagocytosis is shown in Fig. 9.1.

Natural killer cells

Natural killer cells develop from lymphoid progenitor cells, but unlike the other types of lymphocytes (T cells and B cells; see Chapter 10), their function mainly lies in the innate immune response. NK cells use cell-surface receptors to identify virally modified or cancerous cells. Similar to macrophages, NK cells do not require T-cell help to kill pathogens but function more effectively when T-helper cells secrete IFN-γ. One set of receptors activates NK cells, initiating killing; others inhibit the cells:

- Activating receptors include calcium-binding C-type lectins, which recognize certain cell-surface carbohydrates.
- Inhibitory receptors include killer-cell immunoglobulin-like receptors (KIRs). KIRs are members of the Ig gene superfamily (see Chapter 10) and recognize class I MHC molecules on other cells.

Because the C-type lectin receptors are activated by carbohydrates on normal host cells, the KIR system acts to prevent NK cells from attacking the host. Conversely, a cell that is not expressing class I MHC molecules will not activate the KIR system and so would be attacked by NK cells. This is useful in eliminating body cells that have downregulated class I MHC because of viral infection (e.g., herpes) or mutation; the lack of MHC I in these infected or mutated cells evades attack from T cells but this same MHC I deficiency causes NK cells to attack.

NK cells can also destroy antibody-coated target cells irrespective of the presence of MHC molecules, a process known as antibody-dependent cell-mediated cytotoxicity (ADCC). This occurs because killing is initiated by cross-linking of receptors for the Fc portion of IgG1 and IgG3.

NK cells are not clonally restricted, have no memory and are not very specific in their action. They induce apoptosis in target cells (Fig. 9.2) by:

- Ligation of Fas or TNF receptors on the target cells; NK cells produce TNF and exhibit Fas ligand (FasL). This initiates a sequence of caspase recruitment and activation, resulting in apoptosis.
- Degranulation by NK cells, which releases perforins and granzymes. Perforin molecules insert into and polymerize within the target cell membrane. This forms a pore through which granzymes can pass. Granzyme B then initiates apoptosis from within the target cell cytoplasm.

The induction of apoptosis is a crucial tool for the immune system. It can be used for targeted killing of infected or mutated cells and is also a key part of the development of the adaptive immune system (see Chapter 10).

HINTS AND TIPS

Fas receptors are found on human cells. Once they bind to the FasL, they stimulate apoptosis.

Degranulating cells

Mast cells and basophils (Chapter 1: Basophils)

Mast cells and basophils have similar functions but are found in different locations; basophils comprise <1% of circulating white cells, whereas mast cells are resident in the tissues.

High concentrations of mast cells are found close to blood vessels in connective tissue, skin and mucosal membranes. The two types of mast cells – mucosal and connective tissue – differ in their tissue distribution, protease content and secretory profiles.

Mast cells function by discharging their granule contents (such as histamine, serotonin, bradykinin, prostaglandins and

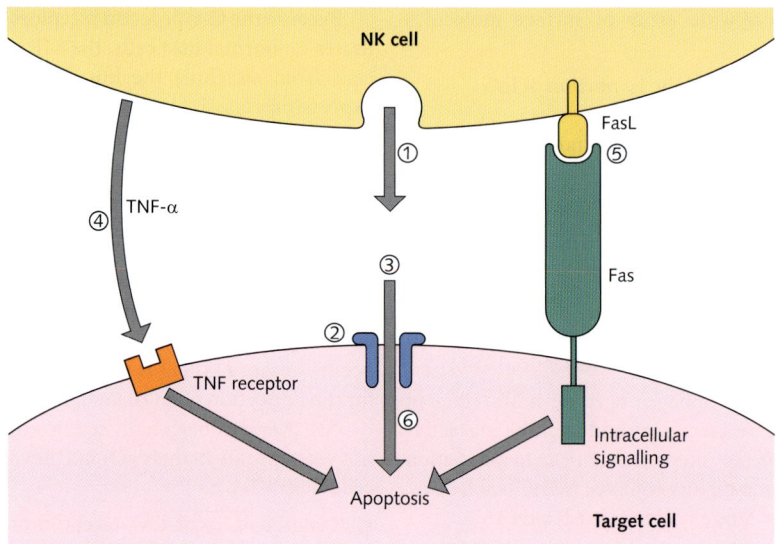

Fig. 9.2 Mechanism of killing by natural killer (NK) cells. Activation of NK cells in the absence of an inhibitory signal results in degranulation. (1) Perforins form a pore in the target cell, allowing entry of granzymes (2) (3). Tumour necrosis factor (TNF) produced by NK cells acts on the target cell's receptors (4). Fas ligand (FasL) interacts with target cell Fas (5). Intracellular signalling from Fas TNF receptors and granzymes results in apoptosis (6).

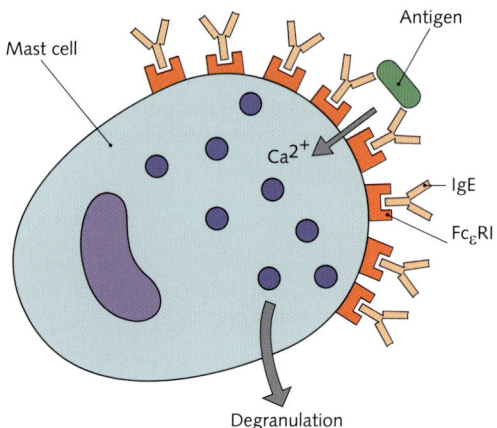

Fig. 9.3 Activation of mast cells by immunoglobulin E (IgE). IgE, produced by plasma cells, binds via its Fc domain to receptors on the mast cell surface. Cross-linking of these receptors by an antigen causes an influx of calcium ions (Ca^{2+}) into the cell. Calcium ions cause a rapid degranulation of inflammatory mediators from the mast cell. $Fc_{\varepsilon}RI$, High-affinity IgE receptor.

leucotrienes). Degranulation is triggered by cross-linking of high-affinity receptors for the Fc portion of IgE (Fig. 9.3). Cross-linkage results in an influx of calcium ions into the cell, which induces release of pharmacologically active mediators from granules. This mechanism allows mast cells to attack larger organisms living in lumens, such as tapeworms, which otherwise would evade immune attack. Mast cell activation releases leukotrienes, which attract eosinophils to the site of parasitic infection. This plays an important role in the development of an episode of a type I hypersensitivity, with the mast cells and basophils providing the early phase response and the eosinophils mediating the late phase response. This underlies the allergic response (see Chapter 12).

HINTS AND TIPS

During severe allergy (anaphylaxis, see Chapter 12: Anaphylaxis), mast cell tryptase levels increase for a few hours (median half-life 90 minutes). This is a useful diagnostic test for anaphylaxis. However, the immediate diagnosis of anaphylaxis is based on clinical symptoms and examination (breathlessness, chest tightness, face or tongue swelling, difficulty swallowing, anxiety, dizziness/loss of consciousness). Tryptase testing may be done after treating the allergic reaction (approximately 4–6 hours) in order to confirm the diagnosis (symptoms of anaphylaxis similar to other medical emergencies, such as acute myocardial ischaemia and exacerbation of asthma).

Eosinophils Chapter 1: Eosinophils

Eosinophils comprise 1% to 3% of circulating white cells and are found principally in tissues. They are derived from the colony-forming unit for granulocytes, erythrocytes, monocytes and megakaryocytes (CFU-GEMM) and their maturation is similar to that of the neutrophil (see Chapter 1). They are important in the defence against parasites and cause damage by extracellular degranulation. Their granules contain major basic protein, cationic protein, peroxidase and perforin-like molecules. Peroxidase generates hypochlorous acid, major basic protein damages the parasite's outer surface (as well as host tissues) and cationic protein acts as a neurotoxin, damaging the parasite's nervous tissue.

Dendritic cells

Dendritic cells constitute the major APCs, serving as an essential link between the innate and the adaptive immune system. As cells of the innate immune system, they are able to detect invading pathogens due to their expression of molecules sensing for pathogen-derived components (such as the Toll-like and NOD-like receptors). However, instead of destroying them directly (like phagocytes), they internalize and process pathogen-derived proteins yielding antigenic peptides, which are then loaded onto the MHC-class I or II molecules in order to be presented to naïve T cells. These cells are then activated and induced to become effector (cytotoxic) cells. DCs also express co-stimulatory molecules (such as CD80 and CD86), potentiating the T-cell responses and produce stimulatory cytokines (such as IL-12) that are required for T-cell activation. This way DCs communicate with the adaptive immune system, initiating a long-lasting, antigen-specific response.

Dendritic cells are also responsible for maintaining immune homeostasis under a steady state, by protecting against the T-cell recognition of self-antigens. This is mediated by the DC-induction of immunosuppressive T-regulatory cells (Tregs) that prevent the initiation of an immune response against self- or nonpathogenic environmental antigens.

SOLUBLE PROTEINS

The soluble proteins that contribute to innate immunity (Table 9.1) can be divided into antimicrobial serum agents and proteins produced by cells of the immune system.

Acute phase proteins

The acute phase response is a systemic reaction to inflammation, where macrophages and monocytes release cytokines IL-1, IL-6, IFN-γ and TNF. These cytokines alter the production of certain proteins, the acute phase proteins (APPs), by the liver. APPs are defined as proteins whose plasma concentration is altered (increased or decreased) by at least 25% during an inflammatory process. APPs with a positive impact include the CRP, ceruloplasmin, serum amyloid A, fibrinogen, α1-antitrypsin,

Table 9.1 The soluble proteins of innate immunity

	Protein	Notes
Secreted agents	Lysozyme	Bactericidal enzyme in mucus, saliva, tears, sweat and breast milk Cleaves peptidoglycan in the cell wall
Innate antimicrobial serum agents	Lactoferrin	Iron-binding protein that competes with microorganisms for iron, an essential metabolite
	Complement	Group of 20 proenzymes activation leads to an enzyme cascade, the products of which enhance phagocytosis and mediate cell lysis. Alternative pathway can be activated by nonspecific mechanism
	MBL	Activates the complement system
	C-reactive protein	Acute phase protein, produced by the liver Binds C-polysaccharide cell wall component of bacteria and fungi Activates complement via classical pathway Opsonizes for phagocytosis
Proteins produced by cells of the innate system	IFN-α	Produced by virally infected cells
	IFN-β	Induces a state of viral resistance in neighbouring cells by: Inducing genes that will destroy viral DNA Inducing MHC class I expression
	IFN-γ	Mainly produced by activated NK cells. Activates NK cells and macrophages

IFN-γ, interferon-γ; MBL, mannan-binding lectin; MHC, Major histocompatibility complex; NK, natural killer.

haptoglobin, hepcidin, ferritin, procalcitonin, complement components and others; those with a negative impact include albumin, transferrin and transthyretin.

Clinically, the APP levels are particularly useful, as they indicate the presence (and intensity) of an inflammatory process and can be used for the diagnosis and monitoring of disease activity or as prognostic markers. However, none of the APPs are specific, nor can they be used to distinguish between infection and other causes of inflammation. CRP and erythrocyte sedimentation rate (ESR) constitute the most widely used APPs. The change in plasma concentration of APPs is accompanied by fever, leucocytosis, thrombocytosis, catabolism of muscle proteins and fat deposits. Symptomatically, this change contributes to what is described as severe fatigue –'malaise'.

C-reactive protein

Levels of CRP rise within hours of tissue injury or infection. The actions of CRP are outlined in Table 9.1. CRP elevation can be slight (e.g., cerebrovascular accident), moderate (e.g., myocardial infarction) or marked (e.g., bacterial infections).

HINTS AND TIPS

Tumour necrosis factor-α, IFN-γ, IL-1 and IL-6 released by macrophages and monocytes stimulate the liver to produce the APPs.

Erythrocyte sedimentation rate

The ESR is an indirect measure of the acute phase response and is defined as the rate at which the red cells in blood fall when placed in a vertical tube. It is especially representative of the concentration of fibrinogen, although other constituents of the blood may influence its levels, such as the α-globulins. Elevated ESR is associated with acute and chronic infection, anaemia, pregnancy, renal disease, multiple myeloma and obesity, whereas decreased levels can be found in hypofibrinogenaemia, heart failure, cachexia, extreme leucocytosis and abnormalities of red cells (such as sickle cells, spherocytosis, acanthocytosis).

HINTS AND TIPS

In chronic inflammation, high CRP and ESR persist. The resulting catabolism of muscle and fat may lead to severe weight loss.

The acute phase response: The acute phase response provides us with chemical markers of inflammation that can be measured. In a child presenting with abdominal pain, a CRP level can aid the clinician in their diagnosis. A normal CRP can allow more conservative management, whereas a raised CRP would indicate an inflammatory response and necessitate urgent treatment, such as surgery in differentiating the abdominal pain of constipation from that of appendicitis. The ESR takes more time than CRP to become elevated – CRP rises within 2 hours of the insult and falls within a day after the insult resolves, making it a more sensitive and therefore preferable test (Fig. 9.4). The neutrophil count is often used to monitor inflammation; both neutrophil count and CRP level are simple, cheap and fast to measure.

For these reasons the neutrophil count and CRP are often used, in conjunction with clinical signs, to see if inflammation is taking place and when it has recovered. The white cell count and ESR are useful markers measured in chronic inflammatory diseases. Some hospitals now measure plasma viscosity instead of ESR. However, ESR levels are still crucial for the diagnosis and monitoring of rheumatologic conditions such as giant cell (temporal) arteritis and systemic lupus erythematosus.

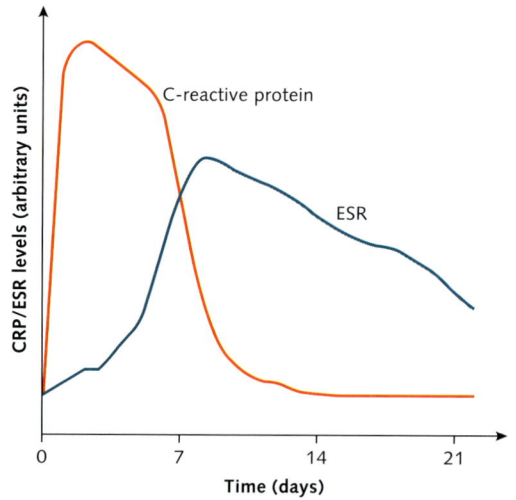

Fig. 9.4 Comparison of the change in C-reactive protein (CRP) levels and erythrocyte sedimentation rate (ESR) following an inflammatory stimulus.

The complement system

The complement system (so-called because its actions are complementary to the function of antibody) is, in fact, much older in evolutionary terms than antibody and is equally as important.

Complement is a collection of over 20 serum proteins, produced mainly by the liver, that are always at high levels in the blood of the healthy individual. The reason for the large number of proteins is to allow amplification; many of the components of complement are proenzymes that, when cleaved, activate more complement. This is similar to the amplification of clotting factors in the coagulation cascade seen in Chapter 6.

The primary goal of the complement is the rapid elimination of a pathogen, which is accomplished through deposition of C3b peptides on the target (opsonization). This promotes its phagocytosis by cells that bear complement receptors. Furthermore, opsonization stimulates the adaptive immune system through antigen presentation, leading to the generation of memory cells. Another goal of the complement is the expansion of the inflammatory response, through the generation of the peptides C3a and C5a, known as anaphylatoxins.

The three pathways that activate the complement system are the classical, the alternative and the lectin. All pathways result in the activation of the complement component C3 to C3 convertase, which leads to the engagement and activation of a common terminal pathway, called the 'membrane attack complex' (MAC). An overview of the complement system is given in Fig. 9.5. To simplify, the complement pathway is divided into three steps: attachment (initiation), activation and amplification (C3 convertase formation) and the formation of MAC.

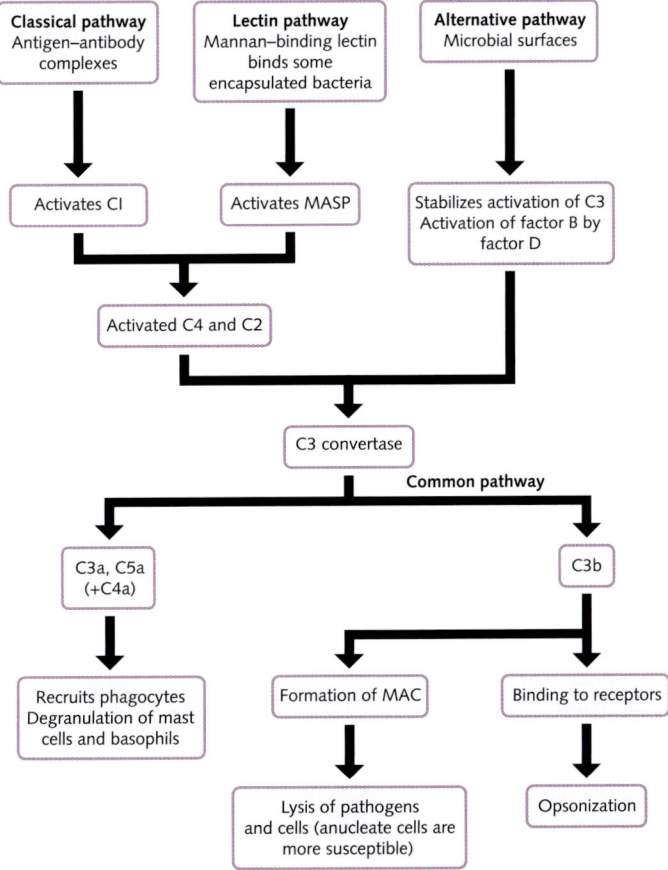

Fig. 9.5 Overview of the complement system. Cell lysis by complement is caused by formation of the membrane attack complex (MAC). This is formed when C5b, C6, C7, C8 and C9 bind together to form a 10-nm pore in the cell surface. *MASP*, MBL-associated serine protease.

The classical pathway

The classical pathway is triggered by the presence of antibodies on the surface of a pathogen.

IgM is particularly good at activating complement as it is a pentamer (has five Fc portions):

- Fc activates C1
- C1 activates C2 and C4
- C2 and C4 activate C3 (C3 convertase)

The alternative pathway

The alternative pathway does not require the presence of an antibody or prior contact with a pathogen to function. It can be triggered when autoactivated C3 ('C3 tickover') is amplified by the presence of a molecule embedded in the membrane of an invading pathogen or by the lack of a complement inhibitory protein. C3 is an unstable molecule and without inhibition, spontaneously breaks down to the very reactive C3b. C3b then binds factor B, which undergoes proteolytic cleavage by factor D, creating the fragments Ba and Bb. The latter binds to the alternative pathway C3 convertase (C3bBb), generating an amplification loop, which leads to a large deposition of C3b on the target.

The lectin pathway

The lectin pathway is activated by two PRMs, the ficolins and the collectins. The latter is comprised of the mannan-binding lectin (MBL), which is a normal component of serum, that binds to carbohydrates found on the cell wall of certain bacteria and fungi (e.g., *Salmonella, Neisseria, Candida albicans*). MBL also binds to MBL-associated serine proteases (MASP), which bear structural homology to the C1 complex. MASP then acts on C4 and C2 to generate the C3 convertase of the classical pathway.

C3 convertase

With the production of C3 convertase, all three pathways converge. C3 convertase has enzymatic effects against C3 and enables the production of large quantities of C3b, thus producing a major amplification step in the complement pathway.

Effectors of complement

C5 is now cleaved into C5a and C5b. C5b then triggers the activation of C6–C9. These form the MAC. The MAC attacks pathogens by inserting a hole in their cell membrane; the pathogen then dies via osmotic lysis. The MAC appears to be the only way the immune system has of killing one family of bacteria, the *Neisseria* (a family that includes meningococcus and gonococcus).

The cleaved fragments C3a and C5a are anaphylatoxins which are chemoattractants for other immune cells which follow the concentration gradient to the infection. Complement also opsonizes bacteria as macrophages have receptors for C3b.

These functions are summarized in Table 9.2.

Inhibitors of complement

As previously discussed, complement can activate spontaneously through the alternative pathway (so-called C3 tickover, which refers to the constant autoactivation of a small amount of C3). This offers a surveillance mechanism by constantly monitoring the environment for possible pathogens. Complement is regulated by inhibitory molecules which are necessary to prevent complement-mediated damage of healthy cells. There are nine complement inhibitors which act at various levels throughout the pathway:

- Membrane cofactor protein, complement receptor type 1, C4b-binding protein and factor H: these prevent assembly of C3 convertase
- Decay accelerating factor (CD55): this accelerates decay of C3 convertase
- C1 inhibitor: inhibits C1
- Factor I and membrane cofactor protein: cleave C3b and C4b
- CD59 (protectin): prevents the formation of the MAC

Table 9.2 Functions of complement	
Function	**Notes**
Cell lysis	Insertion of MAC causes lysis of gram-negative bacteria Nucleated cells are more resistant to lysis because they endocytose MAC
Inflammation	C3a, C4a, C5a cause degranulation of mast cells and basophils C3a and C5a are chemotactic for neutrophils
Opsonization	Phagocytes have C3b receptors, which means phagocytosis is enhanced when pathogens are coated in C3b
Solubilization and clearance of immune complexes	Complement prevents immune complex precipitation and solubilizes complexes that have already been precipitated. Complexes coated in C3b bind to CR1 on red blood cells. The complexes are then removed in the spleen

MAC, Membrane attack complex.

Deficiency in any one of these inhibitory components can result in disease:

- Hereditary angioedema: deficiency of C1 inhibitor leads to unbalanced, spontaneous activation of the early complement pathway, causing life-threatening swellings.
- Atypical haemolytic-uraemic syndrome: genetic deficiency in a complement inhibitor called Factor I leads to activation of the late complement cascade, leading to red cell destruction.
- Paroxysmal nocturnal haemoglobinuria (PNH): It is caused by a mutation in the *PIGA* gene that leads to a deficiency in the GPI-linked complement regulators (CD55 and CD59) on the membrane of haematopoietic cells, rendering them susceptible to complement-induced cell lysis. Intravascular haemolysis, increased tendency for thrombosis and bone marrow failure constitute the hallmark features of the disease.

Therapeutic complement inhibition

It is now evident that the complement system constitutes a key player in maintaining and regulating immune reactions. Its contribution to a variety of autoimmune and inflammatory diseases makes it a very attractive candidate for therapeutic intervention. The approval of the first complement inhibitor, eculizumab (an antibody against complement component C5), in 2007 was a major breakthrough in the field, which changed the outcome in PNH and other diseases.

To date, various therapeutic agents have been developed in an effort to inhibit the complement, such as:

- Inhibitory monoclonal antibodies: C5 inhibitors (eculizumab, ravulizumab, etc.)
- Small molecule inhibitory peptides: target C5 (nomacopan), Factor B (iptacopan) and Factor D (danicopan)
- Aptamers (single-stranded DNA or RNA molecules): siRNA for C5 inhibition (cemdisiran)
- Recombinant complement inhibitors

However, inhibition of the complement pathway comes with side effects, such as an increased risk of encapsulated bacteria (particularly *N. meningitidis*). For that reason, patients who are due to be started on such therapy are required to be appropriately vaccinated prior to treatment commencement.

A number of other complement inhibitors are currently under investigation in an effort to minimize the side effects (such as the breakthrough haemolysis in PNH) and offer a better quality of life (e.g., by using a subcutaneous instead of an intravenous formulation) to patients requiring such treatment.

INNATE IMMUNE SYSTEM PATTERN RECOGNITION MOLECULES

Pattern recognition molecules are required for the detection and elimination of pathogens. We have already come across the recognition molecules MBL and C1b in the complement system and

seen how they function to defend the body. These are found in solution in the serum and are classified as collectins, being composed of collagen-like and lectin portions. Lectins are any protein that binds sugar molecules, usually on the surface of bacteria; for example, MBL binds to the sugar mannose.

Nucleotide-binding and oligomerization domain (NOD) is a pattern recognition molecule found across the body, including in epithelial cells in the gut. It recognizes certain bacterial cell wall components and stimulates an immune response. The *NOD* gene is mutated in some individuals with Crohn disease.

Toll-like receptors (TLRs) are a family of about a dozen PRMs. When they bind their ligand, they send a signal to innate immune system cells which then secrete cytokines. They have a few important clinical roles. In sepsis, TLR-4 is stimulated by vast amounts of lipopolysaccharide found on bacterial cell walls. This causes release of large amounts of TNF from macrophages, which in turn activates nitrous oxide synthase causing a fall in blood pressure and organ perfusion.

Drugs designed to bind and stimulate TLRs are being used in situations where it is helpful to stimulate a more powerful immune response, for example, in some vaccines and cancer treatments.

CLINICAL NOTES

Sepsis: Sepsis is when the body's immune response to infection becomes dysregulated, putting the body at risk of organ failure and death. This can be caused by infection, most commonly bacterial but also viral. The role of overactivation of the innate immune system in sepsis has been detailed earlier, with the example of Toll-like receptor–4 receptor activation leading to a fall in blood pressure.

It is important to identify and treat sepsis as fast as possible; Fig. 9.6 shows a typical scenario in which a patient develops sepsis. Sepsis should be suspected in any patient that develops signs of systemic infection (tachycardia, tachypnoea, pyrexia, hypotension, decrease in blood oxygen saturation, decreased level of consciousness) and has a likely source of infection (urinary tract infection, respiratory tract infection, septic arthritis, meningitis, etc.). The 'Sepsis 6' describes the package of management that should be started immediately and aims to prevent organ failure and death:

1. Give high-flow oxygen
2. Take blood cultures and consider other source cultures
3. Give intravenous antibiotics
4. Give a fluid challenge (e.g., 500 mL 0.9% NaCl)
5. Measure serum lactate and other blood tests (full blood count, CRP, urea and electrolytes, blood gases)
6. Monitor urine output

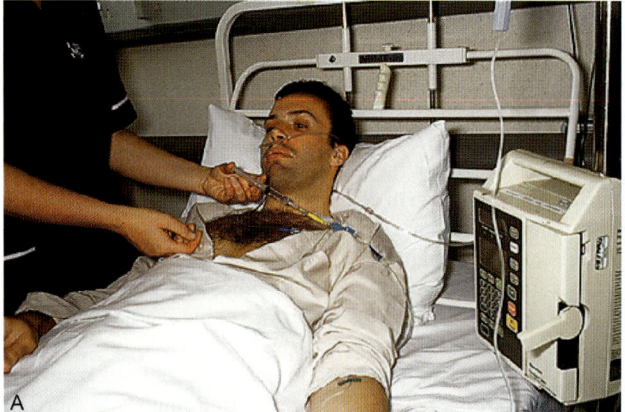
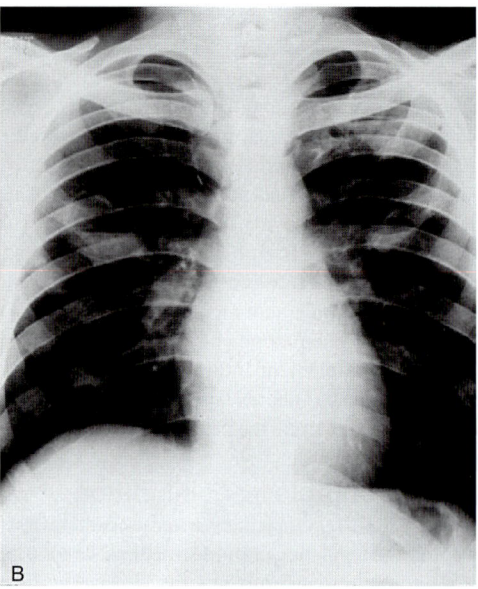

Fig. 9.6 (A and B) A 30-year-old patient is admitted with cerebral oedema following a road traffic collision. He is treated with high-dose corticosteroids, intubated, has a urinary catheter inserted and has multiple venous cannulas inserted. While recovering he develops a productive cough with a respiratory rate of 23 breaths per minute, has a temperature of 38.2°C, a systolic blood pressure of 96 mmHg and a pulse of 124 beats per minute. This patient has sepsis. Many factors in his initial treatment predispose him to this. A chest radiograph shows abscesses typical of Staphylococcal pneumonia, suggestive of a source of infection. The 'Sepsis 6' should be started immediately and a senior review sought. (From Helbert M. *Immunology for Medical Students*. 3rd ed. Philadelphia, PA: Elsevier; 2016).

● Chapter Summary

- The innate immune system provides a broad defence against pathogens. It is made up of barriers to infection, cellular defences and soluble proteins.
- Barriers to infection can be physical, for example, skin, chemical (e.g., stomach acidity) or biological (e.g., gut flora).
- Cells of the innate immune system are phagocytes (e.g., macrophages, neutrophils), NK cells and degranulating cells (e.g., mast cells, eosinophils). Phagocytes generally target extracellular pathogens, NK cells kill virally infected or cancerous host cells, and degranulating cells generally target multicellular pathogens (e.g., worms).
- APPs and the complement system make up the soluble protein fraction of the innate immune system.
  - APPs are produced in response to infection and contribute to the innate immune defence in many ways. They are often measured to aid in diagnosing infection (e.g., CRP).
  - Complement proteins directly attack pathogens and alert the immune system to their presence. The complement system is activated via multiple pathways, either by bacterial cell wall components or antibody bound to pathogens.
- PRMs enable the innate immune system to detect pathogens. Overstimulation of PRMs by large amounts of pathogen contributes to the symptoms of sepsis.

MLA Conditions   **MLA Presentations**
Sepsis

References

1. Hou K, Wu ZX, Chen XY, et al. Microbiota in health and diseases. *Signal Transduct Target Ther*. 2022;7(1):135. doi:10.1038/s41392-022-00974-4.
2. Weiss GA, Hennet T. Mechanisms and consequences of intestinal dysbiosis. *Cell Mol Life Sci*. 2017;74(16):2959–2977. doi:10.1007/s00018-017-2509-x.
3. Lam S, Bai X, Shkoporov AN, et al. Roles of the gut virome and mycobiome in faecal microbiota transplantation. *Lancet Gastroenterol Hepatol*. 2022;7(5):472–484. doi:10.1016/S2468-1253(21)00303-4.
4. Khoruts A, Sadowsky MJ. Understanding the mechanisms of faecal microbiota transplantation. *Nat Rev Gastroenterol Hepatol*. 2016;13(9):508–516. doi:10.1038/nrgastro.2016.98.

The adaptive immune system | 10

The adaptive immune system provides long-lasting immunity, specific to each pathogen that it encounters. Its primary function involves the destruction of invading pathogens and the respective molecules they produce. For that reason, it is crucial to be able to recognize between foreign and self molecules – a feature that is the cornerstone of the adaptive immune system. If this function fails, then the adaptive immune system would recognize, attack and destroy the host's own molecules, leading to autoimmunity. In the same lines, it would be futile to recognize and kill every single foreign molecule, as many of them are harmless. This is prevented by the innate immune system, which activates and recruits the adaptive immune system, only when specific types of molecules found on pathogens (but not on the host), called 'pathogen-associated immunostimulants', are encountered. The inappropriate response to harmless foreign molecules leads to allergic conditions, such as asthma.

Adaptive immune responses are divided into antibody- and cell-mediated immune responses. The antibody responses involve the release of specific immunoglobulins, called antibodies, produced by activated B cells. The cell-mediated immune responses are carried out by T cells, which are activated upon antigen recognition, presented by antigen-presenting cells (APCs).

THE IMMUNOGLOBULIN DOMAIN

Pathogen recognition is central to the functioning of the adaptive immune system. It is largely mediated by a family of proteins that contain very similar amino acid sequences – the immunoglobulin domain. This domain is approximately 110 amino acids in length; the polypeptide chain in each domain is folded into seven or eight antiparallel beta strands. These strands are arranged to form two opposing sheets, linked by a disulphide bond and hydrophobic interactions.

The group of molecules that contain the immunoglobulin domain are referred to as the immunoglobulin superfamily. All molecules in the immunoglobulin superfamily extend from the surface of cells or are secreted from cells.

Members of the immunoglobulin superfamily include:

- B-cell receptors (BCRs) (Fig. 10.1A)
- T-cell receptors (TCR; Fig. 10.2A)
- Major histocompatibility complex (MHC) molecules (Fig. 10.3)
- T-cell accessory molecules such as CD4 (Fig. 10.2B)
- Immunoglobulin (Fig. 10.1B)
- Certain adhesion molecules, for example, ICAM-1, ICAM-2 and VCAM-1

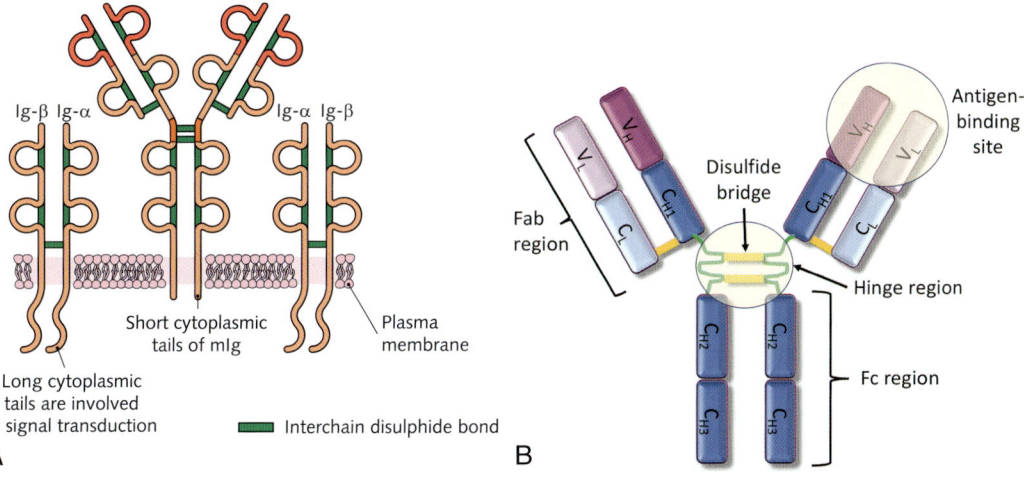

Fig. 10.1 (A) Structure of the B-cell surface receptor. Membrane-bound immunoglobulin (mIg) is nonsignalling. It associates with two Ig-α/Ig-β heterodimers (members of the immunoglobulin gene superfamily), which have long cytoplasmic domains capable of transducing a signal. (B) Structure of IgG. Immunoglobulins are composed from two identical light chains and two identical heavy chains. The chains are divided into domains, each of which is an immunoglobulin fold. The variable domains form the antigen-binding site. Digestion of the immunoglobulin molecule with papain produces an Fc portion (which binds complement) and two Fab portions (which bind antigen). (B, Cann's Principles of Molecular Virology, Seventh Edition, 2024.)

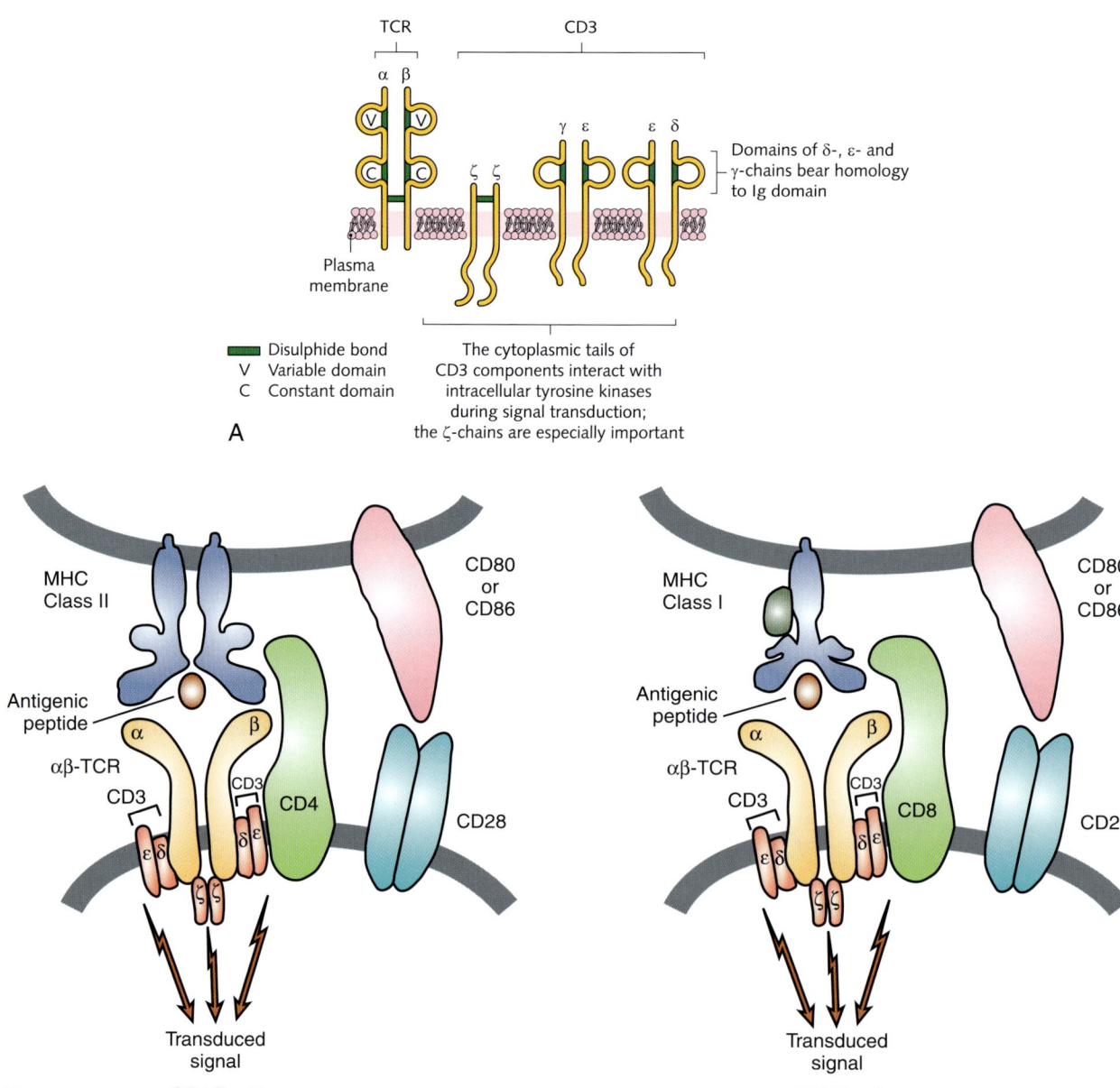

Fig. 10.2 (A) Structure of the T-cell surface antigen receptor. Negative charges on the transmembrane portion of CD3 components interact with positive charges on the T-cell receptor (TCR). This maintains the complex. Antigen is detected by the TCR, but the signal is transduced by CD3. (B) The role of CD4 and CD8 in T-cell receptor–major histocompatibility complex (TCR–MHC) antigen interaction. CD4 or CD8 is closely associated with the TCR complex. They bind MHC in a restricted fashion (CD8 to class I only, CD4 to class II only). Binding is antigen-independent and strengthens the bond between TCR and a complementary peptide–MHC complex. Molecules associated with CD4 or CD8 are then able to transduce a signal. (B, Remington and Klein's Infectious Diseases of the Fetus and Newborn Infant, Ninth Edition, 2025).

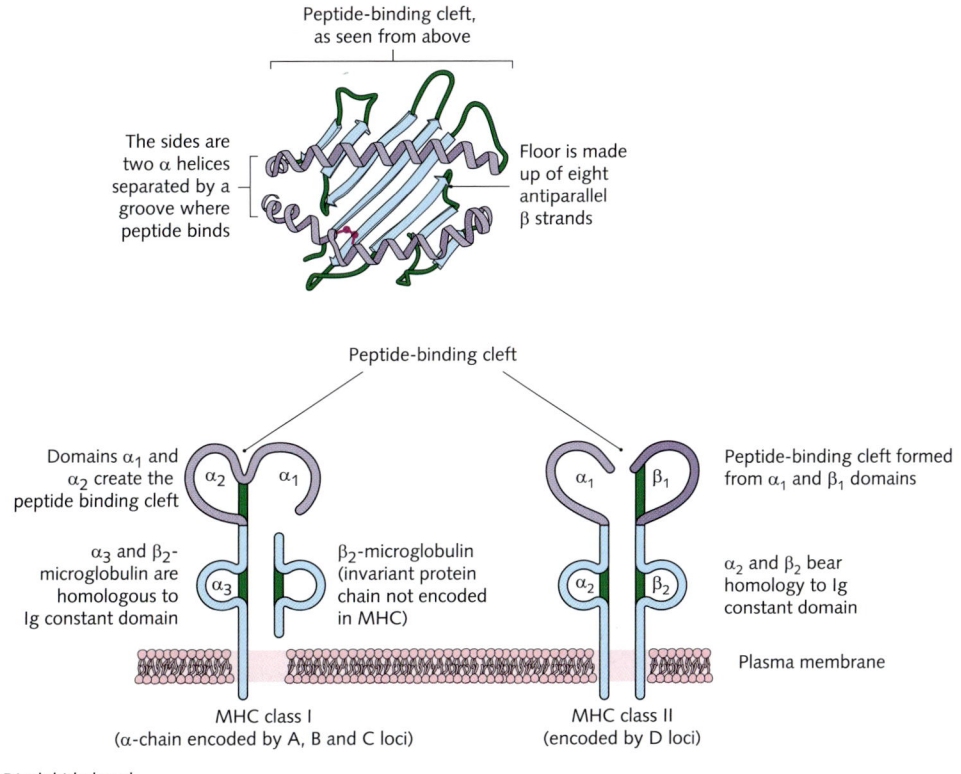

 Disulphide bond

Fig. 10.3 Structure of major histocompatibility complex (MHC) class I and class II molecules. The peptide-binding cleft of a class I molecule is also shown as seen from above.

Structure of B- and T-cell surface antigen receptors

Structure of BCRs

HINTS AND TIPS

The epitope is the part of antigen to which immunoglobulin superfamily molecules, such as immunoglobulin and B-cell surface receptors, bind.

The B-cell surface receptor consists of a membrane-bound immunoglobulin (mIg) molecule associated with two Ig-α/Ig-β heterodimers (also members of the immunoglobulin superfamily). mIg recognizes the conformational structure (shape) of antigenic epitopes while the Ig-α/Ig-β heterodimers are thought to mediate signal transduction (Fig. 10.1A). The role of B cells in adaptive immunity is covered in the section on humoral immunity later in this chapter.

Structure of T-cell surface receptors

Antigen recognition by T cells differs from antigen recognition by B cells. T cells require the antigen to have been processed and presented to them, as opposed to B cells which simply recognize free-floating antigenic epitopes. This processing and presentation of antigen is carried out by APCs, for example macrophages, and involves the MHC, which will be described later.

The T-cell surface antigen receptor is made up of two parts: the TCR and CD3. Both the TCR and CD3 are members of the immunoglobulin superfamily. The TCR recognizes and binds antigen, while CD3 is involved in signal transduction. Therefore, CD3 is functionally analogous to the Ig-α/Ig-β heterodimer in B cells.

The TCR is a heterodimer, comprising α- and β-chains. It is structurally similar to the immunoglobulin Fab region (see the section on Humoral immunity). Each of the α- and β-chains is made up of two immunoglobulin domains, one variable and one constant, linked by a disulphide bond. As in the variable domains of immunoglobulin, three variable regions on each chain combine to form the antigen-binding site.

CD3 is made up of three polypeptide dimers, consisting of four or five different peptide chains. The dimers are γε, δε and ζζ (found in 90% of CD3 molecules) or ζη (Fig. 10.2A).

The major histocompatibility complex

Major histocompatibility complex is a generic term for a group of molecules produced by higher vertebrate species. The MHC molecule functions as a 'window' to the inside of cells; it is the platform on which antigens are presented to the immune system. Human leucocyte antigen (HLA) is the term used to describe human MHC.

COMMON PITFALLS

All nucleated cells express some form of MHC. This enables any infected cell to present antigens from intracellular pathogens to the immune system.

The MHC genes

Major histocompatibility complex genes exhibit considerable diversity; there are more than 100 identified alleles for HLA-B. This means that most individuals will be heterozygous at most MHC gene loci. Therefore, any two randomly selected individuals are very unlikely to have identical HLA alleles. Diversity of the MHC increases the chance that a person will be able to mount an adaptive response against a pathogen. The MHC genetic loci are tightly linked, so that one set is inherited from each parent. A complete set of MHC alleles inherited from one parent is referred to as a haplotype and is found on the short arm of chromosome 6.

The MHC genes are divided into three regions, each region encoding one of the three classes of the MHC: class I, class II and class III. HLA class I and II are further subdivided into three subtypes, namely HLA-A, -B and -C and HLA-DR, -DP and DQ, respectively, which are highly polymorphic. Certain haplotypes have been associated with specific diseases (Table 10.1).

Class I molecules are expressed on the cell surface of all nucleated cells and present peptides from intracellular antigens to CD8+ cytotoxic T cells. Class II molecules are found primarily in APCs (such as monocytes) and present antigenic peptides, generated in the endosomal-lysosomal compartment, to CD4+ T cells.

The MHC alleles exhibit codominance, which means that both alleles are expressed. The HLA haplotype is the main identified genetic factor in autoimmune disease (for more details, see Chapter 12: Role of HLA).

CLINICAL NOTES

Major histocompatibility complex molecules are the main antigens recognized as nonself when graft tissue is used (e.g., in kidney and stem cell transplants), hence the name 'MHC'. To minimize transplant rejection, donors are used whose MHC genes (or HLA types) are similar to those of the patient (see Chapter 13). This illustrates the role of MHC in self versus nonself recognition.

Structure of the MHC

Major histocompatibility complex class I and class II molecules have very similar structures, consisting of cytoplasmic, transmembrane and extracellular portions (Fig. 10.3). MHC class I and class II are both members of the immunoglobulin superfamily, and their primary role is the presentation of peptides to T cells. MHC class III molecules have other roles unrelated to immune function and antigen presentation and are not covered here.

Class I MHC molecules consist of a transmembrane chain, which is folded into three extracellular domains (a1, a2, a3) and an extracellular β2-microglobulin (β2M). MHC class II molecules are heterodimers, consisting of an a and β transmembrane chain. In the class I molecules, the domains a1 and b2M form the antigen-presenting groove, whereas in the class II molecules, this is made up from the a1 and β1 domains. Interestingly, the class I groove is closed, whereas the class II groove is open, allowing for a prolonged lodge of the peptide (longer than the groove itself). These regions are highly polymorphic (hypervariable regions), allowing for a massive variety of peptides to be presented by the HLA groove, in contrast to the rest of the molecule (a3 and B2M in class I and a2 and β2 in class II) which are highly conserved regions.

Table 10.1 HLA subtype association with disease

Disease association with HLA subtypes			
HLA class I	**Disease**	**HLA class II**	**Disease**
HLA-A3	Haemochromatosis	HLA-DQ2/DQ8	
HLA-B8	Myasthenia gravis Graves disease Addison disease	HLA-DR1	Myasthenia gravis Rheumatoid arthritis Schizophrenia
HLA-B16	Multiple sclerosis	HLA-DR2	Multiple sclerosis Systemic lupus erythematosus Goodpasture syndrome Hay fever
HLA-B18	Type I diabetes mellitus	HLA-DR3	Addison Disease Myasthenia gravis Systemic lupus erythematosus Graves disease Rheumatoid arthritis Alopecia areata Antiphospholipid syndrome
HLA-B27	Ankylosing spondylitis Psoriatic arthritis Inflammatory bowel disease Reactive arthritis	HLA-DR4	Rheumatoid arthritis Type I diabetes mellitus
		HLA-DR5	Hashimoto thyroiditis Type I diabetes mellitus Pernicious anaemia Rheumatoid arthritis Antiphospholipid syndrome Alopecia areata
		HLA-DR7	Steroid-responsive nephrotic syndrome

HLA, Human leucocyte antigen

MHC restriction

T cells are only able to recognize antigen in the context of self-MHC molecules (self-MHC restriction), as opposed to B cells, which recognize free antigen. CD8$^+$ T cells recognize antigen only in association with MHC class I molecules (MHC class I restricted). CD4$^+$ cells recognize antigen only in association with MHC class II molecules (MHC class II restricted).

MHC function: antigen processing and presentation

Major histocompatibility complex molecules do not present whole antigen; the antigen is degraded into peptide fragments before binding can occur. There are different pathways of antigen processing for MHC class I and class II (summarized in Fig. 10.4). MHC class I molecules present endogenous antigens, such as those found in cells infected by viruses or intracellular bacteria. Thus CD8$^+$ T cells recognize virally altered cells and destroy them (see Chapter 11).

Major histocompatibility complex class II molecules present exogenous antigen that may have been phagocytosed or endocytosed into intracellular vesicles. Professional APCs process and present antigen to CD4$^+$ T cells in association with MHC class II molecules. These cells express high levels of MHC class II molecules. Professional APCs include:

- Dendritic cells, including Langerhans' cells
- Macrophages
- B cells

The differences between MHC class I and class II molecules are summarized in Table 10.2.

Function of CD4 and CD8

Adaptive immunity relies on the TCR binding of an antigenic peptide bound on an HLA molecule of an APC. However, this is not sufficient to trigger T-cell activation, which requires the participation of the transmembrane glycoproteins, CD4 and CD8. CD4 is expressed on T helper 1 (Th1), T helper 2 (Th2), T

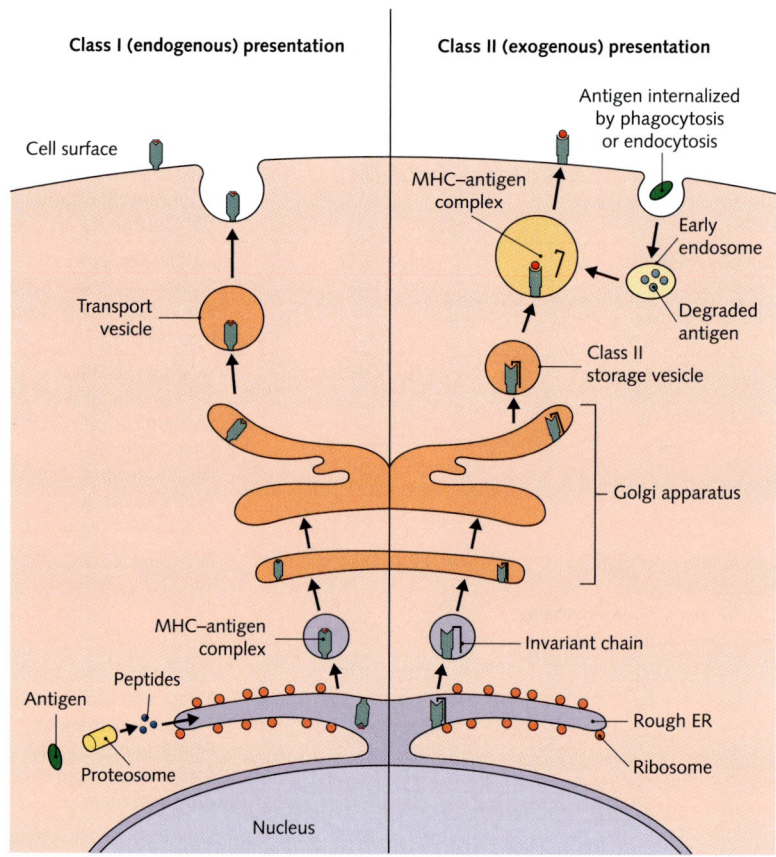

Class I (endogenous) presentation

Class II (exogenous) presentation

Cell surface

Antigen internalized
by phagocytosis
or endocytosis

MHC–antigen
complex

Early
endosome

Transport
vesicle

Degraded
antigen

Class II
storage vesicle

Golgi apparatus

MHC–antigen
complex

Invariant chain

Peptides

Antigen

Rough ER

Proteosome

Ribosome

Nucleus

Fig. 10.4 Routes of antigen processing. Class I molecules present endogenous antigens. Cytosolic antigen is degraded by proteosomes and transported into the rough endoplasmic reticulum (ER), where peptides are loaded onto major histocompatibility complex (MHC) class I molecules. The MHC–peptide complex is transported via the Golgi apparatus to the cell surface. Class II molecules present exogenous antigens that have been phago- or endocytosed into intracellular vesicles. The MHC molecule is transported from the rough ER to the vesicle by the invariant chain (Ii). It is displaced from the MHC molecule by processed antigen, which is then presented at the cell surface.

Table 10.2 Differences between major histocompatibility complex class I and class II molecules

	Class I	Class II
Size of bound peptide	8–9 amino acids	13–18 amino acids (binding cleft more open)
Peptide from	Cytosolic antigen	Intravesicular or extracellular antigen
Expressed by	All nucleated cells, especially T cells, B cells, macrophages, other APCs, neutrophils	B cells, macrophages, other APCs, epithelial cells of the thymus, activated T cells
Recognized by	CD8+ T cells	CD4+ T cells

APCs, Antigen-presenting cells.

helper 17 (Th17) and T-regulatory (Tregs) cells, whereas CD8 is expressed on cytotoxic T lymphocytes (CTLs) and CD8 Tregs.

CD4 and CD8 binding to MHC class I and II molecules, respectively, enhances T-cell responses due to the following effects:

(i) They help to stabilize the weak TCR-MHC interaction and
(ii) They promote and aggregate downstream T-cell signalling, regulating the T-cell activation, proliferation and differentiation.

This interaction also reduces the number of antigenic peptides required for T-cell stimulation and increases the cytokine production by helper T cells.

The role of CD4 and CD8 in antigen–receptor binding is shown in Fig. 10.2B.

COMMON PITFALLS

CD3 is the signal transducer for the T-cell receptor and is found on all T cells.

GENERATION OF ANTIGEN RECEPTOR DIVERSITY

The immune system may encounter approximately 20^8 possible antigens, each requiring a corresponding receptor if host defence is to be effective. The human genome contains only 30,000 genes and so a 'one gene per antigen receptor' code is simply not possible. Instead, this diversity is achieved by genetic recombination, a process in which segments of information are cut and pasted from genes. This enables each gene to produce many different receptors.

TCR and immunoglobulin (i.e., antibodies and mIg) are the only genes to undergo genetic recombination.

HINTS AND TIPS

Rearrangement of gene segments allows antibodies with an immense variety of specificity to be produced from a relatively small amount of DNA.

Genetic rearrangements

Before genetic recombination occurs, the gene segments are in 'germline configuration'. Rearrangement only occurs in the variable domain, which codes for the antigen-binding site of the receptor; the remaining structure must remain constant for the receptor to function. Each variable domain is encoded by a random combination of one of each of the V, D and J exons (nucleic acid sequences). The C exons encode the constant regions.

Following rearrangement, the clonal progeny of each B-cell will produce immunoglobulin of a single specificity. Rearrangement is completed and functional immunoglobulin chains are produced before the B-cell encounters antigen (Fig. 10.5).

The presence of multiple V, D and J gene segments (and the apparently random selection of these segments) generates considerable diversity, which can be calculated (Table 10.3).

A similar process occurs in T cells: α- and γ-chain variable domains have V and J segments; β- and δ-chains have V, D and J segments.

Junctional diversity

The formation of junctions between the various gene segments produces an opportunity for increased diversity, where nucleotides are added or subtracted at random to form the joining segments.

Junctional flexibility and N-nucleotide addition

When exons are spliced, there are slight variations in the position of segmental joining. In addition, up to 15 nucleotides can be added to the D–J and the V–DJ joints. This occurs only in heavy chains and is catalyzed by terminal deoxynucleotidyl transferase (TdT).

Both junctional flexibility and N-nucleotide addition can disrupt the reading frame, leading to nonfunctional rearrangements. However, formation of productive rearrangements increases antibody diversity. The V–J, V–DJ and VD–J joints fall within the antigen-binding region of the variable domain. Therefore, diversity generated at these joints will impact on the antigen specificity of the Ig molecule.

Somatic hypermutation

Somatic hypermutation is a process that increases the affinity of an antibody for its antigen and is also called affinity maturation. This occurs after the immune system is exposed to an antigen. B cells that are dividing by mitosis to increase in number in order to combat infection are allowed to undergo mutation in their variable domain (the only cells in the body permitted to do so). Some mutations decrease the antibody's specificity for the antigen and apoptosis is stimulated in these cells. Other mutations result in antibodies with increased specificity; these B cells are allowed to survive (the mutation is positively selected for). Antibodies produced later in the primary and secondary immune response will therefore have an increased affinity for antigen.

The TCR does not exhibit somatic hypermutation. Diversity is generated only in developing T cells, which undergo apoptosis if they are either self-reactive or nonfunctional.

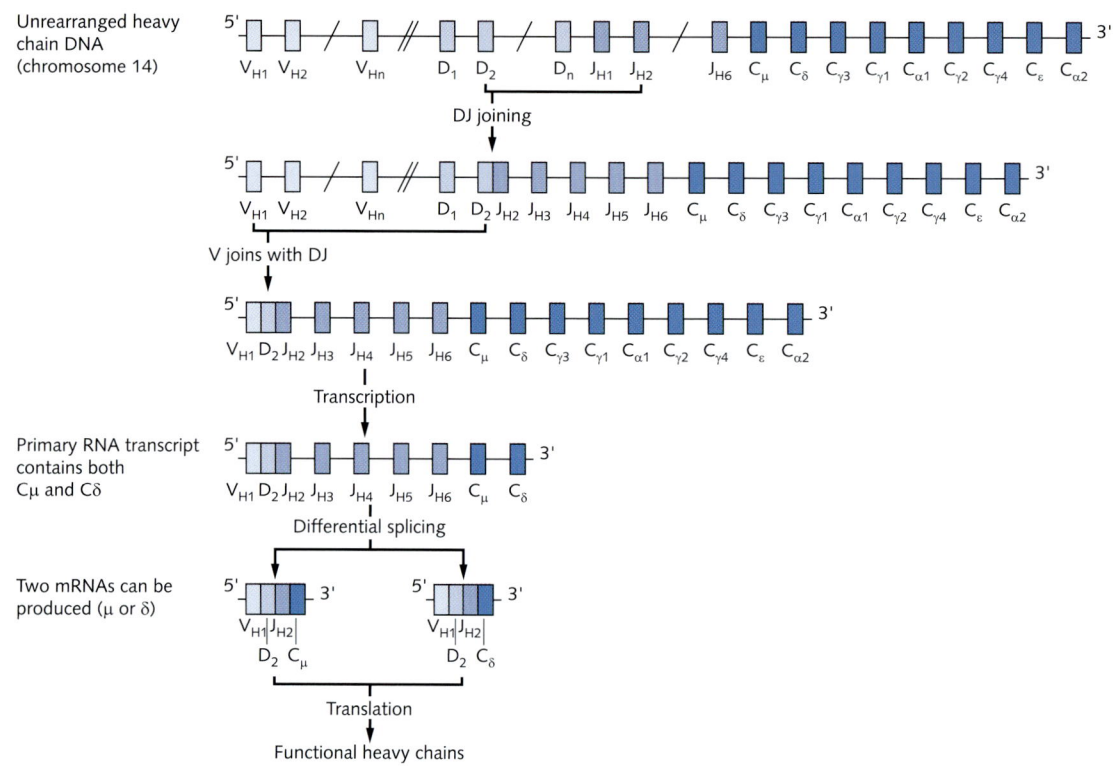

Fig. 10.5 Genetic rearrangement of immunoglobulin genes. Rearrangement of the heavy chain is similar to that of the light chain, although the join between D and J segments occurs first. In an unstimulated B-cell, the heavy-chain mRNA that is transcribed contains both the Cμ and Cδ segments. The mRNA can be differentially spliced such that both IgM and IgD will be produced. They will both exhibit the same antigen-binding specificity.

Table 10.3 Calculation of antibody diversity

Mechanism of diversity	Number of combinations		
	Light chain	Light chain	Heavy chain
Random joining of gene segments	100 × 5 = 500	100 × 6 = 600	75 × 30 × 6 = 13,500
Random chain associations	(500 + 600) × 13,500 = 1.5 × 10^7		

Given that a light chain can associate with any heavy chain and considering the number of gene segments present in germline DNA, it is possible to calculate the number of different molecules that can be produced. The extent of the contribution of junctional flexibility, *N*-nucleotide addition and somatic hypermutation is not known but will be significant.

Class switching

This is the process whereby a single B-cell can produce different classes of immunoglobulin that have the same specificity. The mechanism is not well understood but involves 'switch sites', that is, DNA sequences located upstream from each heavy chain C gene segment. Possible mechanisms include:

- Differential splicing of the primary transcript (Fig. 10.5)

- A looping out and deletion of intervening heavy chain C gene segments (and introns)
- Exchange of C gene segments between chromosomes

This process underlies the class switch from IgM in the primary response to IgG, IgA or IgE in the secondary response. Cytokines are important in controlling the switch.

Recognition molecules and their diversity are crucial for the generation of a specific, adaptive immune response. The adaptive immune response can be humoral or cell mediated.

HUMORAL IMMUNITY

B cells and antibody production

The humoral immune response is brought about by antibodies, which are particularly efficient at eliminating extracellular pathogens. Antigen and therefore pathogens can be cleared from the host by a variety of effector mechanisms, which are dependent on antibody class or isotype (see Tables 10.4 and 10.5):

- Activation of complement, leading to lysis or opsonization of the microorganism
- Antibody-dependent cell-mediated cytotoxicity (ADCC)
- Neutralization of bacterial toxins and viruses
- Mucosal immunity (IgA-mediated)
- Degranulation of mast cells (IgE and IgG mediated)

COMMON PITFALLS

Activated and differentiated B cells are known as plasma cells. It is these plasma cells that produce antibodies.

Abnormal plasma cells are involved in the pathogenesis of multiple myeloma (MM). More specifically, there is increased proliferation of monoclonal plasma cells in the bone marrow (>10% bone marrow cells), resulting in the overproduction of an abnormal protein (called 'paraprotein' or 'M protein') and impaired production of normal immunoglobulins (immunoparesis), leading to recurrent infections. This results in bone destruction, with the characteristic lytic bone lesions, hypercalcaemia, anaemia and renal impairment, giving rise to the diagnostic CRAB criteria (see Chapter 5).

Table 10.4 Properties of the immunoglobulin classes

	IgG	IgA	IgM	IgE
Physical properties				
Molecular weight (kDa)	150	300	900	190
Serum concentration (mg/mL)	13.5	3.5	1.5	0.0003
Number of subunits	1	2	5	1
Heavy chain	γ	α	μ	ε
Biological activities				
Present in secretions	✗	✓	✓	✗
Crosses placenta	✓	✗	✗	✗
Complement fixation	✓	✓	✓✓✓	✗
Binds phagocytic receptors	✓	✗	✓	✗
Binds mast cell receptors	✓	✗	✗	✓
Other features				
Main role	Main circulatory Ig for secondary immune response	Major Ig in secretions	Main Ig in primary immune response	Allergy and antiparasitic response

Ig, Immunoglobulin; IgG, Immunoglobulin G; IgA, Immunoglobulin A.

Table 10.5 Summary of the functions of immunoglobulins

Function	Notes
Opsonization	Phagocytic cells have antibody (Fc) receptors, thus antibodies can facilitate phagocytosis of antigens
Agglutination	Antigens and antibodies (IgG or IgM) clump together because immunoglobulin can bind more than one epitope simultaneously. IgM is more efficient because it has a high valency (10 antigen-binding sites)
Neutralization	Binding to pathogens or their toxins prevents their attachment to cells
Antibody-dependent cell-mediated cytotoxicity (ADCC)	The antibody–antigen complex can bind to cytotoxic cells (e.g., cytotoxic T cells, NK cells) via the Fc component of the antibody, thus targeting the antigen for destruction
Complement activation	IgG and IgM can activate the classical pathway; IgA can activate the alternative pathway
Mast cell degranulation	Cross-linkage of IgE bound to mast cells and basophils results in degranulation
Protection of the neonate	Transplacental passage of IgG and the secretion of sIgA in breast milk protect the newborn

IgA, Immunoglobulin A; IgG, Immunoglobulin G; NK, natural killer; sIgA, Secretory immunoglobulin A.

B cells are activated by antigen in a T-cell–independent or dependent fashion. T helper (Th) cells are primed by APCs, which present antigen to Th cells in conjunction with MHC class II molecules. B cells are stimulated by antigen interacting with BCRs. Primed Th cells interact with B cells that also express antigen–MHC complexes. This interaction induces a sequence of surface receptor binding and cytokine production that results in B-cell activation, proliferation and differentiation. An overview of B-cell activation is given in Fig. 10.6.

HINTS AND TIPS

Primary lymphoid organs (the thymus and bone marrow) are where lymphocytes are created and undergo early development. Secondary lymphoid organs (the spleen and lymph nodes) maintain lymphocytes and are involved in initiating an immune response.

B cells are activated within follicles found in secondary lymphoid structures only if they encounter specific antigen, namely foreign antigen. During proliferation, variable regions of the immunoglobulin genes within B cells undergo somatic hypermutation. Follicular dendritic cells present antigen, to which the B cells with the highest affinity will bind. This causes the expression of bcl-2, which prevents B cells from undergoing apoptosis. Therefore, the highest-affinity B-cell clones are positively selected. B cells require help from T cells to produce antibodies. Activated Th cells provide the help needed by producing cytokines (IL-2, IL-4, IL-5 and IL-6). This acts as a further method of regulation within the immune system, as both B cells and T cells need exposure to the offending antigen in order for a response to be evoked.

The clonal selection of B cells that respond only to foreign antigen is an example of tolerance. This means that B cells that react to autoantigen (and therefore would attack body tissues) are destroyed by apoptosis, that is, B cells 'tolerate' autoantigen. This is explored more in the section on tolerance later in this chapter.

Structure and function of antibody

An antibody is identical to the BCR of the cell it originated from, with the only difference of a hydrophilic C-terminus, allowing its secretion, in contrast to the hydrophobic C-terminus of the BCR.

Antibodies are Y-shaped molecules, composed of two identical heavy and two identical light chains, linked by disulphide bridges. The light chains consist of one variable and one constant domain, while the heavy chain contains one variable and three constant domains. The variable regions (V) are involved in antigen binding and vary between different antibody molecules, whereas the constant regions (C) interact with the effector cells and are less variable. Depending on the C-regions, five different classes of immunoglobulins can be identified: IgM, IgG, IgA, IgE and IgD (Table 10.4).

Digestion of an immunoglobulin molecule (using IgG as an example) with papain (papaya proteinase 1, an enzyme derived from papayas) produces two types of fragment:

(i) Two Fab fragments consisting of the light chain and two domains of the heavy chain (denoted VH and CH1). These fragments bind antigen.

(ii) One Fc fragment consisting of the remainder of the heavy chain (CH2 and CH3), which interacts with the effector cells. This fragment binds complement.

The structure of IgG is shown in Fig. 10.1A.

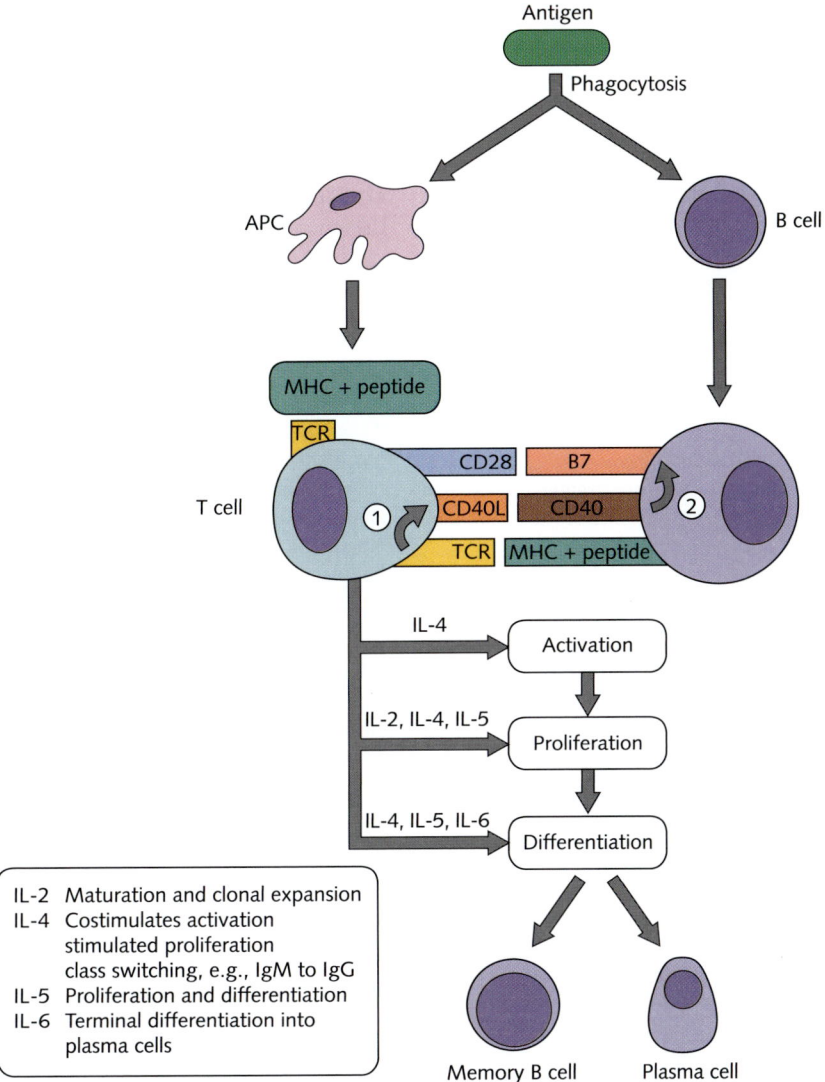

Fig. 10.6 Overview of the humoral immune response. Activated and differentiated B cells, known as plasma cells, produce antibody. B cells are activated by antigen in a T-cell–independent or dependent fashion, as described in the text. (1) Binding of the T-cell receptor (TCR) to major histocompatibility complex (MHC) induces the T cell to produce CD40L, which binds to CD40 on the B cell, producing a major stimulatory signal. (2) CD28 on the T cell then interacts with B7 on the B cell (costimulatory signal). Cytokines are also involved; their actions are shown in the diagram. *APC*, antigen-presenting cells (APCs).

The light chain

There are two types of light chains, termed kappa (κ) or lambda (λ), with no known functional difference. However, an immunoglobulin molecule can either have a pair of κ or λ chains, but never one of each.

The ratio of the two types of light chains varies between species, with humans having an average κ to λ ratio of 2:1. Alteration in this ratio may hinder an underlying clonal disease of B cells

(such as MM), in which case an excess of either κ or λ chains would be noted, due to the secretion of identical light chains from the clonal plasma cells.

The heavy chain

As described above, the class of an antibody, is determined by its heavy chain. Five different classes of immunoglobulins have been identified: IgM, IgG, IgA, IgE and IgD, with different effector

137

functions (Table 10.4). This is owned to the carboxy-terminal part of the heavy chain (the one that is not associated with the light chain).

IgG is the most abundant immunoglobulin in humans and has several subclasses (IgG1, 2, 3 and 4). IgG, IgA and IgD have three constant domains with a hinge region; IgM and IgE have four constant domains but no hinge region. There is little known about IgD that is relevant and it will not be considered.

The variable domain
Each variable domain exhibits three regions that are hypervariable. The hypervariable regions on both light and heavy chains are closely aligned in the immunoglobulin molecule. Together, they form the antigen-binding site and therefore determine the molecule's specificity.

The hinge region
The hinge allows movement and therefore greater interaction with epitopes. The hinge region is also the site of the interchain disulphide bonds.

Classes of antibody
The different properties of the immunoglobulin classes are shown in Table 10.4. Different immunoglobulin classes and subclasses are specific to each species. IgG and IgE are monomeric, while secreted IgA (sIgA) is usually present as a dimer and secreted IgM as a pentamer. The sIgA molecule is made up of two IgA monomers: a J chain and a secretory piece. The IgA dimer (J chain) is produced by submucosal plasma cells and enters the

mucosal epithelial cell via receptor-mediated endocytosis, binding to the poly-Ig receptor. Having passed from the basal to the luminal surface of the epithelial cell, the IgA dimer is secreted across the mucosa, with part of the poly-Ig receptor (the secretory piece) still attached.

The functions of antibodies
The functions of immunoglobulins are shown in Table 10.5.

The lymphatic system

The lymphoid organs are organized tissues, containing lymphoid and nonlymphoid cells. This allows an interaction between the two, which promotes the development, selection and preservation of the lymphoid cells. The lymphoid organs are grossly divided into central or primary, where T lymphocytes mature (B cells mature in the bone marrow), and peripheral or secondary where adaptive immune responses occur and lymphocytes are maintained. The secondary lymphoid organs include the lymph nodes, the spleen and the lymphoid tissues associated with mucosa, such as the gut-associated tonsils, Peyer patches and appendix.

Initiation of adaptive immune responses
Peripheral lymphoid organs are the sites where lymphocytes encounter and interact with antigens, no matter where the pathogen originated. Lymphocytes recirculate continuously through these tissues where the antigens are transferred via APCs (mainly macrophages and dendritic cells) (Fig. 10.7).

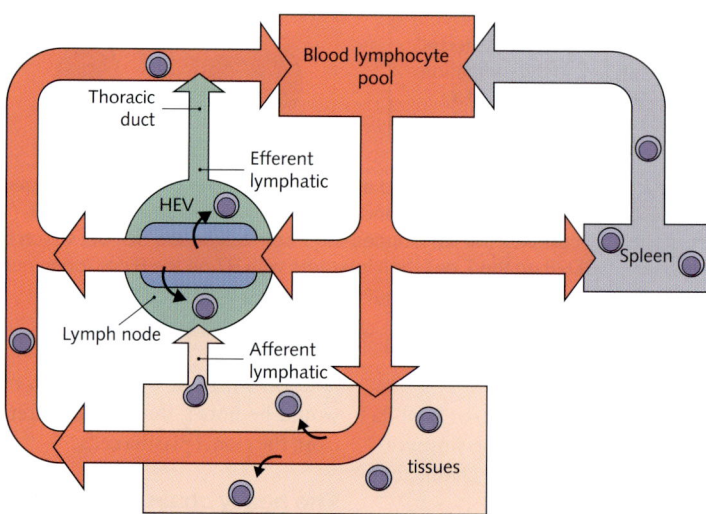

Fig. 10.7 Lymphocyte recirculation. Lymphocytes can enter lymph nodes via specialized high endothelial venules (HEVs) or in lymph. They leave the node in lymph that is returned to the systemic circulation via the right lymphatic duct or thoracic duct. *HEV*, high endothelial venule.

Lymphatic circulation

The lymphatic system acts as a passive drainage system to return interstitial fluid, called Lymph, to the systemic circulation. Afferent lymph vessels carry lymph into lymph nodes. Each node is drained by only one efferent vessel. Lymphatic drainage of the body is not a symmetrical left-right split; the right lymphatic duct drains the right arm and thorax, the rest of the body drains to the left lymphatic duct.

Lymphocytes move continuously between blood and lymph and they tend to recirculate to similar tissues. For example, an activated lymphocyte that has migrated from the skin to a local lymph node is most likely to migrate back to the skin following transport in the blood. This recirculation is governed by the expression of molecules on both the lymphocyte and surface endothelium. These molecules, called integrins, confer specificity to lymphocyte recirculation. This fine tuning of lymphocyte recirculation is known as lymphocyte homing. Areas of endothelium through which lymphocytes migrate are known as high endothelial venules (HEVs).

Lymph nodes

Lymph nodes act as filters, 'sampling' lymphatic fluid (and therefore plasma) for bacteria, viruses and foreign particles. APCs, loaded with antigen, also migrate through lymph nodes. They are present throughout the lymphatic system, often occurring at junctions of the lymphatic vessels. Lymph nodes frequently form chains and may drain a specific organ or area of the body.

Lymph nodes act as sites for initiation of the adaptive immune response. Antigen is sampled, processed and presented by several professional APCs (macrophages and dendritic cells). It is in the lymph nodes that B and T cells first encounter antigen and hence where they are activated and initiate the adaptive immune response.

Lymph nodes can become enlarged (lymphadenopathy) for several reasons, including infection. The causes of lymphadenopathy are outlined in Chapter 1.

Spleen

The organization of the spleen resembles that of the lymph node, although the antigens enter the spleen from the blood rather than from the lymph. The vast majority of the spleen consists of red pulp, which is punctuated by lymphoid white pulp. The red pulp is where the red cells are destroyed. The white pulp is formed by lymphocytes, which surround the arterioles entering the spleen. The inner part forms the periarteriolar lymphoid sheath (PALS), which is where the T-lymphocytes and antigen-loaded dendritic cells come together. The spleen may be enlarged in various clinical situations, which are discussed in Chapter 1.

Mucosal-associated lymphoid tissue

Mucosal-associated lymphoid tissue (MALT) consists of unencapsulated subepithelial lymphoid tissue found in the gastrointestinal, respiratory and urogenital tracts (Fig. 10.8).

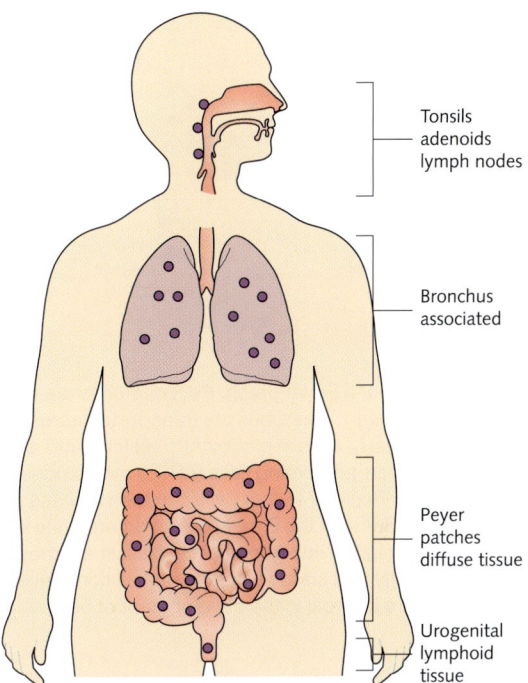

Fig. 10.8 Anatomical location of mucosal-associated lymphoid tissue (MALT). MALT is found in the nasal cavity, throat, respiratory tract, gastrointestinal tract and urogenital tract. Immune cells activated in MALT will return only to other mucosal sites.

It can be subdivided into:

- Organized lymphoid tissue, for example tonsils, appendix, Peyer patches
- Diffuse lymphoid tissue located in the lamina propria of intestinal villi and lungs

Organized lymphoid tissue
Respiratory tract

MALT in the nose and bronchi includes the:

- Lingual, palatine and nasopharyngeal tonsils
- Adenoids
- Bronchial nodules

The respiratory system is exposed to a large number of organisms every day, most of which are cleared by the mucociliary escalator. Microorganisms that are not removed are presented by dendritic cells in the bronchi and stimulate germinal centres.

Gastrointestinal tract

Peyer patches are organized submucosal lymphoid follicles present throughout the large and small intestine, particularly prominent in the terminal ileum. The structure of a Peyer patch is shown in Fig. 10.9.

The tonsils adenoids lymph nodes, Bronchus associated, Peyer patches diffuse tissue, Urogenital lymphoid tissue

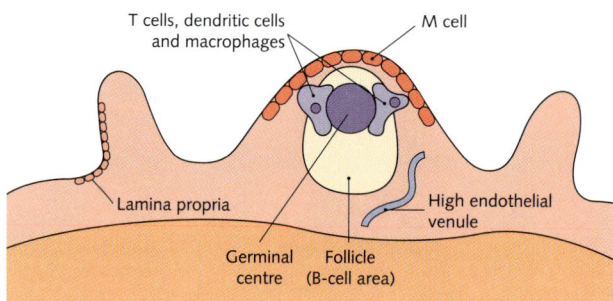

Gut lumen

T cells, dendritic cells and macrophages

M cell

Lamina propria

High endothelial venule

Germinal centre

Follicle (B-cell area)

Fig. 10.9 Structure of a Peyer patch. Peyer patches are found in the gastrointestinal tract. Microbes are transported across specialized epithelial M cells in pinocytotic vesicles into a dome-shaped area. Antigen-presenting cells (APCs) then process and present antigen to T cells. T helper cells can then activate B cells within the follicle. Some of the B cells do not differentiate into plasma cells, but migrate into germinal centres where they undergo high affinity and class switching maturation. Peyer patches also play a key role in the development of oral tolerance.

Food and harmless bacteria living in the gut contain many potentially antigenic substances. The immune system generally does not react to these. This is referred to as oral tolerance and is at least in part mediated by epithelial cells in gastrointestinal MALT, which secrete transforming growth factor β (TGF-β). This has a suppressive effect on local T cells, which is thought to prevent an immune response to peptides in food.

CELL-MEDIATED IMMUNITY

Cell-mediated immunity is mediated by T lymphocytes, macrophages and natural killer (NK) cells. The cell-mediated immune system is involved in the elimination of:

- Intracellular pathogens and infected cells (mainly viruses, mycobacteria and fungi)
- Tumour cells
- Foreign grafts

The thymus plays an important role in cell-mediated immunity because it is the site of T-cell maturation (hence they are called 'T' cells!).

T-cell development and the thymus

The aim of T-cell development and maturation is to select for T cells with receptors that can recognize foreign antigen in conjunction with self-MHC, while also destroying any that do not bind to self-MHC or any that bind to proteins in the body (autoantigens). This process occurs in the thymus.

The thymus is a gland with two lobes, located in the anterior part of the superior mediastinum, posterior to the sternum and anterior to the great vessels and upper part of the heart. Each lobule is divided into two regions (Fig. 10.10):

- An outer cortex
- An inner medulla

T lymphocyte differentiation begins in the bone marrow (see Chapter 1: Lymphocytes) before early precursor cells migrate to the thymus, specifically the cortex. In the thymus, immature T lymphocytes undergo random recombination of their TCR genes (see the section on Generation of antigen receptor diversity). Some of the resulting TCRs will be specific for pathogens and others for normal autoantigens. These developing T cells then migrate towards the medulla where they encounter specialized epithelial cells. These epithelial cells express MHC class I and class II molecules. Developing T cells that are able to bind self-MHC to some extent (as required for their function) will proliferate, resulting in positive selection. Furthermore, T cells that interact with MHC class I lose their CD4 (they are now CD8 T cells) and T cells that interact with MHC class II lose their CD8 (becoming CD4 T cells); this is MHC restriction. T cells that do not interact with the MHC molecules undergo apoptosis, as they do not receive a protective signal as a result of the TCR–MHC interaction. The thymic epithelial cells also have a unique mechanism for expressing many of the body's proteins (e.g., insulin) and peptides from these proteins are displayed on MHC class I and class II molecules. T cells that recognize this autoantigen can be forced to undergo apoptosis – this is central tolerance (see section on Tolerance later in this chapter).

A much smaller and more mature group of thymocytes survive to enter the medulla. Thymocytes continue to mature in the medulla and eventually leave the thymus as mature, antigen-specific, immunocompetent T cells. In total, only 1–5% of thymocytes in the thymus reach maturity, the remainder undergoing programmed cell death (apoptosis). The T cells that leave the thymus have been selected because they can recognize self-MHC, but those that recognize self-MHC plus autoantigen have been deleted. This process is summarized in Fig. 10.11.

T lymphocytes

Functions of different T-cell phenotypes

The different types of T cells can be differentiated by cell-surface molecules and function. There are two different types of TCR, which

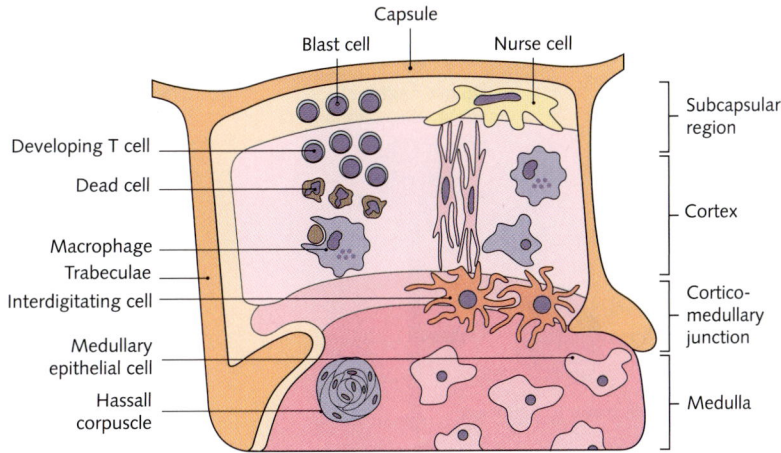

Fig. 10.10 Structure of a thymic lobule. Developing T cells (thymocytes) move from the subcapsular region to the medulla of the thymus during maturation. Several different types of stromal cell support them. Many thymocytes undergo apoptosis (particularly in the cortex) and are phagocytosed by macrophages.

have different functions. T cells expressing αβ-TCRs account for at least 95% of circulatory T cells. They become cytotoxic, helper or suppressor cells and, unless specified otherwise, account for all the T cells mentioned in this book. T cells expressing a γδ-TCR are present at mucosal surfaces and their specificity is biased towards certain bacterial and viral antigens (such as tetanus toxoid, staphylococcal enterotoxin A, listeria monocytogenes and HSV glycoprotein I).

T-helper cells

T-helper (Th) cells play a key role in the development of the immune response. They determine the epitopes to be targeted by the immune system. This is achieved through their interactions with processed antigen, as presented by APCs in conjunction with MHC class II molecules. They also determine the nature of the immune response directed against target antigens, for example, cytotoxic TCR or antibody response. Finally, they are required for normal B-cell function (see 'B cells and antibody production' earlier in this chapter). Overall, they orchestrate the immune response according to the nature of the threat faced.

Most Th cells are CD4+ and can be divided into five subsets on the basis of the cytokines they secrete and hence the actions they have:

1. Th0
2. Th1
3. Th2
4. Th17
5. Regulatory T cells (Treg)

Th0 cells arise as a result of initial short-term stimulation of naïve T cells and are capable of secreting a broad spectrum of cytokines. Prolonged stimulation of Th0 cells results in the

emergence of Th1 and Th2 subsets. The cytokines released by the Th1 and Th2 subsets modulate one another's secretion. The different cytokine profiles of the Th1, Th2 and Th17 subsets reflect their different immunological functions (Table 10.6).

Most immune responses involve more than one subset of T cells. For example, staphylococcus (an extracellular bacterium) stimulates both Th2 and Th17 responses. On the other hand, some responses become very polarized. For example, the immune system relies almost exclusively on Th1 cells to respond to mycobacterium tuberculosis, an intracellular pathogen.

The fifth type of Th cell, Treg, has two main regulatory roles. The first is to dampen the immune response once an infection has been brought under control. The second is to regulate self-reactive T cells that have not developed central tolerance in the thymus. Their action is via cytokines, including TGF-β and IL-10. Tregs also have a role in oral tolerance (described in the section on tolerance later in this chapter).

Cytotoxic T cells

Most cytotoxic T (Tc) lymphocytes are CD8+ and recognize antigen in conjunction with MHC class I molecules (endogenous antigen). Therefore, they are involved in defending against intracellular pathogens, that is, viruses and some bacteria. They lyse target cells via the same mechanisms as NK cells (see Chapter 9: NK cells).

T-cell activation

T cells are activated by interactions between the TCR and peptide bound to MHC. Activation also requires a 'second message' from the antigen-presenting cell. This process, termed costimulation, is shown in Fig. 10.12.

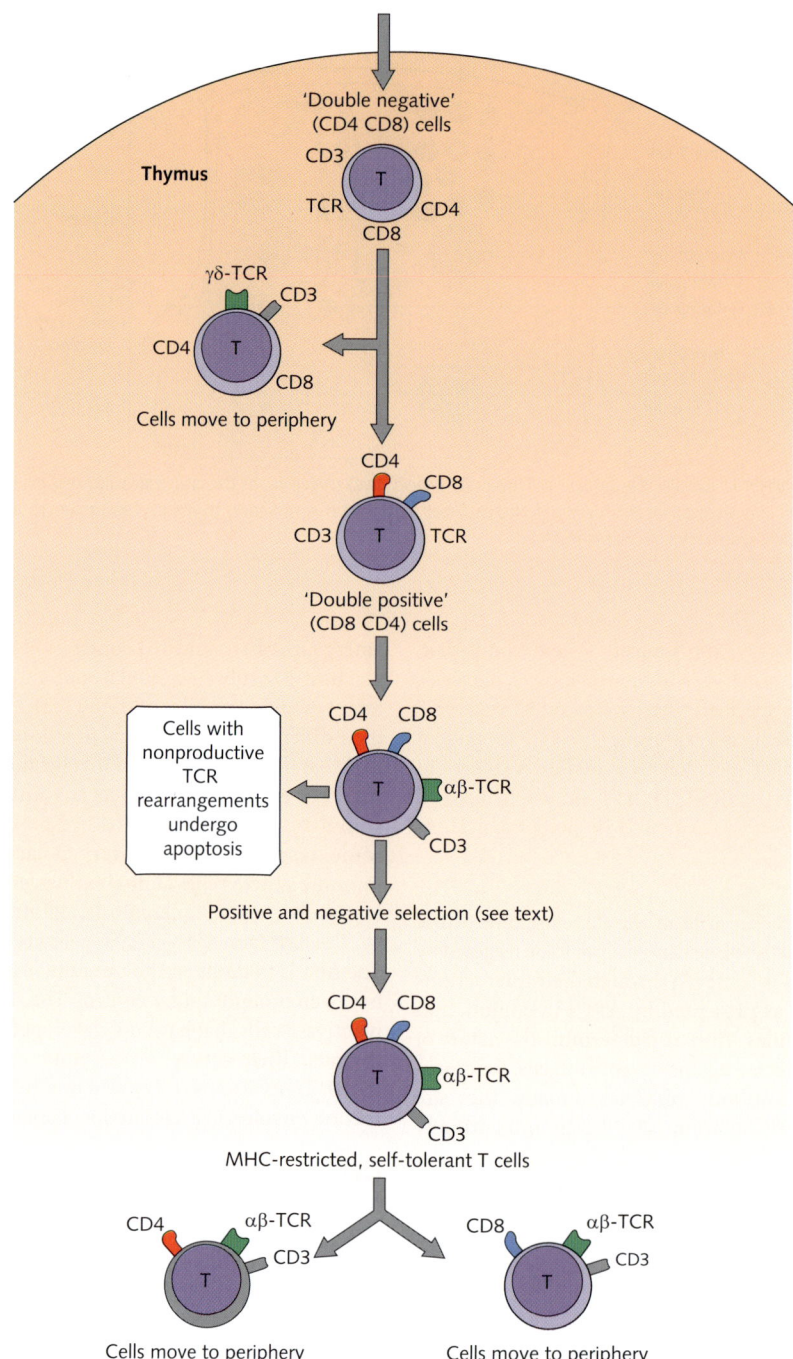

Fig. 10.11 Development of T cells in the thymus. Cells entering the thymus to become T cells are negative for CD4, CD8, CD3 and the T-cell receptor (TCR). Rearrangement of the genes encoding the TCR will produce three cell lines: (1) CD4+ αβ-TCR; (2) CD8+ αβ-TCR; and (3) CD4−CD8− γδ-TCR. The β- or γ-chain genes rearrange first. If a functional β-chain is formed, both CD4 and CD8 are upregulated and the α-chain gene rearranges. The resultant T cells are positively selected if their TCR is functional, but negatively selected if they react too strongly. The majority of thymocytes will undergo apoptosis due to positive or negative selection. *MHC*, major histocompatibility complex.

Table 10.6 Differences between the T helper 1, T helper 2 and T helper 17 cell subsets

Cytokines secreted	Th1 cells *IL-2, IFN-γ, TNF-β*	Th2 cells *IL-4, IL-10*	Th17 cells *IL-17*
Functions	• Responsible for classical cell-mediated immunity reactions such as delayed-type hypersensitivity and cytotoxic T-cell activation • Involved in responses to intracellular pathogens; for example, viruses, some protozoa and fungi, and some bacteria • Activate macrophages	• Promote B-cell activation • Involved in allergic diseases and responses to helminthic infections	• Promote neutrophil activation and migration • Involved in responses to extracellular bacteria and fungi

Th1, T helper 1; Th2, T helper 2; Th17, T helper 17.

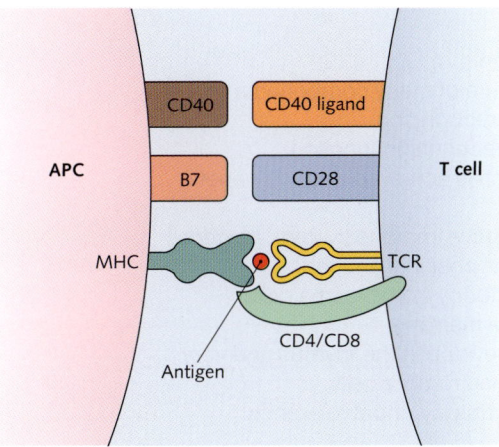

Fig. 10.12 Activation of T cells. Several interactions with antigen-presenting cells (APCs) are required to activate T cells. The T-cell receptor (TCR) and CD4 or CD8 bind to major histocompatibility complex (MHC) and antigens. CD28 on the T-cell binds to B7 on the APC, providing a co-stimulatory signal.

Superantigens

T cells can be activated in a nonspecific fashion by superantigens. Superantigens cross-link between the V-β domain of the TCR and an MHC class II molecule on an APC. Cross-linking is independent of the peptide-binding cleft but depends on the framework region of the V-β domain. This means that one superantigen is able to activate about 5% of T cells, far more than a normal antigen. Staphylococcal enterotoxin is an example of a T-cell superantigen, causing toxic shock syndrome (TSS) (see 'Clinical notes').

CLINICAL NOTES

Toxic shock syndrome: Toxins produced by staphylococci and streptococci can act as superantigens, producing the clinical picture of TSS, where a seemingly innocuous stimulus such as a graze can lead to fever, a diffuse macular rash and sepsis.

There is an association between tampon use and *Staphylococcus aureus* TSS with many known deaths as a result. Management of TSS is the same as that of sepsis (see Chapter 9). Antibiotic therapy should cover *S. aureus* and *Streptococcus pyogenes*.

TOLERANCE

Tolerance is the ability of the immune system to ignore certain peptides that have the potential to trigger an immune response. The need for 'self-tolerance' is logical; immune activation by endogenous peptides would be damaging to tissues. Tolerance also includes harmless environmental antigens such as food or pollen. A breakdown in tolerance to either endogenous or environmental antigens can result in autoimmune disease or allergies (covered extensively in Chapter 12).

Central tolerance

Central tolerance is achieved through negative selection. As previously described, T cells (in the thymus) and B cells (in the bone marrow) are eliminated if they are self-reactive. Central tolerance is not complete: only the most self-reactive lymphocytes are deleted, ensuring that a wide lymphocyte repertoire is maintained. Additionally, some self-reactive T cells develop into regulatory T cells (Tregs) instead of being eliminated.

Peripheral tolerance

In the periphery, self-antigens do not generally elicit an immune response. Several mechanisms prevent autoantigen reactive T cells from causing autoimmune disease. These include:

- Lack of the costimulation required for T-cell activation: costimulatory molecules such as CD40 or CD28 are found on APCs but not on other body tissues.
- Tregs secrete IL-10 and TGF-β in the presence of autoantigen reactive T cells. These cytokines suppress surrounding T cells.

Oral tolerance

A degree of tolerance is required because the gastrointestinal tract is full of antigens that have the potential to trigger an immune response. Epithelial cells in the gastrointestinal tract secrete TGF-β, causing any T cell that recognizes an antigen found in food or on harmless gut bacteria to become a Treg specific to that antigen. These Tregs also play a role in the peripheral tolerance to the harmless gastrointestinal antigens.

CLINICAL NOTES

Oral tolerance is emerging as a way to treat allergies and autoimmune disease. Grass pollen allergy (hay fever) can be managed by long-term sublingual administration of grass pollen. The Th2 cells that mediate the allergy are effectively switched off by Tregs created during the oral administration of grass pollen antigen.

Chapter Summary

- The immunoglobulin domain is the underlying basic structure of many components of the adaptive immune system and provides a basis for antigen recognition.
- B- and T-cell surface antigen receptors serve this antigen recognition function.
- B- and T-cell antigen receptors require huge diversity, which is achieved through genetic rearrangement.
- MHC provides a means of antigen presentation to the adaptive immune system. Its genes vary from person to person, encompassing the spectrum of possible antigen.
- Humoral immunity is concerned with the production of antibody from plasma cells (activated and differentiated B cells, which develop in bone marrow).
- Cell-mediated immunity is coordinated by T cells. These develop in the thymus and vary in their function, generally tackling intracellular infections and tumour cells.
- Self-reactive B and T cells are eliminated in development. This is central tolerance.

MLA Conditions

Toxic shock syndrome (TSS)

MLA Presentations

RESPONSE TO TISSUE DAMAGE

Inflammation is a nonspecific response evoked by tissue injury. The aims of the process are:

- Removal of the causative agent, for example, microbes or toxins
- Removal of dead tissue
- Replacement of dead tissue with normal tissue or scar formation

CLINICAL NOTES

Inflammation is defined clinically by four cardinal signs: rubor, dolor, calor and tumour (redness, pain, heat and swelling). These are key observations in almost every clinical examination and are often best found by comparing one side with the other, for example, feeling the temperature of both legs simultaneously when looking for cellulitis.

Acute inflammation

Acute inflammation is the immediate response to cell injury. It is of short duration (a few hours to a few days) and is triggered by a range of insults, including physical trauma, chemical or thermal damage and infection. Both innate and adaptive immune cells initiate the acute inflammatory response. Infection is sensed by resident macrophages through Toll-like receptors, which then release cytokines, attracting neutrophils to the site of infection. In other instances (such as parasitic worm infection), inflammation is initiated by resident mast cells, which tend to attract eosinophils. CD4+ T lymphocytes play a central role in acute inflammation: they are activated by macrophages and produce many of the chemical mediators of acute inflammation (Table 11.1). Once inflammation has been initiated, several changes occur in vascular endothelium to allow attachment and extravasation of leucocytes – primarily neutrophils but also monocytes and lymphocytes. Attachment and extravasation require the presence of surface molecules on both the endothelium and leucocytes.

Vascular changes

Tissue injury and the ensuing immune response result in the release of chemical mediators (cytokines, chemokines and histamine) that act on local blood vessels. The main changes that occur are:

- Vasodilatation: causing increased blood flow and therefore redness and heat
- Slowing of the circulation and increased vascular permeability: formation of an inflammatory exudate results in swelling
- Entry of inflammatory cells, especially neutrophils, into the tissues

Leucocyte extravasation

The majority of cells that respond in acute inflammation are neutrophils, required for their phagocytic behaviour. Neutrophils adhere to the vessel wall and then pass between the endothelial cells into the tissues, where they follow the increasing chemokine concentration gradient to the site of inflammation (chemotaxis). This is a multistep process involving:

- Margination: adherence of neutrophils to the vessel wall. There are two phases to margination. The first is 'tethering and rolling' and the second is 'activation and strengthening'. Neutrophils adhere to vessel walls via cell adhesion molecules (CAMs).
- Diapedesis (extravasation): neutrophils move between endothelial cells into the tissue.
- Chemotaxis: due to the release of several chemotactic agents (Table 11.1).

Cell adhesion molecules are either members of the immunoglobulin superfamily, the selectin family or the integrin family. Integrin molecules allow immune cells to target specific sites, a process known as homing (as seen in Chapter 10). To interact

Table 11.1 Overview of the mediators of acute inflammation

Action	Mediators
Increased vascular permeability	Histamine, bradykinin, C3a, C5a, LTs C_4, D_4, E_4, PAF
Vasodilatation	Histamine, PGs, PAF
Pain	Bradykinin, PGs
Leucocyte adhesion	LTB_4, IL-1, TNF-α, C5a
Leucocyte chemotaxis	C5a, C3a, IL-8, PAF, LTB_4, fibrin and collagen fragments
Acute phase response	IL-1, TNF-α, IL-6
Tissue damage	Proteases and free radicals

IL, Interleukin; LT, leukotriene; LTs, leukotrienes; PAF, platelet-activating factor; PGs, prostaglandins; TNF, tumour necrosis factor.

successfully with the extracellular matrix, neutrophils must express β_1-integrins, a set of adhesion molecules that can bind to collagen and laminin.

Once neutrophils reach a site of inflammation, they phagocytose foreign particles and release enzymes (see Chapter 9). Leucocytes can release proteases and metabolites during chemotaxis and phagocytosis, which are potentially harmful to the host. Neutrophils die during this process, creating pus.

CLINICAL NOTES

Pus is created during acute infections with certain bacteria, termed pyogenic bacteria. These include *Staphylococcus* (causing skin abscesses, septic arthritis, etc.), *Streptococcus* (causing purulent sputum) and *Neisseria gonorrhoeae* (causing genital discharge), among many others.

Molecular mediators of inflammation

A variety of molecular mediators are produced during an inflammatory response. They usually have short half-lives and are rapidly inactivated by a variety of systems, enabling a timely offset of inflammation once the cause has been removed. A summary of their actions is given in Table 11.1.

Cell membrane phospholipid metabolites

Prostaglandins (PGs) and leukotrienes (LTs) are derived from the metabolism of arachidonic acid, a constituent of cell membranes. PG metabolism is the target of nonsteroidal antiinflammatory drugs (see Chapter 13). Platelet-activating factor (PAF) is also an important mediator of inflammation.

Cytokines

Cytokines are molecular messengers between cells. In inflammation they attract and stimulate different cell types, coordinating the inflammatory response. The cytokine response is generated by CD4$^+$ T cells and macrophages or eosinophils.

Cytokines such as IL-6, IL-8, IL-1, interferon-gamma (IFN-γ) and tumour necrosis factor-α (TNF-α) act to:

- induce expression of CAMs on the endothelium, thus enhancing leucocyte adhesion
- attract neutrophils to the area of injury
- induce prostacyclin (PGI$_2$) production
- induce PAF synthesis
- mediate the development of the acute-phase response
- stimulate fibroblast proliferation and increase collagen synthesis

The complement system

The function of complement in acute inflammation includes attracting and activating white cells and directly attacking pathogens. This is discussed in Chapter 9.

The kinin system

Bradykinin is released following activation of the kinin system by clotting factor XII, which occurs in trauma. Bradykinin increases vascular permeability and mediates pain by modulating afferent neurones.

The coagulation system

The coagulation system is activated at sites of vascular injury (see Chapter 6), so its role in mediating inflammation relates to its activation in tissue damage. Fibrinopeptides produced during coagulation are chemotactic for neutrophils and increase vascular permeability. Thrombin also promotes fibroblast proliferation and leucocyte adhesion.

The fibrinolytic system

Plasmin (see Chapter 6) has several functions in the inflammatory process, including:

- Activation of complement via C3.
- Cleavage of fibrin to form 'fibrin degradation products', which may increase vascular permeability.

Results of acute inflammation

There are several possible outcomes resulting from acute inflammation. These include:

- Regrowth and resolution of tissue following trauma or infection
- Healing by collagenous scar formation if the tissue cannot regenerate, for example, myocardium
- Abscess formation: a pyogenic bacterial infection within a tissue
- Chronic inflammation

CLINICAL NOTES

The differential diagnosis of neutrophilia is rather broad and includes infection, inflammation, medications, cigarette smoking, asplenia, stress/exercise, obesity, endocrine causes (such as thyrotoxicosis or eclampsia), myeloproliferative neoplasms, nonhaematologic malignancies, Down syndrome, etc. A patient with neutrophilia should be evaluated by history taking, thorough clinical examination, medication history, laboratory assessment (such as total white cell count (WCC) and peripheral blood film, renal and liver function, ESR and CRP, coagulation testing) and blood or sputum cultures, as appropriate. Specialized testing (such as bone marrow aspirate and trephine, flow cytometry and molecular/genetic testing) may be required in certain patients, depending on clinical findings and suspicion.

The urgency of referral for evaluation is dictated by the clinical condition of the patient, the degree and rate of neutrophil rise and the findings on peripheral blood film (e.g., blasts or fragments mandate an urgent referral).

Patients with clinical instability (such as hypotension, hypoxia, loss of consciousness) require urgent referral to exclude an acute process (such as acute infection or malignancy), whereas asymptomatic, mild or chronic neutrophilia may be monitored and evaluated in an outpatient setting.

White cell count of >100 x 10^9/L (hyperleukocytosis) warrants urgent haematological assessment for consideration of emergency leukapheresis, in order to prevent hyperviscocity-associated complications, such as vaso-occlusive events.

Leukaemoid reaction refers to a total WCC of >50 x 10^9/L from nonleukaemic causes (such as infections, asplenia, and drugs), with the majority of cells being left-shifted neutrophils and other precursors.

Chronic inflammation

Chronic inflammation arises as a result of prolonged acute inflammation, usually when the causative agent cannot be eliminated so antigenic persistence occurs. This may be due to deficiencies in the host response to certain pathogens or the nature of the pathogen itself, for example, *Mycobacterium tuberculosis*, which has evolved to evade the immune response. Chronic inflammation also occurs in persistent autoimmune disease such as rheumatoid arthritis; the body is incapable of fully clearing autoantigens.

CLINICAL NOTES

Anaemia of chronic disease (ACD) is the second most prevalent cause of anaemia, following iron deficiency anaemia. It is found in patients with an underlying immune/inflammatory condition, such as systemic inflammatory disorders (e.g., rheumatoid arthritis, systemic lupus erythematosus (SLE), inflammatory bowel disease, vasculitis), infections (bacterial, viral, parasitic and fungal), malignancy (multifactorial anaemia), chronic disorders (such as chronic obstructive pulmonary disease, chronic kidney disease) and ageing.

Typically, patients present with progressive anaemia in the context of a known underlying (inflammatory) illness. The anaemia is normochromic/normocytic (i.e., normal mean cell volume [MCV]), mild to moderate in severity and is associated with inappropriately low reticulocyte counts. The white cell and platelet counts are usually normal, unless affected by the underlying disorder.

Anaemia of chronic disease is thought to result from a defensive mechanism protecting the host from iron-binding invading microbes. It is characterized by raised hepcidin, a key regulator of iron homeostasis, which leads to retention of iron within the cells of

reticuloendothelial system (Fig. 11.1A). This, in turn, limits the availability of iron for erythroid progenitor cells, creating the combination of low circulating iron, low total iron binding capacity (TIBC), low transferrin saturation (Tsat) and normal/high iron storage, along with raised ferritin and CRP (acute phase proteins), which constitute the hallmark features of the disease.

Some of these features are also noted in iron deficiency anaemia (low serum iron and low Tsat), complicating the diagnosis of concomitant iron deficiency anaemia. In this case, soluble transferrin receptor levels (sTfR) and serum hepcidin may help to discriminate between the two. Low/absent bone marrow iron stores and low reticulocyte haemoglobin concentration also support a concomitant diagnosis of iron deficiency (Fig. 11.1B). Finally, if the distinction between the two conditions cannot be made with confidence, a clinical response to a short course of iron supplementation (e.g., 2 weeks of oral iron) may confirm the coexistence of true iron deficiency.

The management of ACD involves the following:

(a) Treatment of the underlying disorder
(b) Identification and treatment of other causes of anaemia (e.g., iron/folate/B12 deficiency, haemolysis, impaired renal function)
(c) Avoidance of red blood cell transfusion, unless patient is symptomatic or has life-threatening anaemia

The key cells of chronic inflammation are macrophages, lymphocytes and plasma cells. This is in marked contrast to acute inflammation, which is characterized primarily by a neutrophilic inflammation. Ongoing inflammation is associated with tissue destruction, as well as healing.

In chronic inflammation, macrophage numbers are increased because they are recruited by chemotactic factors (e.g., platelet-derived growth factor [PDGF] and C5a) and are prevented from leaving by migration inhibition factor. The overall maintenance of inflammation at a local level is thought to be due to TNF, secreted by macrophages. When it is secreted at high levels, it has systemic effects, including weight loss (through fat catabolism and appetite inhibition) and fatigue. Other macrophage secretory products mediate characteristic features of chronic inflammation:

- Tissue damage via proteases and oxygen radicals
- Revascularization via angiogenic factors
- Fibroblast migration and proliferation via growth factors (e.g., PDGF) and cytokines (IL-2, TNF-α)
- Collagen synthesis via growth factors (e.g., PDGF) and cytokines (IL-1, TNF-α)
- Tissue remodelling via collagenases
- Simulation of T-cell activity by secretion of IL-12

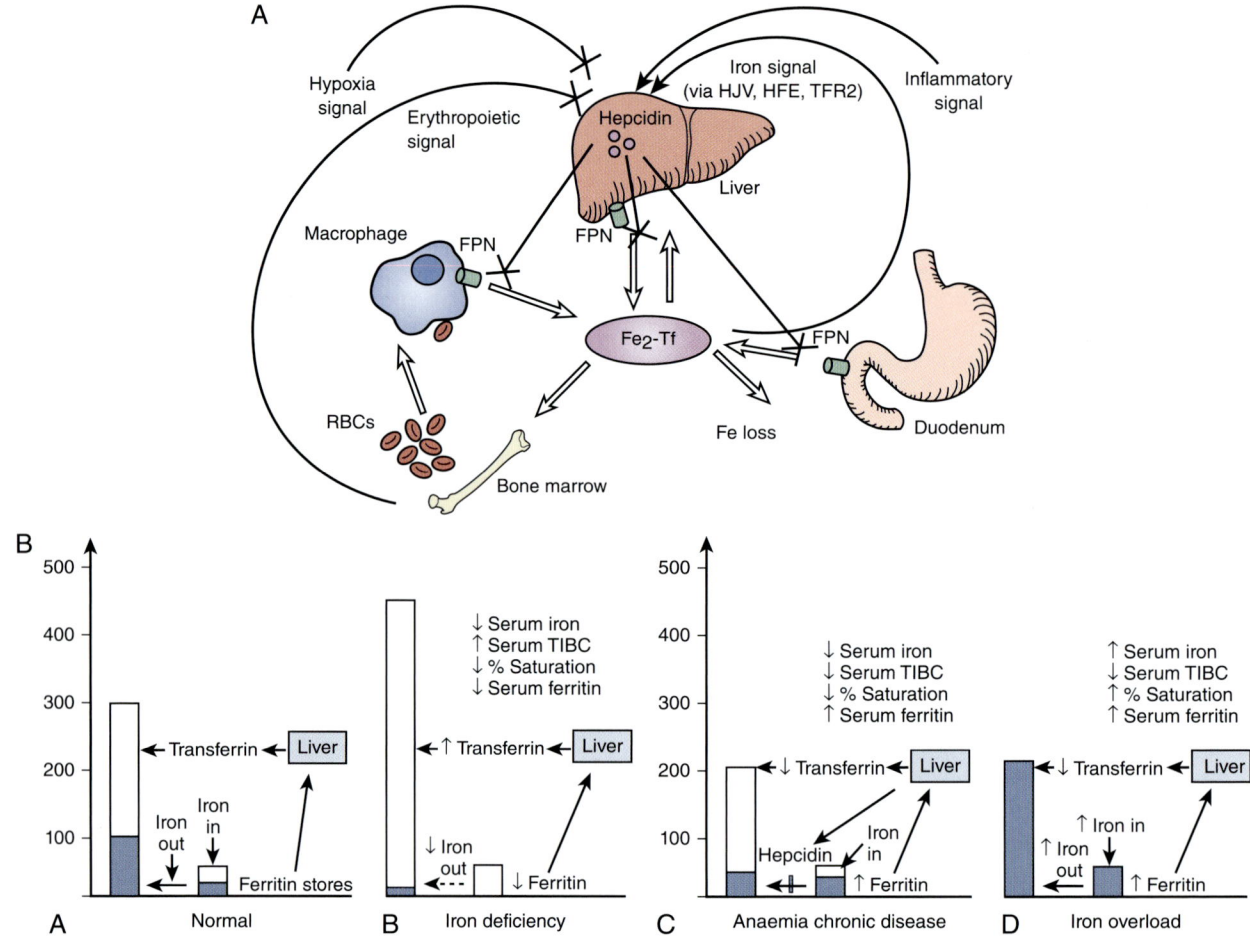

Fig. 11.1 (A) Overview of the influence of inflammation on iron homeostasis. Hepcidin is elevated in chronic inflammatory states resulting in iron retention and subsequent reduction of circulating iron levels. (B) Summary of changes in different iron markers in Anaemia of chronic disease (ACD) vs. iron deficiency. Notably, in the former, ferritin levels are elevated but Tsat is reduced in keeping with reduced iron circulation. (A, From Babitt JL, Lin HY. Molecular mechanisms of hepcidin regulation: implications for the anemia of CKD. *Am J Kidney Dis*. 2010;55:726–741; B, From Alfrey, A. (*Rapid Review Pathology*. 6th ed. Elsevier; 2024).

Lymphocytes and plasma cells are also present at the site of inflammation. In the case of chronic infections, both macrophages and T cells are required to control infection. An overview of chronic inflammation is given in Fig. 11.2.

Inflammation in disease

Inflammation is intended to protect the host but can, under certain circumstances, prove destructive. Antigenic persistence results in the continued activation and accumulation of macrophages and T cells. Macrophages develop into epithelioid cells (modified macrophages) and in turn this forms a granuloma.

TNF-α is required for granuloma formation and maintenance. IFN-γ, secreted by activated T cells, is also required for the transformation of macrophages into epithelioid cells. IFN-γ also stimulates the production of multinucleate giant cells, which arise from the fusion of several macrophages. The granuloma is surrounded by a cuff of lymphocytes and the subsequent migration of fibroblasts results in increased collagen synthesis.

Granuloma formation is the immune response to 'frustrated' or ineffective phagocytosis; the nature of the damaging stimulus determines the type of granuloma formed. Examples of granulomatous disease include:

- Microorganisms such as *M. tuberculosis:* these induce a persistent, delayed-type hypersensitivity response (see Chapter 12: Type IV hypersensitivity), resulting in granuloma formation in the lung. While harmful to the host,

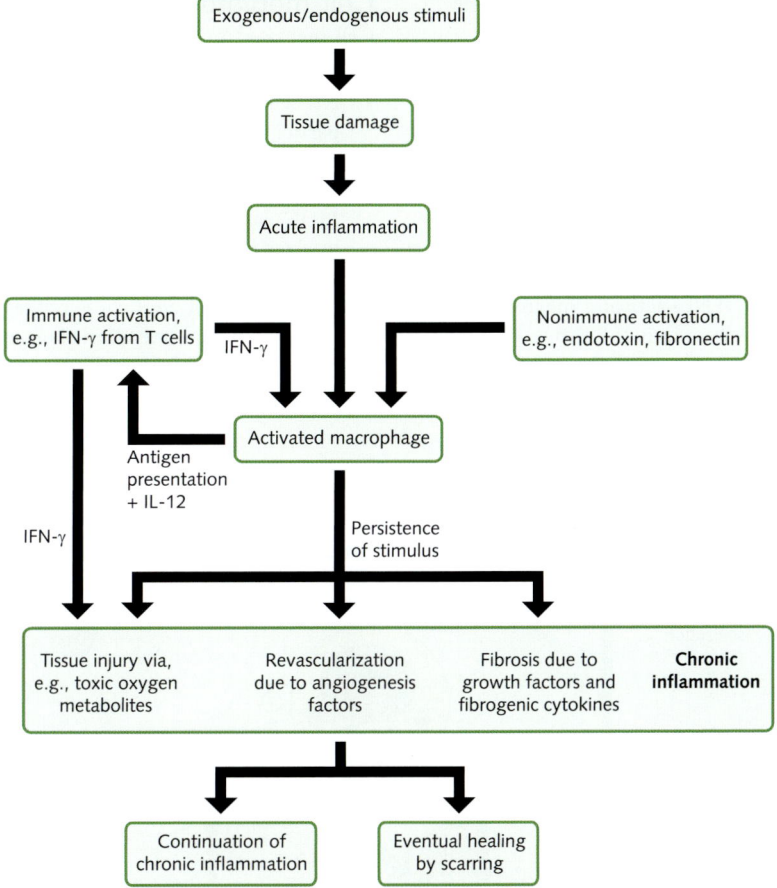

Fig. 11.2 Overview of chronic inflammation. Macrophages can be activated by T cells or by nonimmune mechanisms. Activated macrophages persist at sites of chronic inflammation because of persistent stimulation. They release a number of molecules, which produce the characteristic features of chronic inflammation. Macrophages act as antigen-presenting cells to T cells, which can then activate further macrophages.

this prevents the spread of infection. Caseous necrotic areas (dry, 'cheese-like' white mass of degenerated tissue) might be present in the centre of a *M. tuberculosis* granuloma.

- Foreign body inhalation (e.g., silica): this induces a granuloma that is predominantly surrounded by macrophages.
- Sarcoidosis: this is an idiopathic multisystem granulomatous disorder, most commonly affecting the lungs.

IMMUNE RESPONSE TO PATHOGENS

Immune response to viral infection

Viruses do not always kill host cells, but budding and release of new viral particles often causes the cells to lyse. The immune system can act to prevent infection or the spread of infection or to eliminate an intracellular target once infection has occurred.

Humoral immunity to viruses

The humoral response is involved in preventing entry to, and viral replication within, cells.

Antibody

Antibodies can:

- Bind to free virus, preventing their attachment and entry into cells. This is referred to as neutralization of free virus particles. For example, IgG neutralizes the hepatitis B (HepB) virus on entering the bloodstream and IgA neutralizes the influenza virus entering the nasal mucosa.
- Bind to viral proteins, which are expressed on the surface of infected cells as a result of viral replication within the cells. Antibodies bound to infected cells can initiate antibody-dependent cell-mediated cytotoxicity (ADCC), mediated mainly by natural killer (NK) cells, and

complement activation and also act as an opsonin (see Chapter 9).

Responses directed against free virus are considered to be the most important in vivo. Antibodies are important early in the course of infection to prevent the spread of virus between cells.

Interferon

IFNs are produced by virally infected cells. IFN-α and IFN-β act on neighbouring uninfected cells by inhibiting transcription and translation of viral proteins. IFN-γ activates macrophages and NK cells and enhances the adaptive immune response by upregulating expression of major histocompatibility complex (MHC) class I and class II molecules.

Cell-mediated immunity to viruses

Cell-mediated mechanisms are important for eliminating a virus once infection is established. The cells involved include:

- NK cells: these are cytotoxic for virus-infected cells and participate in ADCC.
- Cytotoxic CD8+ T cells: viral peptides are presented to CD8+ T cells on the surface of infected cells in association with MHC class I molecules. CD8+ T cells can destroy these infected cells.
- CD4+ T cells: T helper (Th) cells coordinate the generation of antibody and cytotoxic T-cell responses and the recruitment and activation of macrophages.

An overview of the immune response to viruses is given in Fig. 11.3.

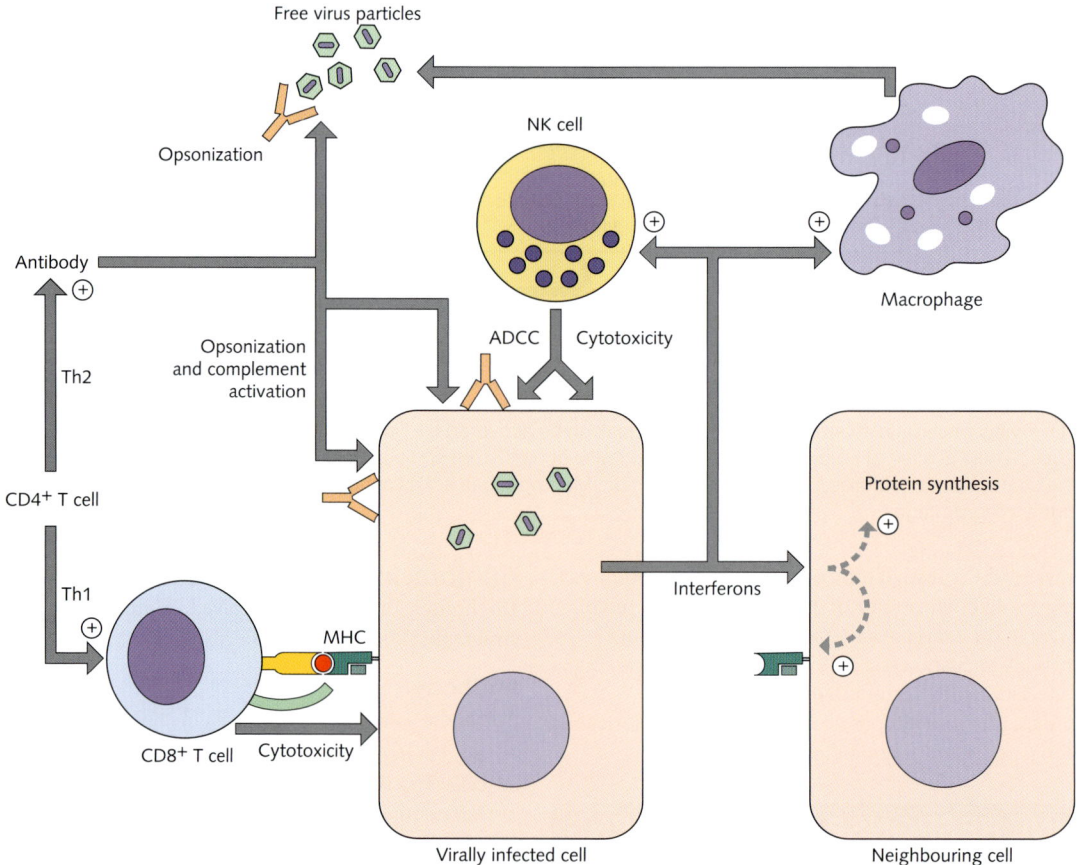

Fig. 11.3 The immune response to viruses. Interferons (IFNs), produced by virally infected cells, have three important actions: induction of an antiviral state in neighbouring cells (IFN-α and IFN-β), macrophage and natural killer (NK) cell activation and major histocompatibility complex (MHC) molecule upregulation IFN-γ. NK cells kill virally infected cells, macrophages phagocytose opsonized free virus and cell fragments and produce further IFN. CD8+ (cytotoxic) T cells sense viral peptides presented by MHC class I molecules and destroy the cell. CD4+ (helper) T cells help to activate macrophages and are involved in the generation of antibody and cytotoxic T-cell responses. *ADCC*, Antibody-dependent cell-mediated cytotoxicity.

Examples of viral infection strategies

Viral infections are common, and most are self-limiting. Some, particularly those that can evade the immune response, can be chronic and are potentially fatal (e.g., Human immunodeficiency viruses [HIV], see Chapter 12; Hepatitis B, see Clinical notes earlier in this chapter). Different viruses use different strategies to evade the host's immune response:

Antigenic shift and drift: for example, influenza. These are mechanisms of genetic and therefore antigenic variation. This circumvents immunological memory because the virus expresses different immunological targets over time.

Polymorphism: for example, adenovirus, rhinovirus. This also causes antigenic variation.

Latent virus: for example, herpes simplex virus (HSV), varicella zoster (see Clinical notes).

Modulation of normal immune effector functions, principally MHC class I. downregulation: for example, cytomegalovirus (CMV), adenovirus, Epstein–Barr virus (EBV), HSV, HIV. Viruses can also interfere with IFN or produce inhibitory cytokines.

Infection and subsequent death of lymphocytes, for example, HIV, measles, CMV, EBV. This reduces the ability of the immune system to combat viral infection.

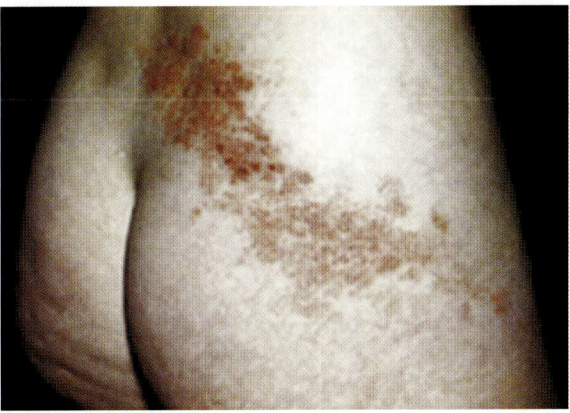

Fig. 11.4 Shingles rash. The rash is characteristically erythematous and vesicular. Its spread is limited to the area that the affected nerve supplies. In this case, it is a dermatome in the lower back/buttock.

CLINICAL NOTES

By becoming latent, a virus 'hides' from the immune system. Varicella zoster virus, of the herpes virus family, causes chickenpox. After initial infection, the virus becomes latent, residing in neuronal cells. This can later reactivate when the immune system is compromised, suggesting that there must be some interaction between the immune system and the virus even when it is latent. Reactivated varicella zoster is known as shingles and characteristically produces a painful vesicular rash that remains within the dermatome of the nerve that it has reactivated from (see Fig. 11.4).

Immune response to bacterial infection

Bacteria are prokaryotic organisms, which can be broadly classified according to their shape (spheres, spiral or rods) or to their cell surface properties. Their cell membrane is surrounded by a peptidoglycan cell wall. Many bacteria also have a capsule of large, branched polysaccharides. Only a small minority of bacteria are able to infect and cause disease in humans, attaching to cells via surface pili. Some 'benign' bacteria have the potential to cause disease in immunocompromised patients; these are called 'opportunistic pathogens'.

Bacteria use a different mechanism from the host machinery for DNA replication, protein translation and metabolism. This has enabled the generation of antibiotics, the majority of which are small proteins that target variable parts of the bacteria machinery (e.g., bacterial enzymes, cell-wall synthesis) that are absent in the host.

Different immune mechanisms operate, depending on whether the bacteria are extracellular or intracellular.

Extracellular bacteria

The majority of pathogenic bacteria do not require the intracellular environment to replicate and spread. Common extracellular bacterial pathogens include *Staphylococcus aureus*, *Streptococcus* spp., *Haemophilus influenzae* and *Pseudomonas aeruginosa*.

Humoral immunity to extracellular bacteria

Complement. Bacteria activate complement via the lectin or alternative pathways (see Chapter 9). Activated complement products play a role in the elimination of bacteria, especially C3b (an opsonin), C3a and C5a (anaphylatoxins that recruit leucocytes) and the membrane attack complex (MAC), which can perforate the outer lipid bilayer of gram-negative (but not gram-positive) bacteria such as *H. influenzae*.

Antibody. This is the principal defence against extracellular bacteria. Initially, sIgA binds to bacteria and prevents their binding to epithelial cells, for example, in the respiratory mucosa. If this response is sufficient, sIgA can prevent the pathogen from entering the body. Antibodies also:

- Neutralize bacterial toxins
- Activate complement
- Act as an opsonin

While plasma cells are responsible for the production of antibody, CD4+ T-cell help is still required for the generation of antibodies in response to bacterial infection. This is predominantly through Th2-mediated activation of B cells. Remember, these Th2 cells are themselves activated by the presentation of bacterial antigen by antigen-presenting cells, in association with MHC class II.

Cell-mediated immunity to extracellular bacteria

Phagocytic cells, predominantly neutrophils, kill most bacteria, by a process called opsonization (refers to the binding of acute phase proteins, such as C3b protein, and antibodies to the cell surface of bacteria, rendering them 'visible' by host immune cells). The process of killing opsonized bacteria is called phagocytosis. Opsonization is particularly important, as it facilitates killing of gram-positive bacteria (such as *Staphylococcus*), which are resistant to killing by MAC. After phagocytosis, bacterial antigens are processed and presented to CD4+ T cells, through MHC class II molecules. As discussed in Chapter 10, there are two major groups of helper T cells, Th1 and Th2, each producing a different set of cytokines. Briefly, Th1 cells produce mainly IFN-γ, promoting cell-mediated responses, whereas Th2 cells activate B cells and promote humoral immunity, primarily through IL-4.

An overview of the immune response to extracellular bacteria is given in Fig. 11.5.

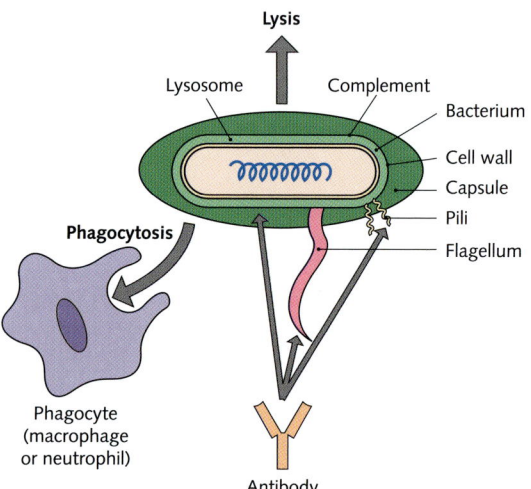

Fig. 11.5 The immune response to extracellular bacteria. The first line of host defence against bacteria is lysozyme. This, together with complement, leads to bacterial lysis. Antibody is produced against flagella (immobilizing the bacteria) and pili (preventing attachment). Capsular polysaccharides can induce T-cell–independent antibody. Antibodies aid complement activation and phagocytosis of bacteria.

Intracellular bacteria
Humoral immunity to intracellular bacteria

The humoral mechanisms that are employed against extracellular bacteria may be used to try to prevent bacteria causing intracellular infection. However, they will not be effective once the infection is intracellular.

Cell-mediated immunity to intracellular bacteria

Cell-mediated immunity is very important in the defence against intracellular bacterial infections, such as those caused by *M. tuberculosis*:

- Macrophages attempt to phagocytose the bacteria. If the organisms persist, chronic inflammation will ensue. This can lead to delayed (type IV) hypersensitivity (see Chapter 12).
- Cells infected with bacteria can activate NK cells, which cause cytotoxicity and can activate macrophages.
- CD4+ T cells release cytokines that activate macrophages. This is predominantly Th1 cells, in contrast to the chiefly Th2 cell response to extracellular bacteria.
- CD8+ T cells recognize bacterial antigens presented in conjunction with MHC class I molecules on the surface of any infected nucleated cell and lyse these cells.

Examples of bacterial strategies to avoid immunity

Bacterial strategies to avoid the immune response must allow one of the following:

1. Escape from phagocyte responses

Examples include: (i) the inhibition of phagocytosis by capsule formation (e.g., *S. pneumoniae*, *Haemophilus*), (ii) toxin-mediated cell destruction (e.g., *Staphylococcus*), (iii) reduction of leucocyte infiltration (e.g., *P. aeruginosa*), (iv) stimulation of pro-apoptotic pathways (e.g., *Shigella* and *Salmonella*), (v) disruption of host cell cytoskeleton, preventing bacterial intake (e.g., *Yersinia*), etc.

2. Resistance to humoral defence mechanisms

This is achieved by inhibition of the release of chemotactic molecules and formation of MAC (e.g., *S. pyogenes* and *Streptococcus pneumoniae*) and by secretion of proteases that degrade complement factors (such as C1q, C3, C4 and C5-9).

3. Bacterial interference with cytokine secretion

A great example is mycobacteria, which produce immunosuppressive molecules, such as IL-10 and TGF-β, inhibiting T-cell activation. They also promote the generation of T-regulatory cells, which further suppress immune responses.

4. Bacterial interference with antigen presentation

This is achieved by expressing proteins that are inefficiently presented by MHC (e.g., *S. enterica*) and by downregulating expression of MHC class II and CD1 molecules (e.g., *Mycobacteria* and *Chlamydia*).

5. Inhibiting T- and B-cell effector functions

This is achieved by: (I) induction of FAS-FASL medicated apoptosis on T cells (e.g., *H. Pylori*), (ii) inhibiting/dysregulating host receptor signal transduction machinery (e.g., *Neisseria gonorrhoeae*).

Immune response to protozoal infection

Protozoa are microscopic, single-celled organisms. Fewer than 20 types of protozoa infect humans, although malaria, trypanosomes and *Leishmania* cause significant morbidity and mortality globally. Protozoa cause intracellular infection, have marked antigenic variation and are often immunosuppressive. They have complex life cycles with several different stages and, therefore, present the immune system with a variety of challenges. Protozoal infection is often chronic, as the immune system is not very efficient at dealing with these organisms. Most of the pathology of protozoal disease is caused by the immune response.

Humoral immunity against protozoa

Complement and antibody are important during the extracellular stage of infection. This opsonizes the protozoa and can cause lysis or prevent infection.

Cell-mediated immunity against protozoa

- *Phagocytosis* by macrophages, monocytes and neutrophils is an important part of the immune response against protozoa.
- *CD4+ T cells* are activated in response to protozoal infection. Th1 cytokines, such as IL-2, IFN-γ and TNF-β, are considered protective.
- *Cytotoxic CD8+ T cells* are important in destroying protozoa that replicate within cells, for example, the sporozoite stage of *Plasmodium falciparum* (which causes malaria).
- *NK cells and mast cells* are often activated in protozoal infection.

Examples of protozoal infection and evasion of the immune response

Protozoa have good mechanisms to prevent the initiation of an immune response. Strategies include:

- Escape into the cytoplasm following phagocytosis, for example, *Trypanosoma cruzi*
- Prevention of complement actions, for example, *Leishmania* spp.
- Gene switching to create antigen variation, for example, trypanosomes
- Immunosuppression, for example, trypanosomes

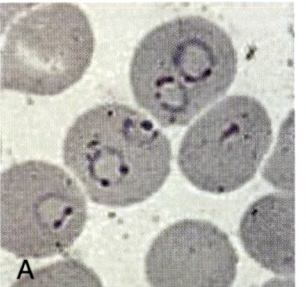
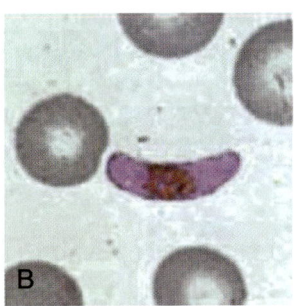

Fig. 11.6 Blood film showing presence of *Plasmodium falciparum* within the red blood cells. (A) Small ring forms. (B) A crescentic gametocyte with centrally placed chromatin. (From Pedigo RA, Blair TE, O'Connell TX. *USMLE Step 3 Secrets*. 2nd ed. Elsevier Inc.; 2023).

CLINICAL NOTES

Systemic protozoal infection normally presents with nonspecific symptoms: *Plasmodium* infection (malaria) can present with malaise, fever (classically in bouts on alternating days), headache, vomiting and diarrhoea (Fig. 11.6). The key feature of the history is recent travel to regions in which malaria is endemic, highlighting the importance of taking a comprehensive history!

Immune response to worms

Multicellular parasites and worms pose a different problem to the immune system, as they are too large to be phagocytosed by macrophages and neutrophils. These worms tend to live on mucosal surfaces and the immune system tries to dispose of these parasites by facilitating their expulsion. The immune system does this by secreting toxic chemicals onto mucosal surfaces, stimulating an increase in mucus secretion and smooth muscle contraction, which together result in expulsion of the worm.

Mast cells are stationed in tissues and have a similar sentinel purpose as macrophages for other types of infection. Mast cells contain preformed granules and when they recognize parasitic infection through cross-linkage of IgE or possibly Toll-like receptors, they degranulate, releasing their preformed granules. They also release proinflammatory cytokines that recruit eosinophils and basophils.

Mast cell preformed granules contain:

- Histamine: causes smooth muscle in the walls of the gut to contract (expel the worm) and smooth muscle of blood vessels to relax.
- Proteolytic enzymes: activate the complement system including anaphylatoxins.

Mast cells also rapidly synthesize chemicals including PGs and LTs, both of which cause vasodilatation and contraction of smooth muscle in gut and bronchial walls.

Eosinophils secrete chemicals similar to those secreted by mast cells, excluding histamine. In addition, they secrete:

- Peroxidase, which generates hypochlorous acid

- A cationic protein, which damages the worm's outer layers and paralyzes its nervous system
- A basic protein that also attacks the outer layers of the worm

Mast cells can be activated by IgE and, although this likely evolved to deal with worm infections, it mediates allergy (type I hypersensitivity).

CLINICAL NOTES

When viewing the results of a full blood count, the WCC is often used as a gross marker of infection or inflammation in disease. The WCC differential, detailing the levels of each type of white blood cell, can give further information on the nature of the disease. For example, a raised neutrophil count (neutrophilia) in the presence of an acute illness would point to a bacterial infection, particularly a pyogenic infection (see Clinical notes on pyogenic infection in this chapter). A raised eosinophil count could be due to a parasitic infection or allergy. It is therefore important to remember the context of the illness in question.

● Chapter Summary

- Acute inflammation is triggered in response to physical/chemical damage or the detection of pathogens. It involves multiple cells and molecules, with the aim of healing and removal of the stimulus.
- Chronic inflammation occurs following incomplete resolution of acute inflammation, with the persistence of antigen. The cells involved are different from acute inflammation and can result in an array of chronic inflammatory diseases.
- The immune system prevents viruses entering body cells (humoral immunity) and kills virally infected body cells (cell-mediated immunity, humoral immunity aids in detection of infected cells).
- The immune response to bacterial infection depends on the nature of the pathogen. Extracellular bacteria are predominantly killed by humoral components and phagocytes. Intracellular bacteria require greater macrophage and T-cell involvement.
- Both humoral and cell-mediated branches of the immune system are involved in responding to protozoal infection, due to both intracellular and extracellular lifecycle stages.
- Multicellular parasites require a more specialized immune response, with a greater involvement of mast cells and eosinophils.

MLA Conditions

Malaria
Tuberculosis

MLA Presentations

Night sweats

HYPERSENSITIVITY

Hypersensitivity is an excessive and, therefore, inappropriate inflammatory response to any antigen. This inflammatory response results in tissue damage.

Hypersensitivity can occur in response to:

- An infection that cannot be cleared, for example tuberculosis
- A normally harmless exogenous substance, for example, pollen, resulting in allergy
- An autoantigen, for example, thyroid stimulating hormone (TSH) receptors in Graves disease, resulting in autoimmune disease

Classification of hypersensitivity

Hypersensitivity reactions have been classified, by Gell and Coombs, into four types (I, II, III and IV).[1] Types I, II and III are antibody mediated; type IV is cell mediated. In this system, the different types of hypersensitivity are classified by their time of onset after exposure to antigen. Despite the fact that a new classification has been proposed by Sell et al.,[2] reflecting the different immune components involved in each type, the former one has been widely adopted.

TYPE I HYPERSENSITIVITY (IMMEDIATE HYPERSENSITIVITY)

Type I hypersensitivity describes an immediate reaction, involving IgE antibodies against a target antigen. It can be briefly divided into three phases:

(i) Sensitization: This occurs when the immune system is first exposed to an antigen, resulting in the production of IgE antibodies. These antibodies bind to the Fc portion of tissue mast cells and circulating basophils.

(ii) Activation: Reexposure to the same antigen causes cross-linking of the mast cell surface IgE molecules, which triggers the mast cells and basophils to release their granules and initiate the next phase.

(iii) Effector phase: This phase describes the result of the mast cell and basophil degranulation and includes the following:

- dilatation of small blood vessels and bronchoconstriction (histamine)

- inhibition of coagulation (heparin)
- arterial vasoconstriction (serotonin)
- platelet adherence to blood vessel wall
- capillary leak, smooth muscle constriction, platelet activation and attraction of granulocytes (prostaglandin and leukotriene).

The presence of a 'wheal and flare' reaction (red, inflamed skin bumps) is the hallmark of type I (IgE-medicated) hypersensitivity. Other clinical manifestations include bronchospasm and wheezing with hypoxia, rhinitis, abdominal pain/cramping, vasodilation with potential hypovolaemia/hypotension and increased vascular permeability with pulmonary or generalized oedema. As such, affected individuals may experience a wide spectrum of symptoms, from pruritus to asthma attack and systemic anaphylaxis.

COMMON PITFALLS

Allergy is synonymous with type I hypersensitivity, but not all hypersensitivity reactions are allergies, for example, type II, III and IV hypersensitivities are not allergies.

Type I hypersensitivities include:

(i) atopic diseases: they refer to an amplified IgE-mediated immune response (e.g., asthma, rhinitis, conjunctivitis, dermatitis) and

(ii) allergic diseases: they refer to an immune response to an allergen (e.g., food and drug allergies, angioedema, urticaria, anaphylaxis). Common allergens are shown in Table 12.1.

Certain risk factors have been described to predispose to the development of allergic diseases, such as socioeconomic status, geographical distribution and genetic predisposition. This is nicely reflected in the 'hygiene hypothesis', which describes an immune dysfunction resulting from the lack of exposure to antigens and microbes in the natural environment in early life. This reduced childhood exposure to biodiverse microorganisms has resulted in a steady increase in the prevalence of allergic disorders and chronic inflammatory conditions in urban populations.

The immune mechanisms and development of type I reactions are illustrated in Fig. 12.1.

Table 12.1 Summary of allergic reactions

Allergic condition	Common allergens	Features
Systemic anaphylaxis	Drugs (e.g., antibiotics, anaesthetics) Bee and wasp venoms Peanuts	Oedema with increased vascular permeability leads to tracheal occlusion, circulatory collapse and possibly death
Allergic rhinitis	Pollen (hay fever) Dust-mite faeces (perennial rhinitis)	Sneezing, oedema and irritation of nasal mucosa
Allergic asthma	Pollen Dust-mite faeces	Bronchial constriction, increased mucus production, airway inflammation
Food	Shellfish Milk Eggs Fish Wheat	Itching, urticaria and potentially anaphylaxis
Atopic eczema	Pollen Dust-mite faeces Some foods	Itchy inflammation of the skin

CLINICAL NOTES

Atopy is a genetic predisposition to produce IgE in response to many common, naturally occurring allergens, especially inhaled allergens and food allergens. It has a prevalence of 10–30%. Atopic patients can suffer from multiple allergies. Although atopy tends to run in families, the genetic basis of atopy is currently unknown.

When diagnosing type I hypersensitivity, the most important part of the history is the timing of allergic symptoms in response to a trigger, as the effects of allergy occur rapidly – within minutes – and the prior history of allergic reactions and history of atopy or food allergies.

For an allergic reaction to occur, IgE against that specific allergen needs to be present. This can be tested for by using skin prick testing, where a small amount of the suspected allergen is inoculated into the skin together with a positive and a negative control (see Fig. 12.2). A positive reaction will result in an itchy red lesion with a wheal at the centre; the reaction is strongest after

Initial sensitization

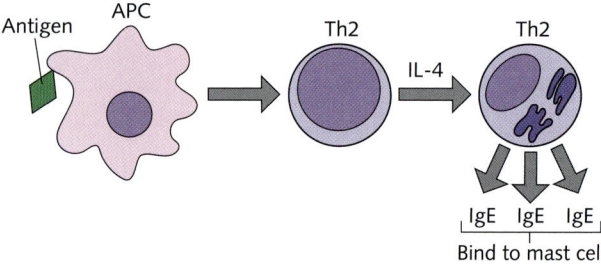

Allergic reaction

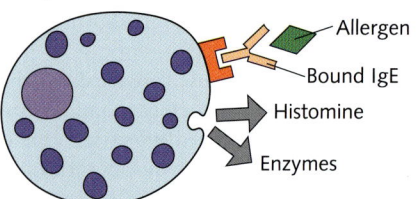

Fig. 12.1 The development and mechanisms of type I hypersensitivity reactions. APCs present antigen to Th2 cells, which in turn stimulate B cells to produce large amounts of IgE for that antigen. This IgE then binds to cell surface receptors on mast cells and basophils. Cross-linkage of this bound IgE results in degranulation.
APC, Antigen-presenting cell; *Th,* T helper.

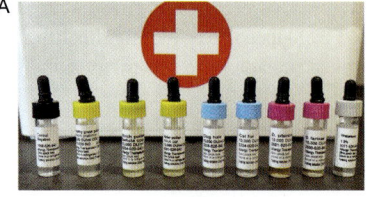

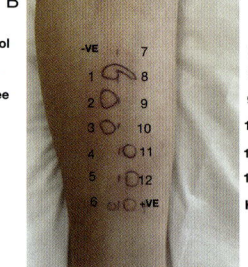

Diluent negative control		
1. Timothy grass		7. Cat
2. Silver Birch tree		8. Cockroach
3. Alder		9. Aspergillus fumigatus
4. Plane tree		10. Alternaria alternata
5. Mugwort		11. Dermatophagoides pteronyssinus
6. Dog dander		12. Dermatophagoides farinae
		Histamine positive control

Fig. 12.2 Skin prick testing. The appearance of an itchy wheal, within a short period of time, indicates a positive result. From this figure, positive and negative controls are visible along with the test for reaction to peanut, almond, hazelnut showing a reaction to peanut. The results should be interpreted in conjunction with the history. Skin prick testing is not advisable in severe allergy. (Source: Encyclopedia of Respiratory Medicine, Second Edition, 2022)

15–20 minutes, indicating that the patient produces IgE to the tested allergen. Serum IgE can also be directly measured using a blood test. A limit of 0.35 kilounits of allergen-specific IgE per litre (kU/L) has been established as the cut-off limit for a positive test result in the clinical use. It is of note that measuring total IgE levels, as opposed to specific IgE, is of little diagnostic value, as various factors, such as viruses, air pollutants, may stimulate the production of IgE, without initiating an allergic reaction.

The type of treatment required for type I hypersensitivities depends on the clinical manifestation and the aetiology of the reaction. More specifically, in the case of anaphylaxis, emergency treatment with epinephrine, bronchodilators, antihistamines and corticosteroids is mandated. Supportive therapy with oxygenation, IV fluids for volume resuscitation and vasopressors for refractory hypotension may also be necessitated with close monitoring of oxygen saturation, blood pressure, heart and respiratory status and urine output (see 'Diseases caused by type I hypersensitivity reactions' for more details).

Diseases caused by type I hypersensitivity reactions

Asthma

Asthma is a chronic inflammatory disorder of the airways, characterized by reversible airflow obstruction. The airways become hyperresponsive and exaggerated bronchoconstriction follows a wide variety of nonimmunological stimuli, for example, exercise or cold air. The symptoms of asthma are dry cough, wheeze, chest tightness and shortness of breath, which tend to be worse at night. Asthma is a common disease and is diagnosed in 5–10% of children. The incidence has risen over the last few decades, particularly in more economically developed countries.

Pollens, house-dust mite faeces and airborne proteins from domestic animals are the most common allergens in asthma. These cause chronic inflammation of the bronchial wall, resulting in the characteristic airway hyperresponsiveness and bronchoconstriction. Histological findings include:

- Infiltration by eosinophils, mast cells, lymphocytes and neutrophils
- Oedema of the submucosa
- Smooth muscle hypertrophy and hyperplasia
- Thickening of the basement membrane
- Mucous plugging
- Epithelial desquamation

Asthma is diagnosed clinically by the presence of the above symptoms, supported by the finding of a reversal in airway obstruction of ≥15% (measured by peak expiratory flow rate or 'peak flow'), either spontaneously or after the administration of an inhaled short-acting β_2-adrenoreceptor agonist (SABA) such as salbutamol. Advice should be given, including avoidance of triggers and how to manage an attack. SABAs are used, as

required, for the short-term improvement of symptoms and inhaled corticosteroids (such as beclomethasone dipropionate) are started as a regular preventative therapy. Other immunosuppressive/antiinflammatory drugs can be considered if symptoms persist or if SABAs are used regularly. This is according to the British Thoracic Society's step-wise approach.[3]

Allergic rhinitis

Nasal congestion, watery nasal discharge and sneezing occur after exposure to allergen. The most common allergens are grass, flower, weed or tree pollens, which cause a seasonal rhinitis (hay fever), and house-dust mite faeces, which can cause a more perennial (year-round) rhinitis. Allergic attacks usually last for a few hours and are often accompanied by itching and watering of the eyes. Skin prick tests can identify the allergen.

The most important treatment is topical (nasal) antihistamines or steroids; additionally systemic antihistamines such as loratadine are used. Avoidance of allergens is advised but is often difficult. Grass pollen immunotherapy is increasingly being used to treat severe seasonal rhinitis (see Chapter 10).

Atopic/allergic eczema

Eczema (dermatitis) is a skin rash that is a result of superficial skin inflammation. It can be triggered by allergens, hence a type I hypersensitivity response, or through sustained contact with other substances, commonly nickel. The latter is termed 'contact dermatitis' and is a type IV hypersensitivity response (see later section on type IV hypersensitivity).

True atopic eczema is most commonly the result of exposure to pollen or house-dust mite faeces. About 10% of children are diagnosed with eczema. The pathophysiology of atopic eczema is thought to be a breakdown in the skin's barrier function, allowing the entry of allergens; atopic eczema is linked to mutations in the filaggrin gene (see later section on development of hypersensitivity). Eczema commonly affects the flexural creases and the fronts of the wrist and ankles. In infancy, the face and trunk are often also involved. Eczematous skin lesions are itchy, erythematous (red), sometimes vesicular and might be dry (see Fig. 12.3). Because of itching, the skin is often excoriated, which can lead to lichenification (thickening of the skin). Eczema is often complicated by superinfection with bacteria, particularly *Staphylococcus aureus*.

The diagnosis of atopic eczema is usually clinical, based on the atopic history and appearance of the rash. Total serum IgE, specific IgE levels and skin prick testing with common allergens are occasionally performed to confirm the diagnosis of atopic eczema. Treatment of eczema is mainly topical, except in more severe cases, when systemic steroids and immunosuppressants are used. Therapies include:

- Emollients: moisturizes dry skin, replacing the lost barrier against allergens
- Topical steroids: antiinflammatory

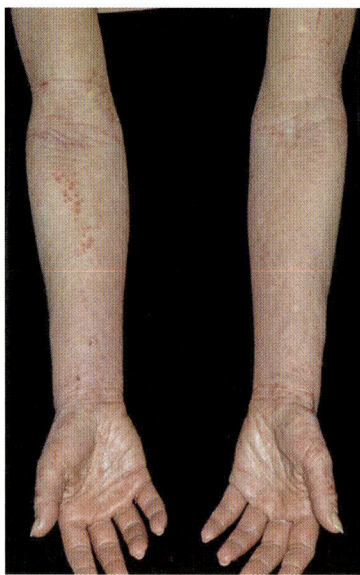

Fig. 12.3 Appearance of an eczematous rash on the arms of an adult. Note the erythematous, raised patches with some excoriation, suggesting itchiness. (Reprinted with permission from Bolognia, JL, Jorizzo, JJ, Schaffer, JV et al. *Dermatology*. 3rd ed. Elsevier.)

- Topical antibiotics or antiseptics: in infected eczema
- Oral antihistamine: reduces itching
- Ciclosporin: resistant cases may require immunosuppression

Anaphylaxis

Anaphylaxis is a life-threatening, generalized hypersensitivity reaction. It is caused by a systemic response to an allergen that is either intravenous (IV) or quickly absorbed. This results in distributive shock and laryngeal occlusion; increased vascular permeability and dilatation lead to a large amount of fluid moving from the circulation into tissues. The subsequent rapid fall in blood pressure and airway occlusion through oedema can be fatal. Many allergens can cause anaphylaxis, but more common environmental causes include bee stings and peanuts. Many cases of anaphylaxis take place in hospital where they may be triggered by antibiotics, latex or anaesthetic drugs. The signs of anaphylaxis are principally the same as those of shock. Signs include:

- Hypotension with tachycardia
- Warm peripheral temperature
- Signs of airway obstruction such as stridor (a harsh and loud sound heard during exhalation)
- Facial oedema and urticaria (often seen)

The management of anaphylaxis, as per the Resuscitation Council (UK) guidelines, should be known by all medical professionals. The initial management of anaphylaxis is resuscitation, that is, attend to life-threatening airway, breathing and/or circulatory problems. Allergens should be removed if possible, for example, by stopping drug infusion. Adrenaline (epinephrine) should be given intramuscularly (IM) as soon as possible. The dose for adults is 500 μg (0.5 mL of 1:1000) and should be repeated after 5 minutes if there is no improvement. Adrenaline should be given intravenously only by a specialist and in environments where monitoring is possible and at a low dose. An IV fluid challenge of between 500 and 1000 mL should be given next to correct hypotension. Chlorphenamine (an antihistamine) and hydrocortisone are also given later (Fig. 12.4). Mast cell tryptase, an enzyme released from degranulating mast cells, is elevated after anaphylaxis. Blood samples taken after an attack can have mast cell tryptase levels measured to confirm the diagnosis of anaphylaxis (see Chapter 9).

The National Institute for Clinical Excellence requires that any patient who suffers from a proven or suspected anaphylactic reaction should be seen in an allergy clinic by a specialist. They should receive advice regarding future attacks, as well as training on how to administer intramuscular adrenaline. They should carry a preloaded adrenaline syringe for such occasions and always wear a MedicAlert bracelet.

TYPE II HYPERSENSITIVITY

Type II hypersensitivity occurs when antibody specific for cell surface antigens is produced, hence it is said to be antibody mediated. Unlike type I reactions where membrane-bound IgE antibodies interact with antigens, type II hypersensitivity circulating antibodies interact with cell-surface antigens. Furthermore, the antigens in type II reactions are rarely harmless. The antibodies are instead produced against infected target cells (microbial antigens) or against self-antigens, leading to autoimmune disorders (such as Goodpasture syndrome and Graves disease). Molecular mimicry refers to similarities between foreign and self-peptides, leading to cross-activation of lymphocytes, complement activation and inflammation. A nice example of molecular mimicry is rheumatic fever, in which the streptococcal antigens structurally resemble ('mimic') cardiac myosin, resulting in cross-reactivity of antibodies against streptococcal and cardiac antigens, leading to heart damage (the mitral valve is the most commonly affected heart tissue).

The most common cause of type II hypersensitivity is medications (such as penicillin, cephalosporins and thiazides). The drug molecule either binds to cell surface, generating a neoantigen or modifies existing epitopes of self-antigens, resulting in immune

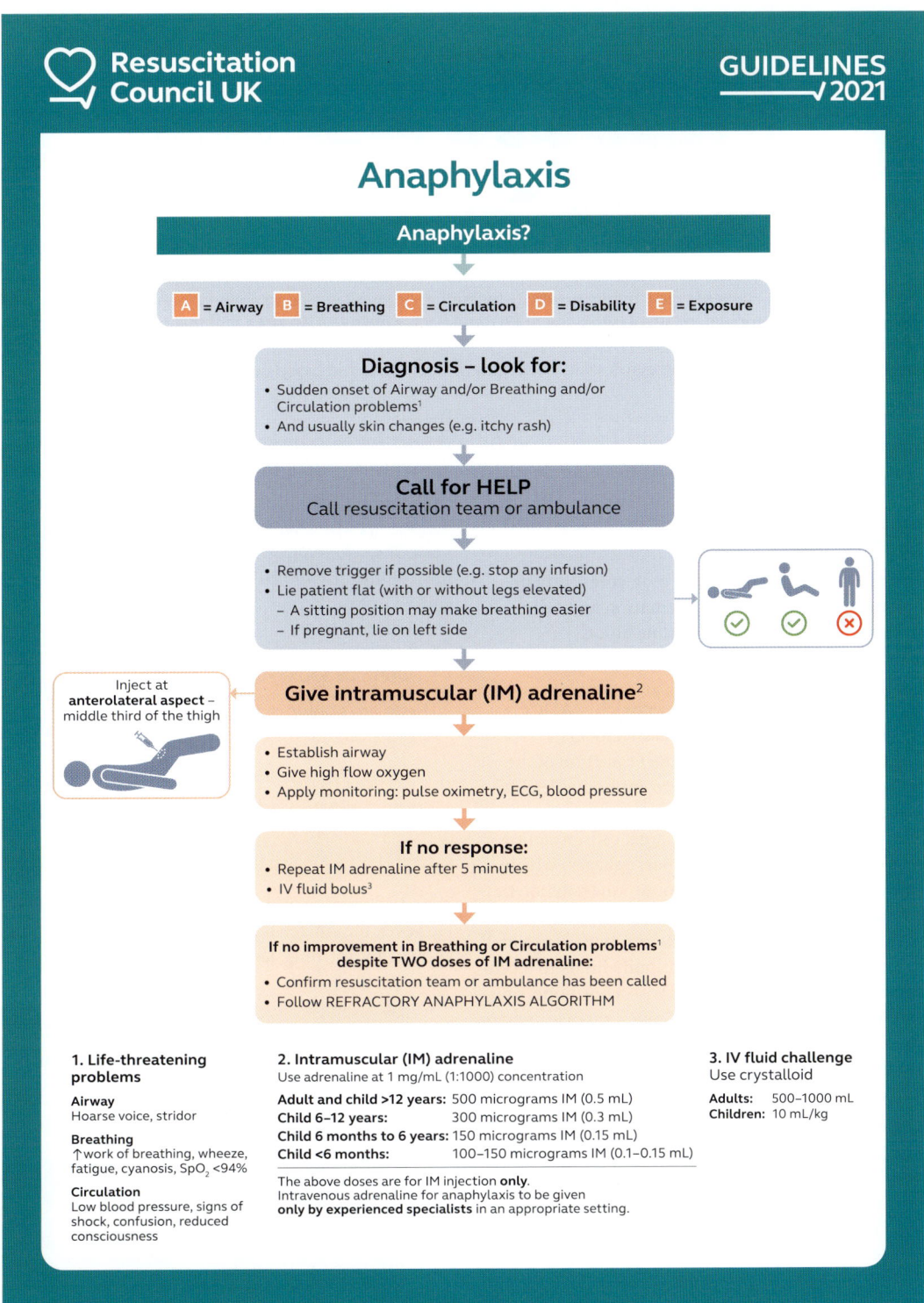

Fig. 12.4 Anaphylaxis algorithm. *ECG*, Electrocardiogram; *IM*, intramuscular; *IV*, intravenous. (Reproduced with the kind permission of Resuscitation Council UK)

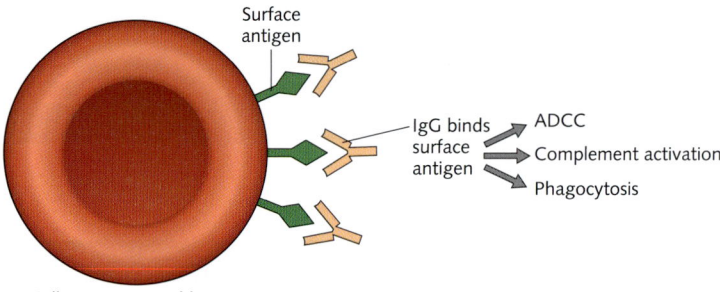

Fig. 12.5 The immune mechanisms of type II hypersensitivity reactions. Antibodies bind to antigen found on the surface of cells resulting in cell death via (1) complement, (2) phagocytes or (3) natural killer cells ADCC. Note that this can also stimulate the cell, as in Graves disease.
ADCC, Antibody-dependent cell-mediated cytotoxicity; *NK*, natural killer; *RBC*, red blood cell.

recognition and attack of these 'modified' antigens. The immune mechanisms of type II hypersensitivity reactions are summarized in Fig. 12.5.

Cell destruction then results via mechanisms discussed in Chapters 9 and 10, including:

- Complement activation: IgG or IgM molecules activate the complement, leading to MAC formation and cell damage. Examples include incompatible blood transfusions (ABO mismatch) and haemolytic disease of the newborn.
- Antibody-dependent cell-mediated cytotoxicity (ADCC): Antibody binding to target cells attracts effector cells (natural killer cells) which recognize the Fc portion of the antibody. Natural killer (NK) binding to antibodies leads to degranulation and cell lysis.
- Phagocytosis: IgG molecules coat the target cell, attracting phagocytes (such as neutrophils and macrophages) which destroy the cell. Examples include autoimmune haemolytic anaemia and immune thrombocytopenia.

However, not all type II hypersensitivity reactions lead to cell destruction. This is the case when the antibody binds to a cell-surface receptor, which normally interacts with a hormone, causing cell dysfunction. An example is Graves disease, where autoantibodies bind to the thyrotropin receptor, driving an over-production of thyroid hormones.

Graves disease

Graves disease is the most common cause of hyperthyroidism. It arises as a result of IgG autoantibody production against TSH receptor in the thyroid gland. The anti-TSH receptor antibody activates the receptor, resulting in increased thyroxine production.

Graves disease affects 1–2% of females. The female:male ratio is 5:1. There is a strong association with human leucocyte antigen (HLA) DR3 in Caucasian people.

CLINICAL FEATURES OF GRAVES DISEASE

Graves disease is associated with the symptoms and signs of hyperthyroidism, as well as some eye signs that occur exclusively in Graves disease (secondary to periorbital inflammation):

- Exophthalmos
- Lid retraction
- Lid lag
- Ophthalmoplegia

These are shown in Fig. 12.6.

TYPE III HYPERSENSITIVITY (IMMUNE COMPLEX)

Type III hypersensitivity reactions are also antibody mediated. However, the antigen is soluble. Antibodies react to soluble (free) antigen by forming lattices of antibody and antigen, termed

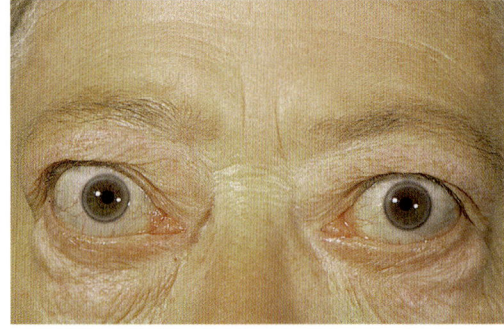

Fig. 12.6 The eye signs associated with Graves disease: lid retraction and exophthalmos.

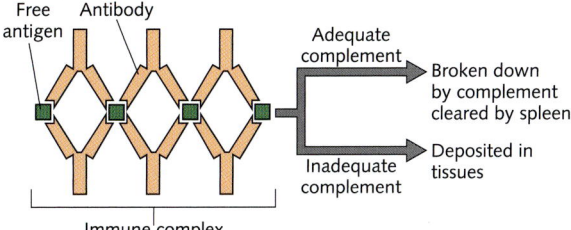

Fig. 12.7 The immune mechanisms of type III hypersensitivity reactions. Immune complexes that are normally broken down by complement and cleared in the spleen are deposited in blood vessels or tissues resulting in severe damage via complement and neutrophils.

'immune complexes'. This is a physiological response and is use-ful, for example, in the removal of soluble bacterial exotoxin.

If there is a rapid influx of soluble antigen or if there is a sig-nificant amount of antigen, the clearance mechanisms can become overwhelmed. The remaining immune complexes are deposited in tissues, such as skin, joints, kidneys (glomeruli) and vessels and activate the complement (classical pathway). This in turn leads to recruitment of inflammatory cells (particularly monocytes and neutrophils) that release cytokines and enzymes, causing tissue damage (Fig. 12.7).

Diseases caused by type III hypersensitivity reactions

The most common examples of type III hypersensitivity reaction include serum sickness, post–streptococcal glomerulonephritis, systemic lupus erythematosus (SLE), Farmer disease and rheu-matoid arthritis (RA). As mentioned before, the formation of antigen-antibody complexes in the circulation, prior to tissue deposition constitutes the key difference between type III and the other hypersensitivity reactions.

SERUM SICKNESS

Serum sickness results from the formation of immune complexes between human and heterologous (nonhuman) proteins. The most common causes of serum sickness are medications containing heterologous antigens (such as antithymocyte globulin and immune modulating agents) and vaccinations (e.g., rabies). Serum sickness is characterized by the triad of fever, rash and arthritis (or polyarthralgias). The symptoms typically occur 6–12 days after the exposure to an offensive agent (owing to the time required for antibody production and formation of immune complexes). However, symptoms may develop much faster (within a few days) if a person has been previously exposed to the antigen. Serum sickness is a self-limiting process that usually resolves

within several weeks after discontinuation of the relevant culprit. Thus, treatment is supportive aiming at reducing symptom severity and removing (or reducing the exposure to) the offensive agent. Antihistamines and NSAIDs may be considered for moderate symptoms, whereas for more severe cases a 7- to 10-day course of glucocorticoids (0.5–2 mg/kg) can be helpful.

Serum sickness is not to be confused with a serum sickness-like reaction (caused by medications, such as cephalosporins and penicillin and certain infections, such as streptococcus and hepatitis B) that have similar clinical symptoms, but are not correlated with immune-complex formation (there is no complement activation and C3/C4 levels are normal).

Type III hypersensitivity can occur locally or systemically. Systemic type III hypersensitivity reactions occur when there is a large amount of antigen present throughout the body; this can occur when antigens such as antibiotics are injected into the circulation or if the antigen is an autoantigen (an autoimmune reaction).

POST–STREPTOCOCCAL GLOMERULONEPHRITIS

Post–streptococcal glomerulonephritis is an important, systemic nonautoimmune type III hypersensitivity reaction. Antigen produced by β-haemolytic Streptococcus forms antigen-antibody complexes. These complexes are deposited in the glomeruli, producing an acute glomerulonephritis. This classically presents in children, 1–2 weeks after a sore throat (the source of the Streptococcus antigen), with oedema, hypertension, haematuria and proteinuria (Fig. 12.8).

Systemic lupus erythematosus

An example of a systemic type III autoimmune disease is SLE. Patients with SLE have autoantibodies directed against DNA, histone proteins, red blood cells, platelets, leucocytes and clotting factors. These autoantibodies are also found in other autoimmune conditions; the most specific autoanti-body for SLE is anti–double-stranded DNA (anti-dsDNA). The sheer amount of corresponding autoantigen in the body means the production of large numbers of immune com-plexes is inevitable.

Deposition of immune complexes leads to the varied clinical features of SLE, including:

- Arthralgia (pain due to deposition in small joints)
- Rashes in sun-exposed areas (Fig. 12.9)
- Glomerulonephritis

Nonspecific systemic features such as fever, malaise and depression are often also present.

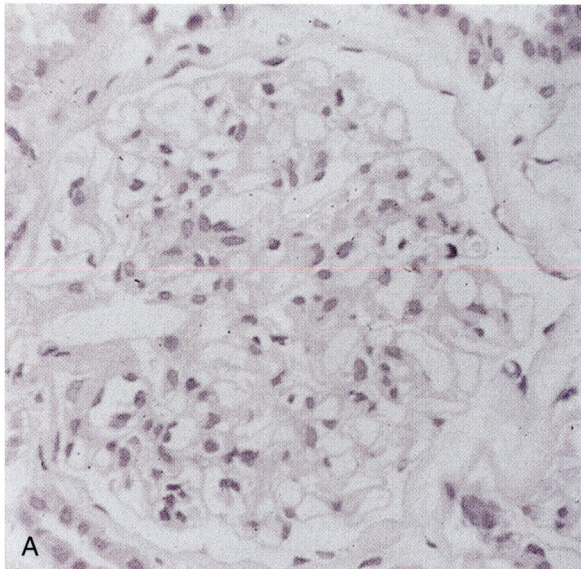

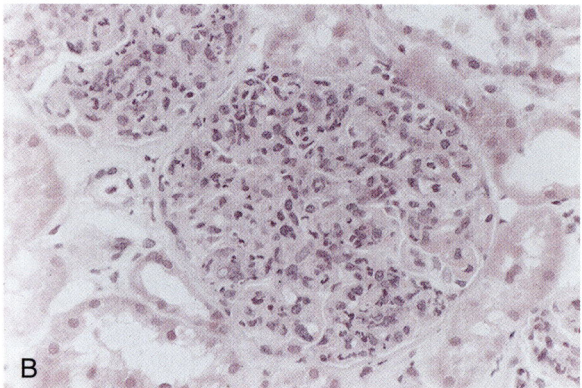

Fig. 12.8 Renal histology from biopsy specimen (light micrographs). (A) A normal glomerulus. (B) A glomerulus from a patient with a diffuse proliferative (poststreptococcal) glomerulonephritis. Note how 'full' the glomerulus appears with a great increase in the number of cells due to inflammation. (Renal Nursing, Third Edition, 2008)

Diagnosis is by antinuclear antibody (ANA) testing. Serum complement levels (C3 and C4) are low in active disease, secondary to their role in breaking apart immune complexes. It is most commonly diagnosed in women in the second or third decade of life.

The aetiology is unknown, but the vast array of autoantibodies present suggests a breakdown in self-tolerance. Genetic factors predispose to the disease; there is an association with HLA-DR2 and HLA-DR3 and with deficiencies of complement proteins, especially C2 or C4 (reduced complement levels result in a decreased ability to clear immune complexes). Other relevant aetiological factors include drugs such as hydralazine, exposure to ultraviolet light and oestrogens.

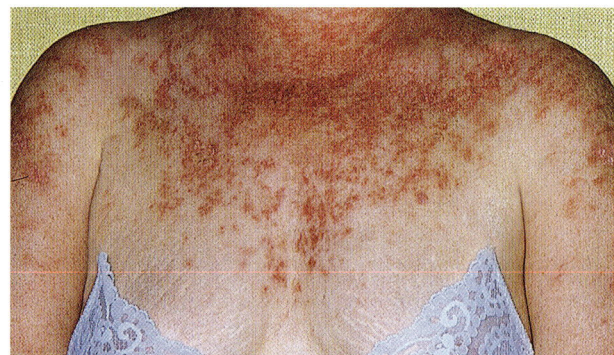

Fig. 12.9 A photosensitive skin rash consistent with systemic lupus erythematosus. (Mosby's Pathology for Massage Therapists, Second Edition, 2009.)

Systemic lupus erythematosus is treated with immunosuppression (aimed at reducing auto-antibody production), steroids, NSAIDs or other antiinflammatory drugs.

HINTS AND TIPS

The more common clinical features of SLE can be remembered with the mnemonic 'A RASH POINts MD':

Arthralgia in the small joints, for example, metacarpophalangeal

Renal disease, for example, glomerulonephritis

Antinuclear antibody: ANA positivity is a nonspecific indicator

Serositis such as pericarditis, pleural effusion

Haematological abnormality: anaemia, lymphopaenia

Photosensitivity: burn easily after UV exposure

Oral ulcers, frequent

Immunological markers such as anti-dsDNA + ve

Neurological disorders such as epilepsy, migraine, ataxia, meningism, psychosis

Malar rash across the cheeks and nose, sparing the nasolabial folds

Discoid rash: erythematous, scaly, round patches

Four or more of these features in a history would be suggestive of SLE.

COMMON PITFALLS

Type II hypersensitivity is based on antibodies (IgG) binding to cell-surface antigens, resulting in cell destruction. However, type III hypersensitivity occurs when antibodies bind free antigen. They form immune complexes that can cause tissue damage if present in excessive amounts.

TYPE IV HYPERSENSITIVITY (DELAYED-TYPE HYPERSENSITIVITY)

Type IV hypersensitivity describes a reaction that takes place days after exposure to antigen. It is primarily mediated by $CD4^+$ T cells, predominantly Th1, and other lymphocytes. Upon first contact with antigen, macrophages present the antigen to Th cells, which are then activated and clonally expanded (this takes 1–2 weeks). Upon subsequent encounter with the same antigen, the sensitized Th cells secrete cytokines. These attract and activate macrophages, which account for more than 95% of the cells involved in type IV hypersensitivity reactions. The type IV reaction peaks at 48–72 hours after subsequent contact with the antigen (time taken for the recruitment and activation of the macrophages), hence it is also termed 'delayed-type hypersensitivity'. An overview of the immune mechanisms involved is given in Fig. 12.10.

Type IV reactions are important for the clearance of intracellular pathogens, such as mycobacteria and fungi. However, if antigens persist, the response can be detrimental to the individual, as the lytic products of the activated macrophages can damage healthy tissues.

There are three subtypes of type IV hypersensitivity reactions:

(i) Contact dermatitis: occurs when allergens penetrate the skin, causing an inflammatory reaction. Clinically, this manifests as an erythematous purpuric rash, with swelling, which may progress to vesicle and bullae formation. When these rupture, a crust is formed. Common culprits include gloves, acrylics and other chemicals, preservatives and clothing (Fig. 12.11a).

(ii) Tuberculin type: occurs after intradermal injection of tuberculin, which causes local induration and redness (Fig. 12.11b).

(iii) Granulomatous type: occurs in response to engulfed antigens that cannot be cleared by macrophages, attracting more macrophages to the site, leading to granuloma (a collection of macrophages with engulfed antigens) formation. Typical examples of this type of hypersensitivity are sarcoidosis and tuberculosis (Fig. 12.11c).

STEVENS-JOHNSON SYNDROME/TOXIC EPIDERMAL NECROLYSIS

This is a rare, acute, life-threatening condition presenting with severe skin and mucosal necrosis (resembling that of a third-degree burn) and hypovolaemic shock, due to third space losses. Medications such as sulpha drugs, anticonvulsants and NSAIDs are the most common implicated agents (>80% cases).

Evaluation includes skin biopsy, full blood count, liver and renal function tests and assessment of pulmonary (CXR) and heart (ECG/echo) function. The treatment requires a multi-disciplinary approach, with admission to an intensive care unit and a focus on supportive care (cessation of the suspected culprit, fluid replacement, pain relief, meticulous skincare with daily examination). High-dose corticosteroids are also given for the first 3–5 days, although it remains unknown whether they offer any benefit. Antibiotics are also given, if there is a secondary infection, but not prophylactically.

As with type I reactions, skin testing is used to detect type IV reactions. Instead of a skin prick, however, patch testing is used to diagnose antigens causing delayed hypersensitivity in contact dermatitis. A selection of sensitizing antigens are normally tested at the same time. They are usually placed in a grid pattern on the upper back and then dressed. Patients are then seen, sometimes more than once, over the next 48–72 hours to assess the response. The response varies from no response to an extreme reaction.

The tuberculin skin test can be used to determine whether a person has been exposed to *M. tuberculosis*. An intradermal injection of purified protein derivative (PPD) is given to the individual. Previous exposure to *M. tuberculosis* or bacille Calmette–Guérin (BCG) vaccination results in a positive response. This is apparent as a firm, red (due to the intense infiltration of macrophages) lesion at the injection site 48–72 hours after the injection. The skin lesions in both contact dermatitis and tuberculin testing are composed of macrophages and T cells.

A summary of the four types of hypersensitivity is shown in Table 12.2 and a summary of important autoimmune diseases is given in Tables 12.3–12.5.

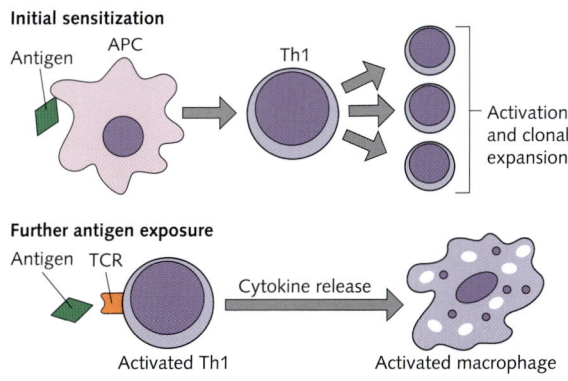

Fig. 12.10 The immune mechanisms of type IV hypersensitivity reactions. Antigens are first presented to Th1 cells, which are then activated. These Th1 cells can then activate macrophages. Type IV hypersensitivity reactions take several days to be initiated because of the various cells that are involved. *APC*, Antigen-presenting cell; *Th*, T helper.

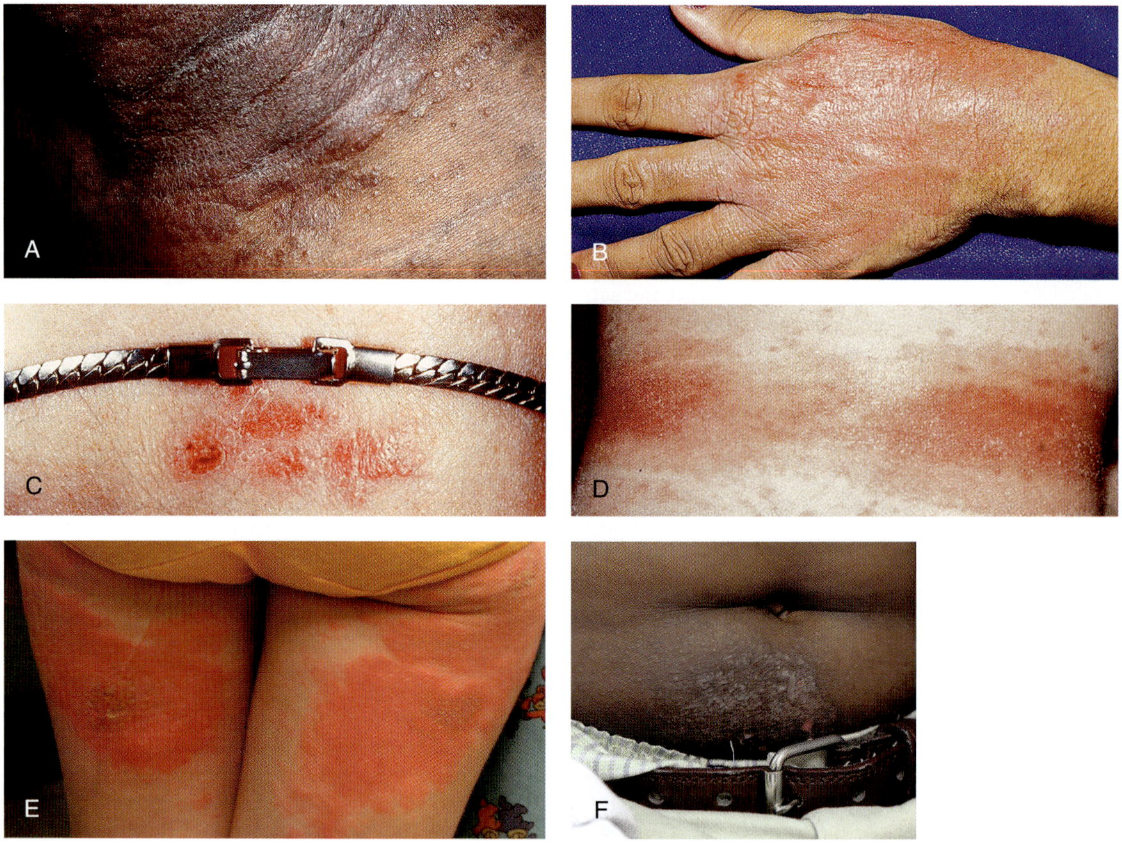

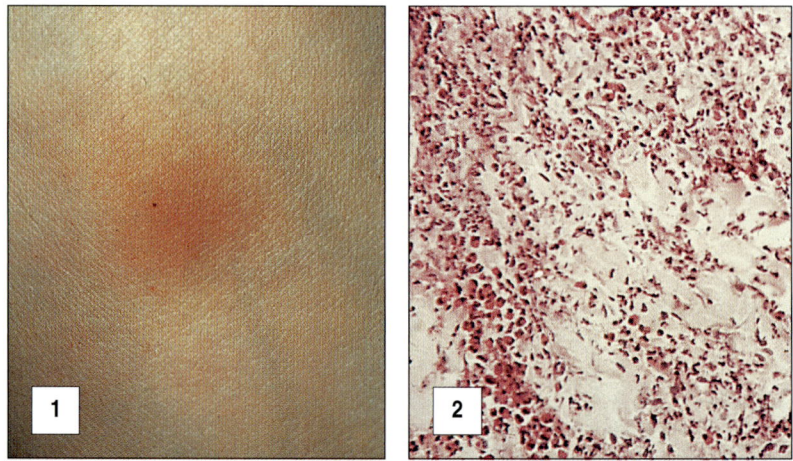

Fig. 12.11a Allergic Contact Dermatitis. Benzocaine reaction on (A) the neck and (B) the top of the hand. Nickel allergy on (C) the wrist. Elastic waistband reaction in (D). The itchy dermatitis in (E) was secondary to school toilet seat. Chronic contact dermatitis from a nickel belt buckle (F). (From Cohen BA, editor. Pediatric Dermatology. 5th ed. Elsevier; 2022.)

Fig. 12.11b Clinical and histological appearances of tuberculin-type sensitivity. The response to an injection of leprosy bacillus into a sensitized individual is known as the Fernandez reaction. The reaction is characterized by an area of firm red swelling of the skin and is maximal 48–72 hours after challenge (1). Histologically (2), there is a dense dermal infiltrate of leukocytes. H&E stain. × 80.

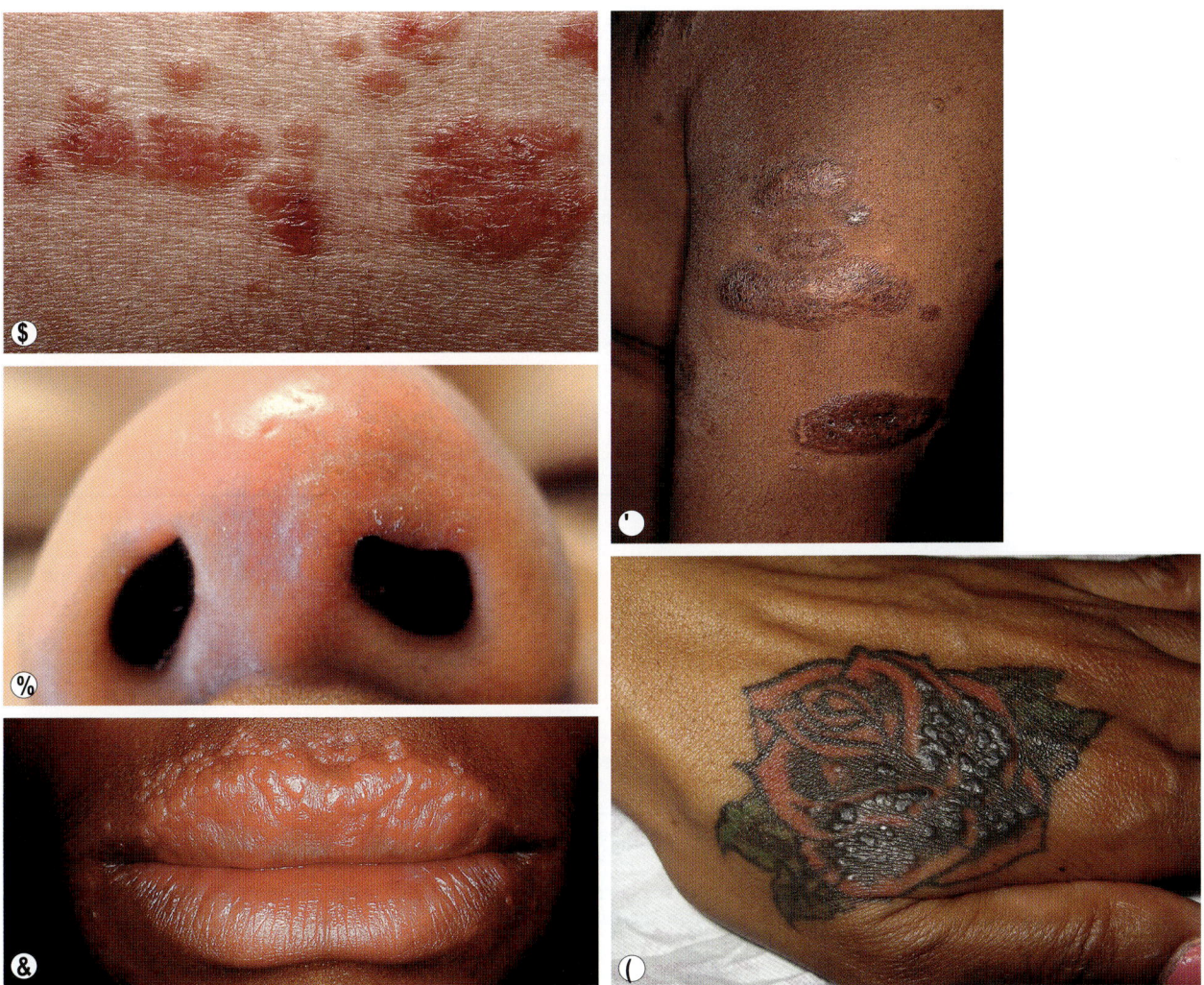

Fig. 12.11c Cutaneous sarcoidosis – papules and plaques. (A) Cutaneous sarcoidosis usually consists of papules and plaques with a typical reddish-brown to violet–brown color. (B, C) Lesions often favor the nose, lips and perioral region. (D) Hyperpigmented plaques, some of which have scale. (E) Papules of cutaneous sarcoidosis arising within a tattoo; the differential diagnosis includes foreign body reaction. (From Jean L. Bolognia, Lorenzo Cerroni, Julie V. Schaffer, *Dermatology: 2-Volume Set*, Fourth Edition, 2018. A , C , D Courtesy of the Yale Dermatology Residents' Slide Collection.)

Table 12.2 Summary of the different types of hypersensitivity

Type of hypersensitivity	Immune mediators	Time of onset	Examples
Type I	IgE, mast cells, eosinophils	Immediate (if IgE is preformed)	Anaphylaxis, asthma, atopic eczema
Type II	Antibody (normally IgG), complement, phagocytes	Rapid (if IgG is preformed)	Haemolytic disease of the newborn, ABO incompatibility
Type III	IgG, complement and neutrophils	Hours	SLE, Farmer's lung
Type IV	Th cells, macrophages	48–72 hours	Contact dermatitis, tuberculin skin test

SLE, Systemic lupus erythematosus; Th cells, T-helper cells.

Table 12.3 Other autoimmune diseases of connective tissues

Disease	Autoantigen	Autoantibodies	Features
Sjögren syndrome	Exocrine glands	Anti-Ro and La	Reduced lacrimal and salivary gland secretion, causing dry eyes and mouth
Myositis	Muscle	ANA (Jo-1)	Muscle weakness and atrophy; mild arthritis and rashes are common
Systemic sclerosis	Nucleoli	ANA (topoisomerase 1 and centromere)	Increased collagen deposition in skin; usually runs an indolent course, but eventual involvement of internal organs occurs in most patients
MCTD		ANA (RNP)	Features of SLE, RA, scleroderma and polymyositis; may not be a distinct entity

ANA, Antinuclear antigen; MCTD, mixed connective tissue disease; RA, rheumatoid arthritis; RNP, ribonucleoprotein; SLE, systemic lupus erythematosus.

Table 12.4 Autoimmune vasculitides

Disease	Diagnostic test[a]	Features
Polyangiitis	pANCA (myeloperoxidase)	Necrotizing inflammation of medium-sized arteries. Any organ or tissue can be affected
Granulomatosis with polyangiitis (previously Wegener granulomatosis)	cANCA (proteinase 3)	Presents with respiratory tract lesions, typically in the lungs and nose, in association with glomerulonephritis

[a]Antineutrophil cytoplasmic antibodies (ANCA) are specific antibodies against neutrophils. pANCA reacts with neutrophil myeloperoxidase and gives a perinuclear pattern on immunofluorescence; cANCA reacts with proteinase 3 in the cytoplasm and gives a diffuse cytoplasmic pattern in immunofluorescence.

Table 12.5 Summary of organ- or cell-specific autoimmune diseases

Disease	Autoantigen	Features
Myasthenia gravis	Acetylcholine receptor	Muscle weakness and fatigue due to impaired neuromuscular transmission; 70% of patients have thymic hyperplasia, 10% have thymic tumour
Goodpasture syndrome	Type IV collagen in the basement membrane of kidney and lung	Pulmonary haemorrhage and acute glomerulonephritis; peak incidence in men aged in their mid-20s
Pernicious anaemia	Intrinsic factor	See Chapter 3: Pernicious anaemia
AI haemolytic anaemia	Erythrocyte membrane antigens	See Chapter 3: Autoimmune haemolytic anaemia
AI thrombocytopenia	Platelet glycoproteins	See Chapter 6: Thrombocytopenia
Hashimoto thyroiditis	Thyroid peroxidase	See earlier in this chapter
Graves disease	TSH receptor	See earlier in this chapter
Type I diabetes mellitus	Islet cell antigens	See earlier in this chapter
Coeliac disease	Tissue transglutaminase	Malabsorption due to villous atrophy in the small bowel. Diarrhoea and anaemia are common. Patients can present at any age. Treated with a gluten-free diet

The organ-specific autoantibodies are caused by similar genes, usually in the HLA complex. Family members therefore tend to have different organ-specific diseases. AI, Autoimmune; HLA, human leucocyte antigen; TSH, thyroid stimulating hormone.

IMMUNE SYSTEM DISORDERS (INSTEAD OF 'DEVELOPMENT OF HYPERSENSITIVITY')

Immune system disorders result from defects in immune pathways. These disorders include:

(i)   Inappropriate immune responses to a pathogen, giving rise to allergies
(ii) Inappropriate immune responses to a self-component, giving rise to autoimmune disorders
(iii) Immune deficiency diseases (such as AIDS)

Allergy

The incidence of allergies has increased dramatically in recent decades and the prevalence is also very high, with up to 40% of the population reporting some form of allergy. This led to the belief that our urban, 'clean' lifestyle has contributed to allergy formation, supported by the fact that allergies are less prevalent in rural populations. It is not clear why this is the case; current theories are that microorganism exposure during certain points of development reduces the incidence of allergy (an advance on the 'hygiene hypothesis'). Allergies run in families, suggesting a genetic influence, but no single genetic polymorphism has emerged that is common to all allergy sufferers. One gene implicated in some cases of allergy codes for the protein filaggrin. This protein normally maintains the skin's barrier function; polymorphisms in the filaggrin gene are highly associated with atopic eczema and allergy.

Ultimately, allergy forms when the initial exposure to an antigen, for example, grass pollen, results in a Th2-cell-biased response, leading to IL-4 production and subsequent IgE overproduction for that antigen. A breakdown in tolerance also contributes to allergy development (see Chapter 10).

Autoimmune disease

Autoimmunity is a state in which the body exhibits immunological reactivity to itself. The need for 'self-tolerance' and the mechanisms of central and peripheral tolerance have already been discussed in Chapter 10: Tolerance. If tolerance breaks down, autoimmunity can develop. Tolerance can break down in the thymus (usually for genetic reasons) or in the periphery (usually as a result of environmental factors such as infection). Autoimmunity is multifactorial; a defect in at least one of the regulatory mechanisms is required before disease develops, such as:

(i)   Alteration of self-antigens: It has been described that the shape of a self-antigen may change and that antigenic components can be attached to self-proteins, generating an immune response, which leads to autoantibody production. An example of this process is the production of rheumatoid factor causing RA.
(ii) Release of 'hidden' self-antigens: When intracellular antigens, that normally are not in contact with circulation, get released into circulation (e.g., as a result of trauma), they are encountered as foreign by immune effector cells.
(iii) Cross-reaction with foreign antigens (molecular mimicry): This occurs when foreign antigens resemble those on normal tissues, resulting in antibody reaction not only with the foreign antigens but also the similar self-antigens, leading to tissue damage. Typical examples include rheumatic fever and the Chagas disease.
(iv) Genetic factors/role of human leucocyte antigen: Many autoimmune diseases have a familial component. The HLA haplotype is the main identified genetic factor. If an individual has inherited an HLA allele that does not bind well to self-antigen in the thymus, reactive T cells are not deleted during development, leading to a loss of 'self-tolerance'. Certain HLA alleles are linked to specific autoimmune processes, for example, HLA-DR4 in RA, and HLA-DQ8 in coeliac disease. However, a certain HLA haplotype does not automatically result in the development of an autoimmune disease; 95% of patients with ankylosing spondylitis have HLA-B27, but only 5% of the population with HLA-B27 have ankylosing spondylitis.
(v)   Infection: Many infections are able to activate T and B cells in a nonspecific fashion. This results in the proliferation of several T- and B-cell clones, which can produce autoreactive autoantibody or mediate autoimmunity.

COMMON PITFALLS

Self-reactive antibodies can be found in the blood of healthy individuals, with no evidence of disease. As such, the identification of autoantibodies is not sufficient to diagnose an autoimmune disorder and should not be used as a diagnostic tool.

The capacity of autoantibodies to cause dysfunction differentiates autoimmune disease from an autoimmune response.

EXAMPLES OF AUTOIMMUNE DISEASES

Type I diabetes mellitus

Type I diabetes mellitus (TIDM) occurs as a result of the destruction of the insulin-producing β cells of the islets of Langerhans of the pancreas. One in 300 people in Europe and the USA are affected. An autoimmune aetiology is very likely. Over 90% of patients with the disease carry either HLA-DR3 or HLA-DR4 or both. HLA-DQ2 is also implicated–this variant appears to prevent pancreatic islet cell autoantigen from binding correctly. Therefore, self-reactive T cells cannot be negatively selected in the thymus and tolerance breaks down. Since not everyone with these HLA alleles develops TIDM, external triggers must also be involved. It is thought that infection may be one of these triggers, causing a degree of inflammation in the pancreatic islets, attracting macrophages and sensitizing self-reactive T cells. This knowledge of the immune basis for TIDM has not previously been useful, but in the next few years it is likely to play a role in the prevention of the disease.

Hashimoto thyroiditis

Hashimoto thyroiditis is the most common cause of hypothyroidism in the developed world. Antigen-specific cytotoxic T cells attack the thyroid gland, leading to progressive destruction of the epithelium. Due to unregulated T-helper cell interaction with B cells, autoantibodies are produced against thyroid antigens such as thyroid peroxidase. Marked lymphocytic infiltration (mainly by B cells and CD4+ T cells) of the thyroid gland is accompanied by migration of large numbers of macrophages and plasma cells, resulting in the formation of lymphoid follicles and germinal centres within the thyroid. Middle-aged females are most commonly affected (female:male ratio as high as 20:1). The disease is associated with the HLA-DR5 haplotype.

Rheumatoid arthritis

Rheumatoid arthritis is a chronic systemic disease that primarily involves the joints, resulting in inflammation of the synovium and destruction of the articular cartilage (Fig. 12.12). Initially, the disease affects the small joints of the hands and feet symmetrically, later spreading to the larger joints. A typical history of RA is joint pain and stiffness on waking, lasting at least 30 minutes and progressive over time. RA also has extraarticular pathology in the lungs, eyes and skin. RA affects approximately 1–2% of the world's population and is most common between the ages of 30 and 55 years. The female:male ratio is 3:1.

A central feature in the immunopathogenesis of RA is the citrullination of proteins. This is the conversion of the amino acid arginine to citrulline in proteins that may not normally contain

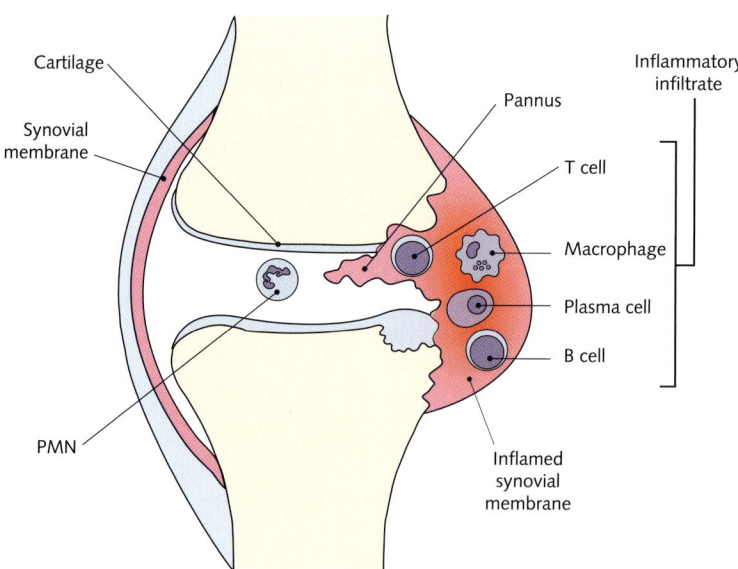

Fig. 12.12 Rheumatoid joint showing pannus formation and cartilage destruction. The synovial membrane is infiltrated by inflammatory cells and hypertrophies forming granulation tissue known as 'pannus'. This eventually erodes the articular cartilage and bone. T cells and macrophages in the inflamed synovium secrete TNF.
PMN, Polymorphonuclear leucocyte; *TNF*, tumour necrosis factor.

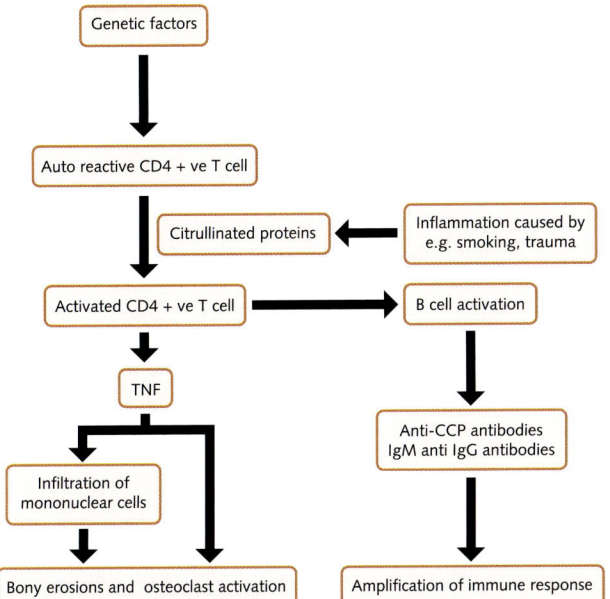

Fig. 12.13 Pathogenesis of RA. Autoreactive CD4+ T cells, which target citrullinated peptides, mediate the pathological changes. Synovial T cells produce a number of cytokines including TNF. These stimulate the acute phase response, synovial inflammation and bone erosion. Activation of B cells can result in the production of anti-CCP antibodies and rheumatoid factor. *CCP*, cyclic citrullinated peptide; *RA*, rheumatoid arthritis.

RHEUMATOID ARTHRITIS INVESTIGATIONS

The blood tests in RA reflect its inflammatory nature; C-reactive protein (CRP) and erythrocyte sedimentation rate (ESR) are raised, indicating an acute phase response. Rheumatoid factor (IgM anti-IgG autoantibodies) is present in approximately 80% of patients and indicates a poorer prognosis than those who are rheumatoid factor negative. Anti-CCP antibodies can also be measured and are thought to be more selective and specific for RA than rheumatoid factor. The overall diagnosis of RA is clinical.

Radiographic features include:

Soft tissue swelling
Juxta-articular osteoporosis
Joint space narrowing
Joint destruction and erosions (see Fig. 12.14)
Subluxation

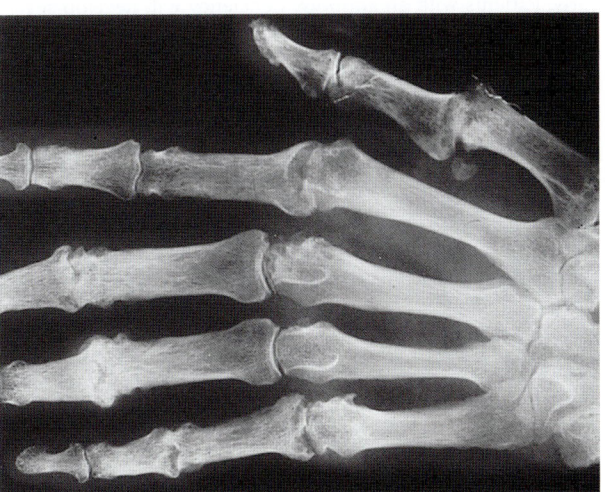

Fig. 12.14 An X-ray of a hand showing joint destruction and erosion due to rheumatoid arthritis.

citrulline. It is thought that citrullinated proteins become a target for autoreactive T and B cells. Additionally, anticyclic citrullinated peptide (anti-CCP) antibodies are found in the serum of most RA patients and in people who will develop RA. Citrullination may occur as a result of inflammation, triggered for reasons such as smoking, which is associated with the development of RA. The overall immunopathogenesis of RA is outlined in Fig. 12.13.

A key event in the pathogenesis of RA is the secretion of tumour necrosis factor (TNF) by T cells and macrophages, which coordinates the neutrophil-mediated joint inflammation and osteoclast-mediated bone erosion.

Once RA is suspected clinically, prompt referral is essential to minimize morbidity associated with this chronic condition. Management is based on the early use of steroids and non-steroidal antiinflammatories (NSAIDs). Specific antirheumatic drugs that modulate the immune response, known as biological disease-modifying antirheumatic drugs (DMARDs), are also used. These biological DMARDs usually target TNF (e.g., infliximab and adalimumab). The anti–B-cell monoclonal antibody rituximab and the anti-IL-6 receptor monoclonal antibody tocilizumab can also be used (see Chapter 13).

IMMUNE DEFICIENCY

Immune deficiency predisposes individuals to infections from opportunistic pathogens (those that do not normally cause disease) as well as normal pathogens, and may increase the risk of developing certain malignancies. Although the cause of the deficiency can be primary or secondary, the part of the immune system that is deficient will determine the sort of infection to which the individual is predisposed. For example, antibody deficits result in extracellular bacterial infection while T-cell deficiencies can result in viral, fungal and intracellular bacterial infections.

Primary immunodeficiencies

Primary immunodeficiencies are intrinsic, usually inherited, defects of the immune system. They can be caused by single gene mutations, genetic polymorphisms or by the interaction of several genes (polygenic). Different components of the immune system can be affected, including:

- Antibodies (Table 12.6)
- T cells (Table 12.7)
- Phagocytes (Table 12.8)
- Complement (Table 12.9)

It is important to recognize primary immunodeficiencies early. Patients with an antibody deficiency will develop severe lung infections that lead to chronic structural changes in the lungs (bronchiectasis) unless given immunoglobulin. Children with T-cell defects can be killed by opportunistic infections or from live vaccines such as BCG.

Neonates do not possess a fully developed immune system at birth. In the neonatal period, infants are normally protected by maternal IgG that crosses the placenta in utero, but this is metabolized during the first months of life. In the first 6 months of life, there is a trough in immunoglobulin levels that makes infants prone to infection. IgA in breast milk can compensate. Babies born prematurely are deprived of maternal IgG and suffer exaggerated neonatal antibody deficiency. Infants normally begin production of their own IgG by the age of 3 months (Fig.12.15). In some individuals, IgG production might not start for up to 9–12 months, possibly due to the lack of help from T cells.

NOD2 AND CROHN DISEASE

Polymorphisms in the gene for the pattern recognition molecule nucleotide-binding oligomerization domain containing 2 (NOD2) are found in many cases of Crohn disease. Normally, NOD2 activates the innate immune response in gut epithelial cells. Therefore, the theory is that Crohn disease is caused by repeated bacterial infection resulting from immunodeficiency rather than autoimmunity.

Secondary immunodeficiencies

Secondary immunodeficiency is acquired, through disease, drugs or malnutrition.

Malnutrition and disease

It is rare that the lack of dietary protein and certain elements (e.g., zinc) predisposes patients to secondary immunodeficiency. Infections such as malaria and measles can also result in immunodeficiency.

Malignancy

Secondary immunodeficiency is particularly common with tumours that arise from the immune system, such as myeloma, lymphoma and leukaemia (see Chapter 5). Many other tumours are immunosuppressive. This is likely to provide the tumour cells with a selective advantage, because they evade destruction by cytotoxic cells.

Steroids, other drugs and radiation

Iatrogenic causes of immunosuppression are common. Immunosuppressive drugs can be given to suppress inflammatory or autoimmune disease or to prevent rejection of transplanted material (see Chapter 13: Transplantation). Radiation and cytotoxic drugs can be used to treat malignancies and frequently cause immunosuppression.

Table 12.6 Primary antibody deficiencies

Disorder	Features
Transient physiological agammaglobulinaemia of the neonate	See Fig. 12.11.
X-linked agammaglobulinaemia of Bruton	X-linked recessive disorder with defective B-cell maturation. Low serum immunoglobulin levels result in recurrent pyogenic infections (seen after about 6 months). Treatment is with immunoglobulin replacement.
Common variable hypogammaglobulinaemia	Heterogeneous group of disorders with normal lymphocyte numbers but abnormal B-cell function; late onset (15–35 years of age) presenting with recurrent pyogenic infections. Treatment is with immunoglobulin replacement.
Selective IgA deficiency	Occurs in 1 in 700 Caucasians but is rarer in other ethnic groups; can be asymptomatic or produce recurrent infections of the respiratory and gastrointestinal tracts.

Pyogenic infections are common due to infections with encapsulated bacteria such as streptococci and staphylococci (not selective IgA deficiency).

Table 12.7 Primary lymphocyte deficiencies

Primary immunodeficiency	Examples

B-cell deficiencies	– X-linked agammaglobulinaemia (Bruton disease):
	  – X-linked
	  – Symptoms present around 5-6 months of age (when maternal IgG disappears)
	  – Reduced levels of all immunoglobulins (due to impaired maturation of pre-B cells to mature B lymphocytes)
	  – Recurrent bacterial infections
	  – Bone marrow transplantation is the only curable therapy
	
	– IgA deficiency:
	  – The most common primary immunodeficiency
	  – Patients are prone to recurrent sinus and lung infections.
	  – Concurrent autoimmune disease in 20%-30% patients
	  – Immunoglobulin replacement should be avoided to prevent hypersensitivity.

T-cell deficiencies	– Congenital thymic aplasia:
	  – Associated with several genetic disorders (such as DiGeorge syndrome)
	  – Absent T cells but normal B cells
	  – Fungal and viral infections are common
	
	– Hyper-IgM syndrome:
	  – Early onset of bacterial infections
	  – High levels of IgM (due to inability of B cells to switch to other classes of antibodies)
	  – Immunoglobulin therapy is recommended
	
	– IL-12 receptor deficiency:
	  – Characterized by recurrent mycobacterial infections

Combined B- and T-cell deficiencies	– Severe combined immunodeficiency disease (SCID):
	  – X-linked
	  – Deficiency of the IL-2 receptor
	  – Characterized by repeated infections, including opportunistic pathogens
	  – Allogeneic stem cell transplantation the only curable option
	
	– Wiskott-Aldrich syndrome:
	  – X-linked
	  – Normal T-cell numbers, but with impaired function (due to WASP deficiency)
	  – Reduced IgM, normal IgG, raised IgA and IgE
	  – Characterized by recurrent infections, eczema and thrombocytopenia
	
	– Immunodeficiency with ataxia telangiectasia
	  – T-cell deficiency
	  – Low B-cell numbers: IgM low/normal, IgG low, IgA considerably low
	  – Associated with ataxia (lack of movement coordination) and telangiectasia (small blood vessel dilatation)
	  – High incidence of malignancy (especially leukaemias)
	
	– MHC deficiency
	  – Low numbers of CD4 and CD8 lymphocytes
	  – Affected antibody production
	  – Individuals prone to recurrent infections.
	
	– Leukocyte adhesion deficiency syndrome:
	  – Autosomal recessive
	  – Poor adhesion and impaired phagocytosis of bacteria
	  – Characterized by pyogenic infections

Viral infections/acquired immunodeficiency syndrome

Acquired immunodeficiency syndrome (AIDS) is caused by severe human immunodeficiency virus (HIV) infection. HIV is a retrovirus (Fig. 12.16), which is able to infect CD4+ T cells and antigen-presenting cells (such as monocytes, macrophages and dendritic cells).

Sexual transmission is the most important route for the spread of HIV. Transmission can also occur through infected

Table 12.8 Primary phagocyte deficiencies

Disorder	Features
Neutropenia	See Chapter 4: Leucopoenia
Leucocyte adhesion deficiency	Lack of β_2-integrin molecules results in impaired adhesion and extravasation of phagocytes.
Chronic granulomatous disease	Most commonly X-linked (can be autosomal recessive) inheritance. Lack of NADPH oxidase impairs killing of ingested pathogens, which therefore persist.

NADPH, Nicotinamide adenine dinucleotide phosphate.

Table 12.9 Primary complement deficiencies[a]

Disorder	Features
Deficiency of classical pathway components	Tendency to develop immune complex disease such as SLE
C3 deficiency	Prone to recurrent pyogenic infections
Deficiency of C5, C6, C 7, C8, factor D, properdin	Increased susceptibility to *Neisseria* infections
C1 inhibitor deficiency	Causes hereditary angioedema

SLE, Systemic lupus erythematosus.
[a]*Deficiencies of almost all complement components have been described.*

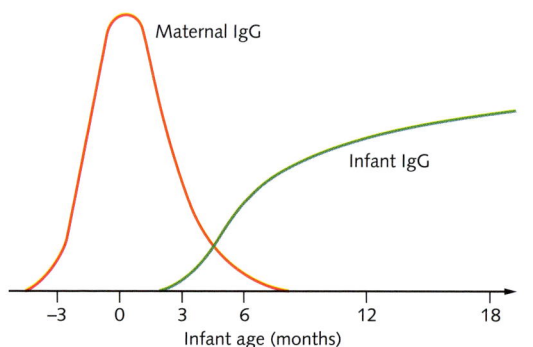

Fig. 12.15 Plasma levels of maternal and neonatal immunoglobulin in the normal-term infant.

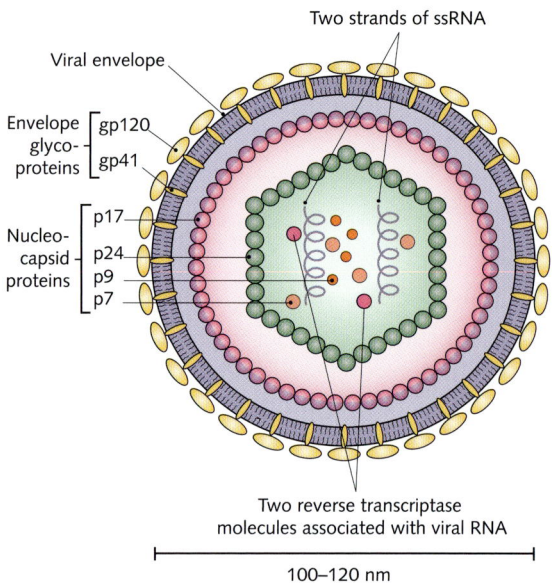

Fig. 12.16 Structure of HIV-1. The envelope glycoproteins gp120 and gp41 are hypervariable. gp120 binds CD4, while gp41 enables entry of the virus into the cell. The viral envelope is a lipid bilayer containing both viral glycoprotein antigens and host proteins.
ssRNA, Single-stranded ribonucleic acid.

blood (such as via blood transfusions), IV drug abuse and needlestick injury (0.3% risk from a single exposure). Vertical transmission is particularly important in developing countries, occurring transplacentally during labour (approximately 25% of cases) or through breast milk. Possible ways to minimize the risk of vertical transmission include: (i) delivery via Caesarean section, (ii) feeding with formula milk rather than breast milk and (iii) early use of antiretrovirals.

Most individuals exposed to HIV sexually become chronically infected. Infected individuals produce antibodies, but this is largely ineffective against intracellular virus. T cells inhibit HIV by interferon secretion or by killing infected cells. Individuals infected with HIV develop symptoms as their body starts to produce antibodies to HIV. This is called 'HIV seroconversion illness'. The patient experiences fever, rash, malaise, sore throat, diarrhoea and arthralgia; lymphadenopathy may also be present. Not all patients experience seroconversion illness and it is often diagnosed retrospectively.

CD4 counts provide a guide of the current immunological status of the patient (Fig. 12.17), whereas HIV RNA levels predict what will happen to the patient over the next few months and years.

HINTS AND TIPS

Each infected individual contains many hundreds of slightly different strains following infection with a single virus, reflecting the ongoing mutation of the virus.

Human immunodeficiency virus can now be treated successfully, offering a life expectancy similar to that of HIV-negative people. The drugs used to combat the virus are called

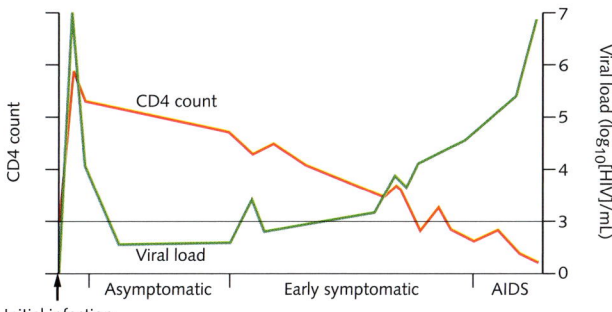

Fig. 12.17 Variation in CD4 count and viral load during the course of HIV infection.

'antiretrovirals' (ARVs) and include classes of drugs that work on the three main elements of the virus (Fig. 12.18):

- Fusion inhibitors prevent attachment to the envelope.
- Reverse transcriptase inhibitors (RTIs) inhibit the production of DNA. There are both nucleotide analogue RTIs (NARTIs) and nonnucleotide RTI (NNRTIs).
- Protease inhibitors prevent the production of viral peptides.

When treating HIV, it is important to remember its ability to mutate and that antiretrovirals could provide a selective advantage for a more resistant strain to develop. For this reason, a combination of at least two classes of drug are used and they are not started until there is evidence of CD4$^+$ ve T-cell decline. This combination of more than one drug is known as highly active antiretroviral therapy (HAART). Antibiotic prophylaxis against infections such as *Pneumocystis carinii* and *Toxoplasma gondii* is advised when the CD4 count is <200/μL.

POSTEXPOSURE AND PREEXPOSURE PROPHYLAXIS

Postexposure prophylaxis (PEP) has long been offered to any person that has recently been exposed to HIV in a high-risk manner, such as unprotected sexual intercourse or exposure to infected bodily fluids in a health care setting. PEP involves a 28-day course of antiretroviral drugs and should ideally be started within 72 hours of exposure.

Preexposure prophylaxis is the regular, long-term use of antiretroviral drugs in populations that are HIV –ve but are at high risk of infection. It aims to prevent the virus from establishing in the host after inoculation.

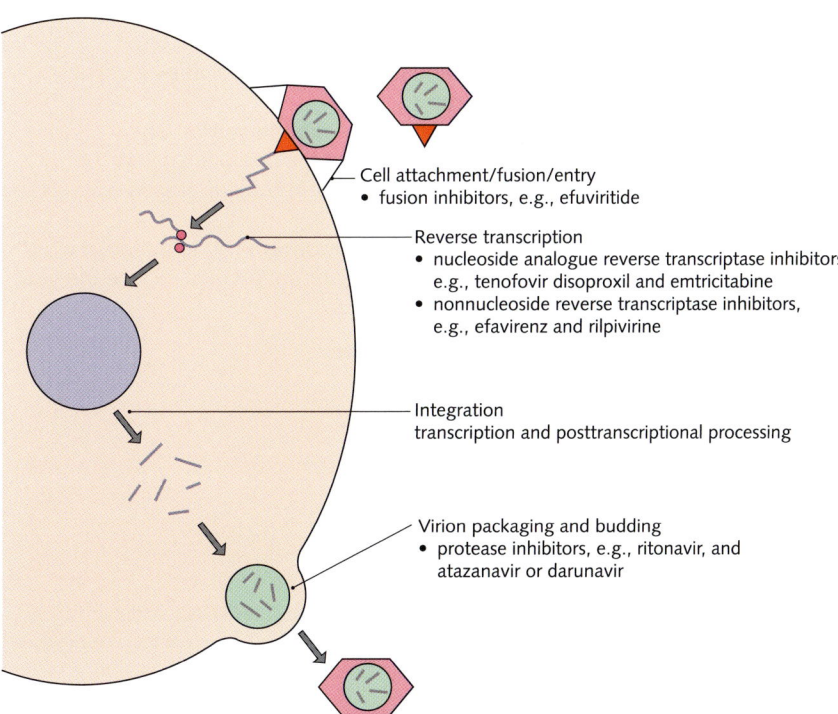

Cell attachment/fusion/entry
- fusion inhibitors, e.g., efuviritide

Reverse transcription
- nucleoside analogue reverse transcriptase inhibitors, e.g., tenofovir disoproxil and emtricitabine
- nonnucleoside reverse transcriptase inhibitors, e.g., efavirenz and rilpivirine

Integration
transcription and posttranscriptional processing

Virion packaging and budding
- protease inhibitors, e.g., ritonavir, and atazanavir or darunavir

Fig. 12.18 Antiretroviral agents in current use and their site of action in the lifecycle of HIV.

INVESTIGATION OF A PATIENT WITH POSSIBLE IMMUNE DEFICIENCY

Immunological investigations

Evaluation of a patient with possible immune deficiency includes the assessment of:

- Immunoglobulins (IgG1-4, IgA, IgE, IgM) and antibody activity (IgG antibodies postimmunization and/or postexposure)
- B- and T-lymphocyte counts and CD4/CD8 ratio
- Lymphocyte stimulation assays (e.g., phytohemagglutinin)

- Quantification of complement components (C3, C4, factor B and C1 inhibitor levels)
- Phagocytic activity

Other important studies are:

- Autoimmune antibodies (ANA, anti-dsDNA, RF, antihistones, anti-Smith, anti-SSA and anti-SSB antibodies)
- Microbiological studies, such as blood cultures, CMV, HIV and HTLV testing, nasopharyngeal swab, stool testing for bacterial, viral or parasitic infections, sputum cultures and CFS fluid, if appropriate.
- Coagulation tests (factor V assays, fibrinogen, PT, aPTT)
- Other tests, as appropriate: bone marrow biopsy, tuberculin test, tumour markers, imaging, DNA testing.

● Chapter Summary

- Hypersensitivity is an excessive immune response to any antigen. Its causes are multifactorial and involve a breakdown in tolerance. It can be classified by type of immune response:
- Type I hypersensitivity involves IgE-mediated mast cell degranulation. Examples include food and pollen allergy, asthma and eczema.
- Type II hypersensitivity is mediated by other immunoglobulins, often followed by complement activation and antibody-dependent cell-mediated cytotoxicity. Examples include Graves disease and ABO mismatch reactions in blood transfusion.
- Type III hypersensitivity is caused by tissue deposition of antigen-antibody complexes. Examples include SLE and Farmer's lung.
- Type IV hypersensitivity is coordinated and mediated by T cells. Examples include contact dermatitis and RA.
- Hypersensitivity is generally managed by avoidance of triggers (if possible), local or systemic immunosuppression, or targeted therapy.
- Immunodeficiency can be intrinsic (primary) or acquired (secondary). Primary immunodeficiency can involve one or many components of the immune system. Secondary immunodeficiency has many causes, including immunosuppressive drugs and infection.
- Acquired immune deficiency syndrome (AIDS) is caused by severe HIV infection, a virus that infects antigen-presenting cells and CD4$^+$ T cells. Treatment aims to reduce the viral load and restore the CD4$^+$ T-cell count.

MLA Conditions	MLA Presentations
Allergic disorder	Allergies
Contact dermatitis	Anaphylaxis
Human immunodeficiency virus	Wheeze
Urticaria	

References

1. Gell PGH, Coombs RRA, eds. *Clinical Aspects of Immunology*. Oxford, England: Blackwell; 1963.
2. Sell S, Rich RR, Fleisher TA et al, eds. *Clinical Immunology: Principles and Practice*. 1st ed. St. Louis, Mo: Mosby-Year Book; 1996:449–477.
3. NICE guideline (NG80). Asthma: diagnosis, monitoring and chronic asthma management. www.nice.org.uk/guidance/ng80

The immune system can be manipulated in various ways, either to enhance its beneficial actions (vaccination) or to suppress any adverse reactions (immunosuppression, antiinflammatory drugs).

IMMUNIZATION

Immunization plays a key role in disease prevention, constituting an essential part of public health. Immunity can be achieved by passive or active immunization (Table 13.1).

Passive immunization

This is a temporary immunity that results from the transfer of exogenous antibody from one person to another. It occurs without prior exposure to the specific antigens. Passive immunity is seen in the foetus when maternal IgG crosses the placenta and in breast-fed babies due to the IgA content of breast milk. Passive immunity can be conferred to individuals who have been exposed to a pathogen to which they are not immune by the injection of immunoglobulins to the antigen specific to that pathogen. These are taken from blood donors immune to the pathogen.

Examples where passive immunity is used include:

- Open fracture management: if tetanus vaccination history is uncertain or incomplete, antitetanus immunoglobulin is given.
- Hepatitis B (Hep B) postexposure prophylaxis: HepB immunoglobulin can be given to unvaccinated individuals, for example, after a contaminated needlestick injury.
- Management of digoxin toxicity with Digibind (immunoglobulin that binds and neutralizes digoxin molecules).

Passive immunization is also indicated in patients who cannot form antibodies (such as the immunocompromised) and in cases where the disease develops before the formation of antibodies (such as in rabies).

Active immunization

Active immunization results from contact with antigens, either through natural infection or by vaccination. Individuals exhibit a primary immune response with clonal expansion of B and T cells and formation of memory cells. Subsequent exposure to the same antigen will induce a more rapid and robust immune response (see Chapter 10). In the absence of vaccination, the first exposure to the antigen might lead to life-threatening consequences before a sufficient immune response can be generated.

Vaccination

Vaccination is a form of active immunization that induces specific immunity to a particular pathogen. The aim is to produce a rapid, protective immune response on re-exposure to that pathogen. An ideal vaccine is:

- Safe, with minimal side effects and free from contaminating substances
- Immunogenic, activating the required branches of the immune system, inducing long-lasting local and systemic immunity
- Heat stable because there are difficulties with refrigeration, particularly in tropical countries
- Inexpensive, an important consideration, especially in developing countries

Despite the fact that vaccination is a key element of public health, prolonging life expectancy and improving quality of life due to disease prevention, it remains a controversial topic. In recent years, antivaccination movements have gained momentum, leading to the emergence and outbreak of previously (nearly) eradicated diseases. Preventive measures, such as patient education, primary care provider engagement and patient reminder systems, are in place to enhance vaccination compliance rates and protect the community.

Types of vaccine

The types of vaccines in current use are listed in Table 13.2. Vaccines can be live attenuated (weakened) organisms, killed organisms or subunit (a protein from the surface of the organism); the features of each are compared in Table 13.3. In general, live vaccines are more potent but risk greater side effects than subunit vaccines. More recently, a novel vaccine type was developed, the messenger RNA (mRNA) vaccine, to deal with the COVID-19 pandemic. mRNA vaccines work by introducing an mRNA that corresponds to an antigenic viral protein (such as the spike protein). Upon cell uptake, the mRNA gets translated to protein in the cytoplasm (does not enter the nucleus and does not alter the DNA) (Fig. 13.1). This protein is recognized as foreign by immune cells, which mount an immune response leading to antibody production. More importantly, once the mRNA has been translated, it breaks down within the cell. Another advantage of these vaccines is that people are not exposed to the virus itself and as such they cannot become infected with it. It is of note that the

Table 13.1 Comparison of passive and active immunity

	Features	Examples
Passive	Preformed immunoglobulins transferred to individual Large amounts of antibody available immediately Short lifespan of antibodies	Antitetanus toxin antibody
Active	Contact with antigen induces adaptive immune response Takes some time to develop immunity Long-lived immunity induced: includes T cells, B cells and antibody	Natural exposure Vaccination

Table 13.2 Different types of vaccine in use in the United Kingdom today

Vaccine	Features	Examples
Live attenuated	Attenuation achieved by repeated culture on artificial media or by serial passage in animals; immunogenicity is retained, but virulence is significantly diminished	Oral polio (Sabin), BCG, MMR
Killed	Intact organisms killed by exposure to heat or chemicals, for example, formalin	Intramuscular polio (Salk), pertussis, influenza
Subunit	Purified, protective immunity-inducing antigenic components; often surface antigens	Nonconjugated pneumococcal, acellular pertussis
Recombinant	Genes encoding epitopes, which elicit protective immunity, are inserted into pro- or eukaryotic cells; large quantities of vaccine are produced rapidly	HepB surface antigen (produced in yeast cells), HPV vaccines
Toxoids	Bacterial toxins inactivated by heat or chemicals	Diphtheria, tetanus
Conjugates	Polysaccharide antigen is linked to protein carrier to enhance immunogenicity	Hib, meningococcal, pneumococcal
mRNA	Introduction of a noninfectious, nonreplicating mRNA that corresponds to an antigenic protein	COVID-19 vaccines

BCG, Bacille Calmette–Guérin; HepB, hepatitis B; Hib, haemophilus influenzae type b; HPV, human papilloma virus; MMR, measles, mumps, rubella; mRNA, messenger RNA.

Table 13.3 Features of live versus killed vaccines

Feature	Live attenuated vaccine	Killed vaccine	mRNA
Level of immunity induced	High: organism replicates at site of infection (mimicking natural infection)	Low: nonreplicating organisms produce a short-lived stimulus	High: production of the target immunogen stimulates both humoral and cellular immune responses
Cell-mediated response	Good: antigens are processed and presented with MHC molecules	Poor	Very good: antigens are processed and presented with MHC I and MHC II molecules
Local immunity	Good	Poor	Good
Cost	Expensive to produce and administer	Cheaper than live vaccines	Cheaper than live and killed vaccine
Reversion to virulence	Possible but rare	No (therefore safe for immunocompromised and pregnant patients)	No (safe for immunocompromised patients, pregnant women and children >6 months of age)
Stability	Heat labile	Heat stable	Highly temperature sensitive
Risk of contamination	Possible, for example, by virus in cell media	N/A	None

The genes of attenuated organisms can differ from the wild type by just a few base pairs. It is relatively easy for them to mutate back to the disease-causing strain. MHC, Major histocompatibility complex; N/A, not applicable.

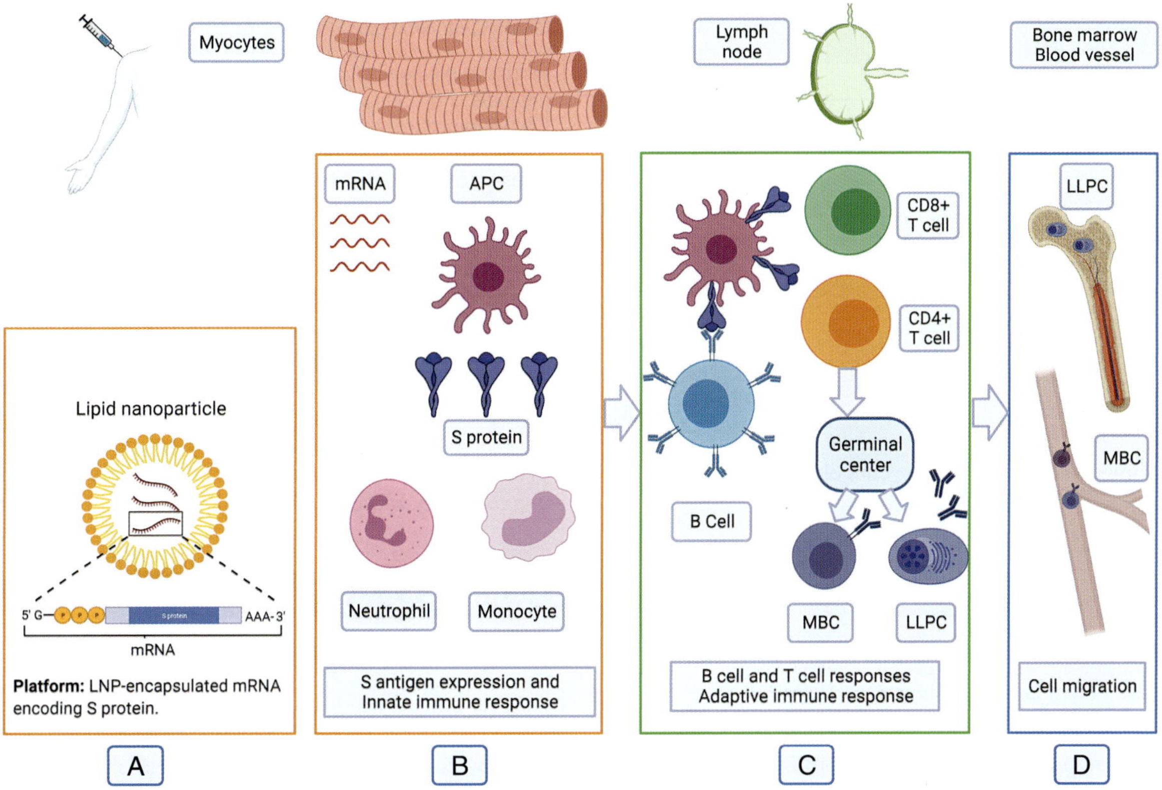

Fig. 13.1 mRNA vaccine immune response. Once injected into the muscle, the lipid nanoparticle (LNP) complex containing the in vitro transcribed mRNA (A) is internalized and reaches the cytoplasm of the myocyte via the endosomes. The local translation of the mRNA generates spike proteins, which trigger an innate immune response (B). The antigen-presenting cells (APCs) in the muscle transport the expressed spike protein to the lymph nodes, where specific B- and T-cell responses are triggered (C). Some of the B cells get transformed into long-lived plasma cells (LLPCs) and memory B cells (MBCs) and migrate (D). (Source: *Textbook of SARS-CoV-2 and COVID-19*, First Edition, 2024).

2023 Nobel Prize in Medicine was awarded to the scientists that developed the mRNA vaccines.

The vaccination schedule changes from time to time as new vaccines become available. For the UK, the Government's website is a good place to look for the most up-to-date schedule and details of individual vaccines: www.gov.uk/government/collections/immunisation. Each country has its own version. It is not necessary to memorize this schedule, but it is worth having a rough idea of what is given and when. A condensed version of the UK's vaccination schedule is given in Table 13.4.

CLINICAL NOTES

A healthy immune system can cope with live attenuated vaccines. However, these vaccines are contraindicated in immunocompromised patients as they can cause severe infection. Anaphylaxis to a certain vaccine is also a contraindication to future treatment. Some vaccines, for example, measles, yellow fever and Bacille Calmette–Guérin (BCG), are contraindicated in pregnancy.

Vaccines are not 100% efficacious. A small proportion of individuals receiving vaccination will not respond adequately. However, by immunizing the majority of the population, nonresponders are unlikely to come into contact with the virus because the viral reservoir is reduced (herd immunity).

You will notice that a number of vaccinations are given simultaneously; this is not just for convenience. Given alone, some of the subunit vaccines would not evoke a sufficient immune response in order for immunity to develop. For example, the diphtheria, tetanus, pertussis (DTaP) vaccination relies strongly on the danger signal produced in response to the killed pertussis organism to develop immunity to the diphtheria and tetanus toxoids.

Table 13.4 Routine immunization schedule used in the United Kingdom

Age	Vaccine
Vaccines for babies under 1 year old	
8 weeks	6-in-1 vaccine (DTaP, polio [IPV], Hib, HepB)
	MenB
	Rotavirus vaccine
12 weeks	6-in-1 vaccine (DTaP/IPV/Hib/HepB)
	PCV
	Rotavirus vaccine
16 weeks	6-in-1 vaccine (DTaP/IPV/Hib/HepB)
	MenB
Vaccines for children 1 to 15 years old	
1 year	MMR
	PCV
	Hib/MenC
	MenB
2 to 15 years	Children's flu vaccine (annually)
3 years 4 months	4-in-1 vaccine (DTaP/IPV)
	MMR
12–13 years (girls only)	HPV types 6, 11, 16 and 18
14 years	3-in-1 vaccine (DT/IPV)
	MenACWY
Vaccines for Adults	
>65 years	Annual influenza
	PPV: one-off
	Shingles
70–79 years	Annual influenza
Any age	Occupation, for example, Hep A, Hep B
	Travel, for example, Yellow fever

DTaP, Diphtheria, tetanus and pertussis; HepB, hepatitis B; Hib, haemophilus influenzae type b; HPV, human papillomavirus; MenB, meningococcal group B; MMR, measles, mumps, rubella; PCV, pneumococcal conjugate vaccine; PPV, pneumococcal polysaccharide vaccine.

It is also possible to enhance the immune response to subunit vaccines by using adjuvants. Adjuvants, for example, aluminium salts and *Bordetella pertussis*, are nonspecific stimulators of the pattern recognition molecules of the innate immune system. When these are present, the innate immune system transmits a 'danger signal' to the adaptive immune system to promote a good response.

CLINICAL NOTES

Vaccination against toxins such as tetanus does not provide immunity against the toxin-producing bacterium (*Clostridium tetani*). Its benefits come from preventing the sequelae associated with the tetanus toxin, that is, tetanus of the masseter muscles (lock jaw).

Contraindications to vaccination, although rare, include allergy to a vaccine or to a component of a vaccine. Furthermore, immunocompromised patients and pregnant women should not be given live attenuated vaccines. In terms of complications, the commonest side effects include B symptoms (fever, fatigue, myalgia) and pain and swelling at the injection site. More serious complications are rare and include anaphylaxis to a vaccine or to one of its ingredients and Guillain-Barré syndrome, a potentially life-threatening condition, which is extremely rare.

TRANSPLANTATION

Human leucocyte antigen typing

Considering that major histocompatibility complex (MHC) is the main antigen involved in foreign tissue rejection, the ideal donor would have identical human leucocyte antigen (HLA) molecules as the recipient. Apart from monozygotic twins, in all other situations, there will be some genetic disparity between donor and recipient. Both donors and recipients are HLA typed and the closest match is used, aiming to minimize the risk of graft rejection.

HINTS AND TIPS

Remember, HLA is synonymous with MHC in humans.

Solid organ transplantation – mechanism of rejection

HINTS AND TIPS

Autologous grafts are grafts moved from one part of the body to another, for example, skin grafts.
Syngeneic grafts are between genetically identical individuals, for example, monozygotic twins.
Allogeneic grafts are between individuals of the same species.
Xenogeneic grafts are between different species.

The immune system presents a challenge for the long-term survival of organ and tissue transplants. Unless the donor and recipient are immunologically identical, the recipient will mount a rejection response against 'foreign' antigens expressed by the graft. The graft antigens responsible for most of the immune response in the recipient are the MHC molecules (see Chapter 10: The MHC). However, even when the donor and recipient are genetically identical at the MHC loci, graft rejection can occur due to differences at other loci, which encode minor histocompatibility antigens. A rejection response can lead to loss of a graft. There are three types of graft rejection:

1. Hyperacute: occurs within hours as a result of preformed antibodies against the donor tissue, a type II hypersensitivity reaction often due to ABO mismatch.
2. Acute: takes several days to develop, a type IV hypersensitivity reaction that develops against incompatible donor MHC and other molecules. It can be reduced by HLA matching and managed with antirejection therapy.
3. Chronic: occurs months to years after transplantation. It can be caused by a variety of mechanisms. It cannot be treated.

T-cell allorecognition constitutes the key event that ultimately leads to graft rejection. Based on the mechanism of T-cell allostimulation, there are two distinct types of allorecognition:

(i) The direct pathway: This involves the direct recognition of allo-MHC molecules on graft antigen-presenting cells (APCs) by recipient's T cells and is responsible for the early alloimmune response, leading to acute graft rejection.
(ii) The indirect pathway: In this pathway, T cells recognize alloantigens presented by host APCs. More specifically, donor MHC molecules are released from the graft, taken up by host APCs and presented to recipient T cells, eliciting an alloreaction which may lead to both acute and chronic rejection.

Haematopoietic stem cell transplantation

Haematopoietic stem cell (HSC) transplants are used in the treatment of various malignant and nonmalignant (e.g., primary immunodeficiencies) diseases. The process involves administration of a conditioning therapy (chemotherapy and/or irradiation) to eradicate the host's haematopoietic system, followed by infusion of either donor's HSCs (allogeneic haematopoietic stem cell transplantation [HSCT]) or patient's own HSCs (autologous transplants). In the case of allogeneic HSCT, the aim of the transplant is to replace a malignant (or dysfunctional) haematopoietic system with a healthy one, whereas in the case of autologous HSCT, the aim is to minimize the duration of pancytopenia, induced by the administration of a mega-dose chemotherapy (e.g., given for the treatment of a malignant disorder). The allo-HSCT provides the added benefit of removing residual malignant (e.g., leukaemic) cells via the graft-versus-leukaemia (GvL)

effect, where the donor lymphocytes recognize and attack the antigenically foreign malignant host cells.

The source of HSCs can be either the bone marrow (BM), peripheral blood (PB) or umbilical cord blood, each one with its own advantages and disadvantages. PB grafts, which involve administration of growth factors, such as the granulocyte colony-stimulating factor (GCSF), promote HSC proliferation and release to circulation (where they are collected from). These have been increasingly used in recent years due to the ease of collection and the potential survival advantage associated with the GvL effect (the PB contains more lymphocytes than the BM). Of course, the type of transplant selected depends on the disease, patient's age, comorbidities and graft availability, among other factors.

One of the most common and more severe complications of allo-HSCT is the development of graft-versus-host disease (GvHD), in which donor T cells recognize host cells and tissues as foreign (most commonly gastrointestinal tract, skin and liver) and initiate an immune reaction and attack, with potentially detrimental (life-threatening) results. GvHD is divided into acute (the first 100 days post–allo-HSCT) and chronic (>100 days after allo-HSCT), each one with a different pathophysiological mechanism, treatment strategy and outcome.

MEDICATIONS USED FOR THE PREVENTION OF IMMUNE REJECTION

Antirejection therapy

Immunosuppressive drugs can be used to prevent rejection by suppressing antibody and T-cell responses. Examples of drugs used include:

- Steroids: these have antiinflammatory effects, as well as directly affecting T-cell and phagocyte function (see 'Corticosteroids' below)
- Antimetabolites (reduce cell division): azathioprine, mycophenolate mofetil and methotrexate
- T-cell signalling inhibitors (calcineurin inhibitors): tacrolimus and ciclosporin

Immunosuppression can also be induced by using monoclonal antibodies against components of the immune system, for example, the anti-IL-2 receptor antibody basiliximab. Due to its potency, basiliximab tends to be used in the short term, such as in treatment of acute transplant rejection.

CLINICAL NOTES

Azathioprine is used in many conditions including rheumatoid arthritis, inflammatory bowel disease and in antirejection therapy. It is metabolized by the enzyme

---

thiopurine methyltransferase (TPMT). There are variations in the TPMT gene that affect its ability to metabolize azathioprine; a patient's TPMT activity levels should be measured prior to starting to take azathioprine to avoid potentially lethal myelosuppression due to build-up of the drug.

The disadvantage of immunosuppressive therapy is that the recipient is at increased risk of opportunistic infections (e.g., cytomegalovirus) and certain malignancies. Most transplant patients will stay on these drugs for life as rejection can still take place many years after transplantation.

Common types of transplantation performed today are summarized in Table 13.5.

Corticosteroids

The adrenal cortex releases several steroid hormones into the circulation. Glucocorticoids affect carbohydrate and protein metabolism and also affect the immune system, acting as immunosuppressive and antiinflammatory agents. Glucocorticoids act primarily on phagocytes. By binding to intracellular receptors and modifying gene expression, they inhibit the production of mediators of inflammation (prostaglandins, cytokines) and prevent antigen presentation. At higher doses they have a direct effect on lymphocytes. Several corticosteroids are available therapeutically, including:

- Hydrocortisone: can be given intravenously in status asthmaticus or topically for inflammatory skin conditions.
- Prednisolone: oral preparations are given in many inflammatory, rheumatological and allergic conditions, as well as in exacerbations of chronic obstructive pulmonary disease.
- Beclomethasone: used as an aerosol in asthma or topically for eczema.

Adverse effects and contraindications

Glucocorticoids cause many adverse effects at the high doses required to produce an antiinflammatory effect and many patients find them difficult to put up with. The clinical features are that of Cushing syndrome. Some important adverse effects are shown in Table 13.6.

Steroids are contraindicated if there is evidence of systemic infection. Long-term high-dose steroid therapy is usually avoided. When they are used long term, there should be regular checks on blood pressure, blood sugar and bone density. Care should be taken when finishing a course of corticosteroid therapy, as endogenous corticosteroid production is suppressed by long-term (>3 weeks) or high-dose therapy. The dose of corticosteroids should be gradually reduced over weeks if a long course or high dose has been used. Failure to do so could result in an Addisonian crisis.

Table 13.5 Common transplants

Transplant	Notes
Kidney	Live or cadaveric donor; the fewer the MHC mismatches, the greater the success rate; must be ABO compatible.
Heart	Matching is beneficial, but often time is a more pressing concern.
Liver	No evidence to suggest that matching affects graft survival; rejection less aggressive than for other organs.
Skin graft	Most grafts are autologous, but allografts can be used to protect burn patients.
Corneal graft	Matching (MHC class II) is required only if a previous graft was vascularized.
Stem cell	HVG or GVH responses possible. The transplant must be well matched and antirejection therapy used. Host immune cells are destroyed by irradiation prior to transplant (avoids HVG). T cells are depleted from the graft (avoids GVH) using *mAb* and complement.

GVH, graft-versus-host; HVG, host-versus-graft; mAb, monoclonal antibody; MHC, major histocompatibility complex.

Table 13.6 Some adverse effects of glucocorticoids and their prevention or treatment

Adverse effect	Prevention or treatment
Diabetes	Regular blood sugar measurements
Osteoporosis	Bone density should be regularly monitored during steroid treatment. Patients, especially the elderly, may need bisphosphonates and calcium supplements.
Peptic ulcer	Proton pump inhibitors may be required.
Thin skin, easy bruising and poor wound healing	No treatment, but early and intensive intervention of wounds is necessary to prevent chronic morbidity.
Adrenal insufficiency	Prevent sudden decreases in dose, increase dose when ill and carry a steroid card. Treatment is resuscitation and steroid replacement.

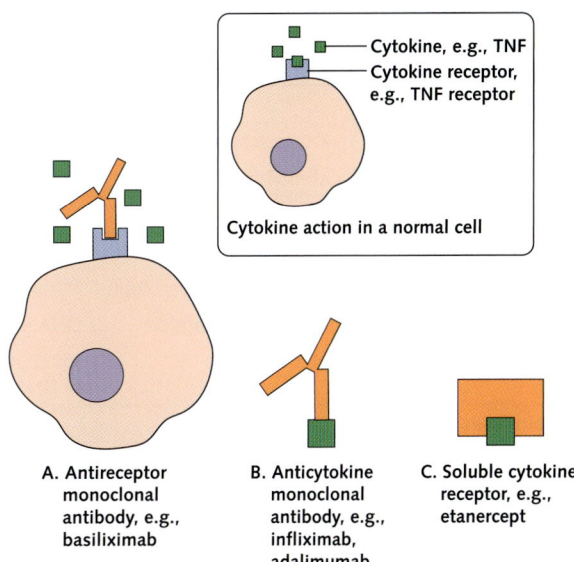

Fig. 13.2 Mechanisms of action of biologics. Monoclonal antibodies can be employed to block receptors, altering cellular function (A). Monoclonal antibodies can also be designed to bind to cytokines directly, attenuating the action of the cytokine (B). Similarly, soluble receptors can be produced, which bind to cytokines, reducing their action on cells (C). While the mechanism of action of anticytokine monoclonal antibodies and soluble cytokine receptors is similar, their molecular components are distinct.

Biologics

Biologics are drugs manufactured in a living system and are very large, complex molecules. Biologics can be designed to block specific parts of the immune system. Typically, they are either monoclonal antibodies against cellular receptors, monoclonal antibodies against cytokines or soluble receptor molecules (Fig. 13.2). There are many different biologics and their use is specialized. It is useful to understand that they also have specific side effects. For example, Rituximab, an anti-CD20 monoclonal antibody (mAb), leads to B-cell depletion, which in turn increases the long-term risk of viral and opportunistic infections. Some biologics boost the immune response to cancers, for example, ipilimumab. Other biologics bypass the immune system entirely and interact with cancer cells directly. For example, trastuzumab (Herceptin) interacts with the human epidermal growth factor receptor 2 on some breast cancer cells. They can also be conjugated with a chemotherapeutic agent, such as brentuximab vedotin (anti-CD30-drug conjugate), facilitating the delivery of the antimitotic agent to malignant cells.

Due to their cost, many of these drugs are used as second- or third-line therapy. Some examples of immunological biologic therapy and the targets involved are detailed in Table 13.7. The field of biologics is rapidly expanding and this is by no means a comprehensive list.

CANCER IMMUNOTHERAPY

Over the last decade, there has been a great progress in cancer immunotherapy, which has translated to improved survival outcomes for cancer patients. A number of approaches to harness the immune system have emerged, such as:

(i) Immune-checkpoint inhibitors: Programmed cell death 1 (PD-1) is an inhibitory molecule expressed on the cell surface of multiple malignant cells, inhibiting tumour cell apoptosis and promoting T-cell exhaustion. Antibodies inhibiting PD-1 and PD ligand 1 (PD-L1), such as pembrolizumab, nivolumab, atezolizumab and avelumab, respectively, are under evaluation for the treatment of a number of malignancies with very encouraging results. Cytotoxic T-lymphocyte-associated protein 4 (CTLA-4) is another immune-checkpoint molecule, the inhibitor of which is under exploration for the treatment of malignant diseases, such as metastatic melanoma.

(ii) Manipulation of T cells: Adoptive cell transfer has transformed the field of immune therapy in the last decade. It refers to the ex vivo manipulation of T cells to render them more reactive and specific against certain (tumour) antigens. This involves:

a. Chimeric antigen receptor (CAR)-T cells: T cells are genetically modified to express the antigen-binding domain from a B-cell receptor, along with the intracellular domain of a CD3 TCR (CD3ζ), (Fig. 13.3). This allows T-cell activation upon recognition of a specific cell surface antigen, independently of MHC.

Table 13.7 Examples of immunosuppressive agents

Drug category	Examples of drugs	Target and mechanism
Corticosteroids		
	Prednisolone	Inhibits antigen presentation, promotes the synthesis of antiinflammatory proteins, affects metabolism and distribution of B- and T-cell lymphocytes
	Methylprednisolone	
Antimetabolites		
	Azathioprine	Antagonist of purine metabolism
	Mycophenolate mofetil	Purine inhibitor
	Cyclophosphamide	DNA alkylation
	Methotrexate	Antifolate antimetabolite (inhibition of dihydrofolate reductase → inhibition of DNA synthesis)
Calcineurin inhibitors		
	Cyclosporin	Inhibits the synthesis of interleukins, including IL-2, which is essential for T-cell activation and differentiation
	Tacrolimus	Inhibits T-cell proliferation by binding to FK506 binding protein
mTOR inhibitors		
	Sirolimus	Form an immunosuppressive complex with the FKBP12 protein, which blocks the activation of the cell-cycle kinase, mTOR → blockage of cell cycle progression
	Everolimus	
Biologic agents		
	Basiliximab	IL2 receptor (CD25a) antibodies: inhibits T-cell proliferation
	Tocilizumab	Anti-IL6 receptor mAb
	Brentuximab vedotin	Anti-CD30 mAb-drug conjugate
	Etanercept	Recombinant human TNF-α receptor fusion protein
	Rituximab	Binds to CD20 receptor on B cells, which are then killed by ADCC
	Pembrolizumab	Blocks PD-1 receptors on T cells. PD-1 activation by cancer cells provides an immune tolerance to the cancer, blocking PD-1 removes this tolerance

PD-1, Programmed cell death 1.

CAR-T cells have been approved for the treatment of haematologic malignancies, such as diffuse large B-cell lymphoma (DLBCL), acute lymphoblastic leukaemia (ALL) and multiple myeloma.

b. Tumour-infiltrating lymphocytes (TILs): This involves the isolation of T-lymphocytes from a freshly resected tumour tissue which recognize specific tumour antigens, followed by in vitro co-culture with IL-2 to promote T-cell activation and expansion. TILs are then reinfused back to the patient following a lymphodepleting regimen (such as cyclophosphamide) to allow in vivo survival and expansion of TILs.

c. Bispecific T-cell engager antibodies (BiTEs): These consist of a protein fragment, recognizing CD3 on one end and a target tumour antigen on the other end, acting as a linker between T cells and tumour cells. Most importantly, they act in an MHC-independent way,

allowing for a broad application without patient-specific processing. An example is blinatumomab, which has specificity for CD19 antigen (found on B cells) and the Fc region of CD3 (found on T cells) and is being used for the treatment of relapsed/refractory ALL.

(iii) Oncolytic viruses: Oncolytic viruses have been employed as antitumour 'agents' in various ways, such as (a) 'APCs' mediating tumour-antigen presentation, (b) engineered to preferentially infect cancer cells and spare normal cells, (c) transduction agents, promoting the expression of immunomodulatory cytokines.

(iv) Vaccines: Vaccine development methods vary significantly, depending on the type or number of antigens, the accompanying adjuvant(s), the administration schedule, etc. Broadly, the principle behind vaccine manufacturing involves using a tumour-associated antigen (which may vary from a simple peptide to a broad range of antigens) to

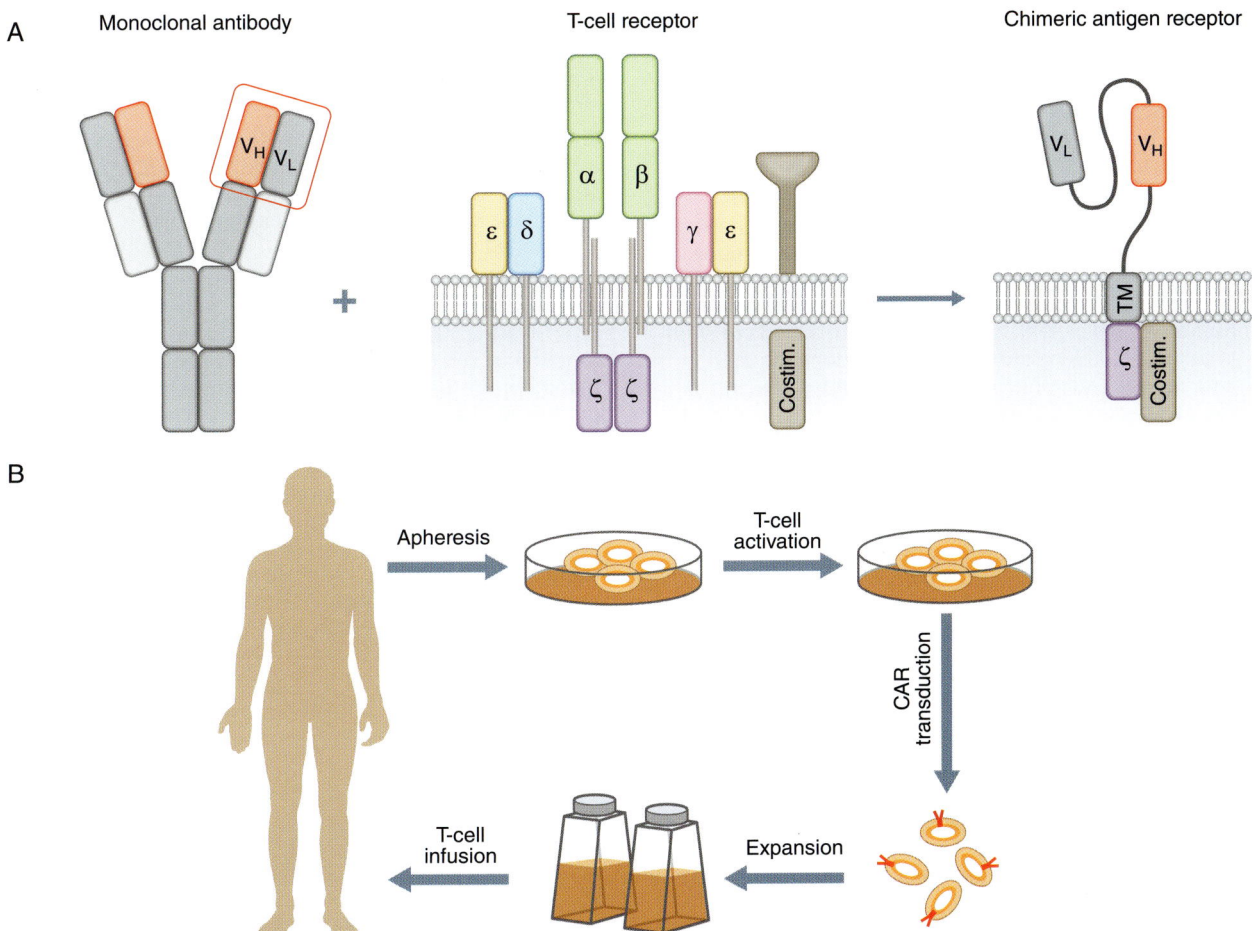

Fig. 13.3 The manufacturing process for CAR-T cells. (A) The chimeric antigen receptor (CAR) is genetically engineered by combining the extracellular antigen receptor–binding domain from a monoclonal antibody (VH and VL are the heavy and light chain variable regions) with the intracellular activation domain from a T-cell receptor (ζ) and a costimulatory subunit (Costim.); they are linked by a transmembrane (TM) component. During the process, the extracellular domain of the T-cell receptor is cleaved and removed (α–e). The new CAR uses the monoclonal antibody binding domain, e.g., anti-CD19, to bind to the target CD19 on the lymphoma cell surface and this can now activate the T-cell effector killing mechanisms via the activation domain, allowing the CAR-T cell to kill the lymphoma cell. (B) The CAR-T cells are manufactured by transducing the new gene for CAR into the patient's T cells. T cells are harvested from the patient by apheresis and then genetically altered in a laboratory process that takes about 4 weeks. The manufactured CAR-T cells are expanded in numbers during this time in tissue culture before being reinfused into the patient. (Source: Modified from Fesnak A O'Doherty U. Clinical development and manufacture of chimeric antigen receptor T cells and the role of leukapheresis. *Eur Oncol Haematol* 2017;13(1):28–34 and Majzner RG, Mackall CL. Clinical lessons learned from the first leg of the CAR T cell journey. *Nat Med 2019*; 25:1341–1355 with permissions.)

train patient's immune system to recognize and attack cancer cells. It is a targeted and personalized therapy, with a huge potential for cancer treatment. However, to date, only one vaccine-based therapy has been approved for cancer treatment, Sipuleucel-T, involving autologous dendritic cells which have been engineered to target prostatic acid phosphatase (PAP) in patients with castrate-resistant prostate adenocarcinoma.

CYTOKINE RELEASE SYNDROME

Cytokine release syndrome (CRS) is a potentially life-threatening complication of CAR-T-cell therapy (most common cause), therapeutic antibodies and other immune therapies (such as antithymocyte globulin). It can also occur after haploidentical stem cell transplantation.

It is an acute, systemic inflammatory response, which occurs 1–14 days post CAR-T-cell therapy (within minutes to hours post antibody administration).

The exact pathophysiological mechanism remains elusive, although an exaggerated immune response has been described, with activation of bystander immune (e.g., macrophages/monocytes) and nonimmune (endothelial) cells and distorted cytokine release (very high levels of IL6, IFN-γ, TNF-α, etc.). This leads to what is called a 'cytokine storm', which overwhelms the counter-regulatory homeostatic responses, leading to the generation of CRS.

Clinically, it presents with fever and multiorgan dysfunction (hypoxia, vascular leak with peripheral and/or pulmonary oedema, hypotension/circulatory collapse, renal failure, cardiac dysfunction), the severity of which specifies the CRS grade (grade 1–4) which in turn guides the management plan. Neuropsychiatric symptoms (such as aphasia, impaired cognitive skills, motor weakness, altered level of consciousness, seizures and cerebral oedema) may also occur (usually 2–4 days after the onset of CRS) and are referred to as 'Immune effector cell-associated neurotoxicity syndrome (ICANS)'.

The differential diagnosis of CRS includes sepsis (such as the CRS-like syndrome induced by COVID-19 infection), tumour progression, heart failure, allergic/anaphylactic reaction and haemophagocytic lymphohistiocytosis (HLH).

As mentioned above, the management depends on the grade of CRS, with moderate/severe cases requiring prompt admission to intensive care unit for close monitoring and organ support. The goal of CRS management is to prevent/treat life-threatening complications of immune therapy while preserving its antitumour effects. Symptomatic management (with fluids, antihistamines, antibiotics, etc.) applies to all patients, whereas for moderate/severe cases (grade 2–4) administration of tocilizumab (anti-IL6 receptor) and glucocorticosteroids is recommended. For refractory cases, agents such as anakinra (IL-1 receptor antagonist), etanercept (anti-TFN-α), alemtuzumab (anti-CD52), ATG and cyclophosphamide have been used.

Chapter Summary

- Immunization is active or passive: each type of immunization can be used in appropriate settings.
- Vaccination is an important form of active immunization; there are different types of vaccine depending on the pathogen targeted.
- Organ transplantation presents an immunological challenge, which can be mediated by HLA matching and using antirejection therapy (which itself presents problems).
- Antiinflammatory drugs are widely used and have important side effects. Steroids cause a range of problems, including cushingoid effects.
- Biologics and immunotherapy have an important role in the future of medicine and allow us to target or change aspects of the immune system.

MLA Conditions

MLA Presentations

Vaccination

SELF-ASSESSMENT

MLA High Yield Association Table

Key findings	Diagnoses
Lacks nucleus, carries oxygen around the body	Red blood cell
Large unpigmented cells, fights infection, immune defence system	White blood cell
Lacks nucleus, haemostasis	Platelet
Granules in cytoplasm	Granulocyte
Multilobed nucleus, granules in cytoplasm, fight bacterial infection	Neutrophil
Bilobed nucleus, pink cytoplasm, orange granules in cytoplasm, parasitic infections, immune reaction	Eosinophil
Bilobed nucleus, dark purple granules in cytoplasm, immunity	Basophil
Large kidney-shaped nucleus, light blue cytoplasm, adaptive immune response	Monocyte
Small cells, round nucleus, dark blue cytoplasm, viral infections	Lymphocyte
Large cells, eccentric nucleus, purple/blue cytoplasm, myeloma	Plasma cell
Development of blood cells, bone marrow, spleen	Haematopoiesis
Destruction of old red blood cells, removal of infection	Spleen function
Left upper quadrant pain, reduced appetite, abdominal distension, early satiety	Enlarged spleen
Acute left upper quadrant pain, fever, hypotension, severe abdominal distension	Splenic infarct/rupture
Left flank scar, history of trauma or lymphoma, previous immune thrombocytopenia, long-term penicillin V prophylaxis	Splenectomy
Recurrent painful crises, anaemia, transfusions, long-term penicillin V	Autosplenectomy due to sickle cell disease
Raised white cells, platelets or red cells; left upper quadrant pain; abdominal distension; thrombosis	Myeloproliferative disorder causing splenomegaly
Fevers, night sweats, enlarged glands, enlarged spleen	Lymphoma with associated splenomegaly and lymphadenopathy
Recent foreign travel, recurrent fevers, abdominal pain	Malaria with splenomegaly
Liver cirrhosis, low platelets, left upper quadrant pain	Cirrhosis with splenomegaly
Enlarged glands	Lymphadenopathy
Sore throat, enlarged neck glands, fevers	EBV-associated lymphadenopathy
Fevers, night sweats, weight loss, enlarged glands	Lymphoma with associated lymphadenopathy
Mature red cells, biconcave discoid shape, no intracellular organelles, lifespan 120 days	Erythrocyte
Carries oxygen, blood pH buffer, vasodilation	Haemoglobin
Red blood cell production	Erythropoiesis
Commits myeloid cells to erythrocyte development pathway	Erythroid burst-forming units (BFU-E)
No haemoglobin, organelles present, large nucleus	Pronormoblast

Continued

Key findings	Diagnoses
Reduction in cell size and nuclear size, accumulation of haemoglobin	Early, intermediate and late normoblasts
Circulate in bloodstream, RNA present, round shape, polychromasia	Reticulocyte
Nucleated red blood cells, polychromasia, sudden drop in haemoglobin, raised bilirubin	Haemolysis
Hormone which raises red cell production	Erythropoietin
High erythropoietin level, weight loss, abdominal pain	Renal cell carcinoma secreting high levels of erythropoietin
Anuria/oliguria, raised creatinine level, anaemia, low erythropoietin level	Renal disease and reduced erythropoietin production
Four globin chains, two α- and two β-globins	Haemoglobin molecule structure
Tetrapyrrole ring, ferrous (Fe^{2+}) centre	Haem
Four molecules of oxygen	Haemoglobin oxygen capacity
≥ 1 haem-bound oxygen	Oxyhaemoglobin (oxyHb)
No haem-bound oxygen	Deoxyhaemoglobin (deoxyHb)
Increased mobility of globin chains, high oxygen affinity	Relaxed Hb (R-Hb)
Reduced mobility of globin chains, low oxygen affinity	Taut Hb (T-Hb)
Low pH, high pCO_2, high 2,3-diphosphoglycerate (2,3-DPG)	Reduced oxygen affinity
High pH, low pCO_2, low 2,3-DPG	Increased oxygen affinity
Graph plotting pO_2 (x axis) against haemoglobin oxygen saturation (y axis), sigmoid curve	Oxygen dissociation curve
Hb with two γ globins and two α globins, higher affinity for oxygen	Foetal haemoglobin (HbF)
Predominant haemoglobin in foetuses and newborns until 6 months	HbF
Sickle cell disease, lower oxygen affinity at low pO_2, abnormal polymerization, vasoocclusion	Sickle haemoglobin (HbS)
Genes encoding ϵ-, γ-, δ- and β-globins	Chromosome 11
Genes encoding ζ- and the α-globins	Chromosome 16
Single globin with single haem group; primarily in muscles	Myoglobin
Dark, leafy green vegetables; red meat	Dietary iron
Ascorbic acid	Enhances iron absorption
Transport protein, carry ferric (Fe^{3+}) ions	Transferrin
Deliver iron to cells; found on erythroblasts, liver and reticuloendothelial macrophages and muscles	Transferrin receptors
Iron storage protein, water soluble	Ferritin
Iron storage protein, insoluble	Haemosiderin
Protein synthesized by liver; limits iron circulation	Hepcidin
Gastrointestinal tract bleeding, menstruation	Iron loss
Multiple blood transfusions; excess intake; haemochromatosis	Iron overload
Autosomal recessive; fail to produce hepcidin; excess iron; heart failure; liver failure; diabetes; thyroid dysfunction; hypogonadism; arthritis	Haemochromatosis
Supports red cell, dense protein	Cytoskeleton
Band 3, glycophorin, cell membrane bilayer	Integral proteins
Spectrin, ankyrin, attached to lipid bilayer	Peripheral proteins

Key findings	Diagnoses
Anchors proteins on red cell surface	Glucosyl phosphatidylinositol (GPI) anchor
Oxidized iron ion (Fe^{3+}) in haemoglobin	Methaemoglobin (MetHb)
Cyanosis, hypoxia, blue-ish discolouration of skin	Methaemoglobinaemia
Blood sample collection	EDTA tubes
Precipitates RNA, identifies reticulocytes	Supravital stain
Low haemoglobin, fatigue, breathlessness, palpitations, syncope	Anaemia
Average size of red cells	Mean cell volume (MCV)
Average mass of haemoglobin per red cell	Mean cell haemoglobin (MCH)
Microcytic anaemia, angular stomatitis, hair loss, koilonychia	Iron deficiency anaemia
Target cells, pencil cells, microcytic cells	Iron deficiency
Microcytic anaemia, weight loss, melaena, PR bleeding, abdominal pain	GI cancer
↓ serum ferritin, ↑ TIBC, ↓ TSAT	Iron deficiency markers
Abnormal, giant red cell precursors	Megaloblastic anaemia
Red cells with high MCV (>100 fL)	Macrocytic anaemia
Hypersegmented neutrophils	Macrocytic anaemia, B12 deficiency, folate deficiency
Macrocytic anaemia, glossitis, neuropsychiatric deficits	Folate deficiency
Anorexia, glossitis, constipation, ascending distal motor weakness, peripheral numbness	B12 deficiency
Antigastric parietal cell antibodies	Pernicious anaemia
Antiintrinsic factor antibodies	Pernicious anaemia
Anaemia, neurological symptoms, premature whitening of hair	Pernicious anaemia
Raised in B12 deficiency; falsely raised in renal disease and bacterial overgrowth	Methylmalonic acid (MMA)
Type 2 diabetes, macrocytic anaemia, low B12	Metformin use
Normocytic anaemia, chronic inflammation	Anaemia of chronic disease
Autoimmune disease, high ferritin, low TSAT, low TIBC	Functional iron deficiency/anaemia of chronic disease
Chronic renal impairment, normocytic anaemia	Reduced Epo
Hypotension, tachycardia, normocytic anaemia, raised reticulocytes, high platelets	Acute blood loss
Nucleated red blood cells, polychromasia, anaemia, spherocytes, low haptoglobin, high LDH	Haemolysis
Haemolysis, enlarged liver, enlarged spleen	Extravascular haemolysis
Haemolysis, urinary haemosiderin	Intravascular haemolysis
Autoimmune haemolytic anaemia	Direct antigen test (DAT)
Haemolysis at body temperature, IgG-mediated	Warm autoimmune haemolysis
Haemolysis at below core body temperature, IgM/C3D mediated	Cold autoimmune haemolysis
Anaemia, young child, viral illness, dark urine	Paroxysmal cold haemoglobinuria (PCH)
Diagnostic test for paroxysmal cold haemoglobinuria	Donath-Landsteiner test
Spherocytes, anaemia, jaundice, defective spectrin	Hereditary spherocytosis
Elliptocytes, defective spectrin	Hereditary elliptocytosis

Continued

Key findings	Diagnoses
Diagnostic test for membrane disorders	EMA binding test
Anaemia, acanthocytes, splenomegaly	PK deficiency
Bite/blister cells, Heinz bodies, high reticulocytes, X-linked disorder	G6PD deficiency
Schistocytes	Microangiopathic haemolytic anaemia (MAHA)
Haemosiderinuria, anaemia, jaundice, fatigue, thrombosis	Paroxysmal nocturnal haemoglobinuria (PNH)
Abnormalities of haemoglobin	Haemoglobinopathies
Sickle cells, target cells, normocytic anaemia, high reticulocytes	Sickle cell anaemia
Glutamine to valine substitution, β-globin gene, abnormal β-globin chains	Sickle cell disease
Stimulates HbF production, used in sickle cell disease	Hydroxycarbamide
Removal of patient's blood and replacement by donor red cells	Exchange transfusion
Sickle cell disease, anaemia, fever, dyspnoea, low pO_2	Acute chest crisis
Anaemia, fever, severe pain, sickle cells	Vaso-occlusive crisis
Deficiency of either α- or β-globins	Thalassaemia
Reduced β-globin chain production	β+ thalassaemia
Absent β-globin chain production	β0 thalassaemia
One abnormal copy of β-globin gene and one normal copy, mild microcytic anaemia	β-thalassaemia trait
Deletion of three α-globin genes; golf ball inclusions, cresyl blue stain, microcytic anaemia	Haemoglobin H disease
Measure migration of molecules by their weight and size	Electrophoresis
Anaemia, reticulocytopenia	Aplastic anaemia
Severe normocytic anaemia, reticulocytopenia, parvovirus B19	Pure red cell aplasia
Increased red cell count above normal levels, raised haematocrit	Polycythaemia
Ratio of volume of red blood cells to total blood volume	Haematocrit (Hct)
White blood cell	Leucocyte
Segmented nuclei; granular cytoplasm	Neutrophil structure
Innate immune system, phagocytosis, release enzymes	Neutrophil functions
Dead neutrophils	Pus
Bilobed nucleus, orange granules in cytoplasm	Eosinophil structure
Attack multicellular parasites; mediate allergic reactions	Eosinophil functions
S-shaped nucleus, purple cytoplasmic granules	Basophil structure
Heparin, histamine, peroxidase, chemotactic factors	Basophil granule contents
Type I hypersensitivity reactions	Basophil function
Large cell, kidney-shaped nucleus, basophilic cytoplasm	Monocyte structure
Phagocytose damaged red cells, pathogens and debris; adaptive immune response; release cytokines	Monocyte functions
Increased proportion immature neutrophils	Left shift
Increased and persistent proportion of mature neutrophils	Right shift
Total white cell count >11 × 10^9/L	Leucocytosis
Fever, unwell, sore throat, raised white cells	Reactive leucocytosis due to infection

Key findings	Diagnoses
Pregnancy, exercise, smoking, steroids	Causes of neutrophilia
Total white cell count <4 × 10^9/L	Leucopenia
Neutrophils <2 × 10^9/L	Neutropenia
Neutrophils <0.5 × 10^9/L	Agranulocytosis
Reduced or ineffective neutrophil production by bone marrow	Inadequate granulopoiesis
Malar rash, joint pains, fevers, fatigue, neutropenia	Autoimmune neutropenia due to SLE
Splenomegaly, neutropenia, joint pains	Felty syndrome
Fatigue, cachexia, previous IVDU, previous blood transfusion, unprotected sexual intercourse, lymphopenia	HIV infection
Smear cells	CLL
Auer rods	AML
Blast cells	AML
Immature leucocytes with occasional blasts and immature red blood cells	Leucoerythroblastic change
History of seizures/epilepsy, leucopoenia	Neutropenia secondary to anticonvulsants (phenytoin/carbamazepine)
History of thyroid goitre, leucopoenia	Neutropenia secondary to antithyroid drugs (carbimazole)
Fevers, night sweats, weight loss	'B symptoms'
Excess proliferation of 1> myeloid progenitors	Myeloproliferative disorders
Abnormal maturation of myeloid cells	Dysplastic cells
Immature myeloid cells	Blasts
Clonal proliferation of immature cells	Leukaemias
Clonal proliferation of lymphoid cells	Lymphomas
Clonal proliferation of abnormal plasma cells	Plasma cell dyscrasias
Fevers, itching, reduced appetite, splenomegaly, high Hb, JAK2 mutation	Polycythaemia
Fever, abdominal distension, splenomegaly, bleeding, high platelets, JAK2/CALR/MPL mutation	Essential thrombocythaemia
Fever, sweats, cachexia, splenomegaly, leucoerythroblastic blood film	Myelofibrosis
Elderly, recurrent infections, easy bruising, weight loss, fatigue	Myelodysplastic syndrome
Blurred vision, headaches, confusion, SOB, CXR infiltrates, high white cell count	Leucostasis due to high white cells in acute leukaemia
Gum swelling and bleeding, fatigue, mouth ulcers	Acute myeloid leukaemia
Lymphadenopathy, hepatosplenomegaly, weight loss, enlarged mediastinum	Acute lymphoblastic leukaemia
Severe bleeding, bruising, coagulopathy, malaise	Acute promyelocytic leukaemia
Fever, sweats, fatigue, malaise, low white cells	Neutropenic sepsis
Replace cancerous marrow cells with healthy donor cells	Allogeneic stem cell transplant
High white cell count, acute renal impairment, cardiac arrhythmias, high uric acid	Tumour lysis syndrome
Elevated white cell count, asymptomatic, insidious onset	Chronic leukaemias

Continued

Key findings	Diagnoses
High white cells, myeloid progenitors on blood film, basophilia, eosinophilia	Chronic myeloid leukaemia
High white cells, 'B symptoms', elderly, recurrent infections, 'smear cells'	Chronic lymphocytic leukaemia
Painless, enlarged lymph nodes; B symptoms; splenomegaly	Lymphomas
Cyclical fever (Pel-Ebstein fever), lymphadenopathy, weight loss, alcohol-induced pain, night sweats, bimodal age distribution	Hodgkin lymphoma
Night sweats, fevers (not cyclical), extranodal disease (GI tract/thymus), low blood counts	Non-Hodgkin lymphoma
Facial swelling, hoarseness, stridor, distended veins on chest wall	SVC obstruction
Specific immunoglobulins secreted by monoclonal plasma cells	Paraprotein
Hypercalcaemia, renal failure, anaemia, bony lesions	'CRAB' criteria for myeloma
Confusion, constipation, abdominal pain, muscle weakness, bony pains	Hypercalcaemia
Lower back pain, saddle anaesthesiae, loss of bowel/bladder control	Cauda equina syndrome
Paraprotein present, plasma cells <10% of marrow, no CRAB	Monoclonal gammopathy of uncertain significance (MGUS)
Restrictive cardiomyopathy, neuropathy, nephrotic syndrome	Amyloidosis
IgM paraprotein, B symptoms, headaches, visual disturbance, dyspnoea	Waldenstrom macroglobulinaemia
Rate at which red cells sediment in 1 hour	Erythrocyte sedimentation rate (ESR)
Cell turnover and metabolic rate; released when cells die	Lactate dehydrogenase (LDH)
Bone marrow aspiration fails to produce marrow cells	'Dry tap'
Visual assessment of chromosomal size and structure	Cytogenetics analysis
Molecular analysis which identifies specific deletions or duplications; identifies translocations associated with specific diseases	Fluorescence in situ hybridization (FISH)
Detects particular antigenic protein structures present on leucocytes; identifies CD markers	Immunophenotyping
Process to limit blood loss	Haemostasis
Time taken for platelet plug to form	Primary haemostasis
Reinforcement of platelet plug with fibrin; Initiated by tissue factor	Secondary haemostasis
Time taken for small cut to stop bleeding	Bleeding time
Platelet production from megakaryocytes	Thrombopoiesis
Hormone produced by liver; stimulates platelet synthesis	Thrombopoietin (TPO)
Calcium adenosine triphosphate, ADP, serotonin, histamine, adrenaline	Platelet dense granule contents
Fibrinogen, von Willebrand factor, factors V, XI and XIII	Platelet alpha granule contents
Thromboxane A2 (TXA2)	Synthesized from arachidonic acid
Vasoconstriction	Thromboxane A2 (TXA2) function
Process of cross-linking between platelets	Aggregation
Cleaved fibrinogen by thrombin; reinforces platelet plug	Fibrin
Prostacyclin (PGI2) and nitric oxide	Inhibit platelet aggregation
Thromboxane A2 synthesis	Cyclooxygenase (COX)
COX inhibition	Aspirin
Platelet activation	ADP

Key findings	Diagnoses
ADP inhibition	Clopidogrel, prasugrel, ticlopidine and ticagrelor
Binds vWF and fibrinogen	GPIIb/IIIA receptor
GPIIb/IIIA receptor inhibition	Abciximab, eptifibatide and tirofiban
Stimulates cyclic AMP degradation; platelet activation	Phosphodiesterase
Phosphodiesterase inhibition	Dipyridamole
Reduced platelet count	Thrombocytopenia
Paraesthesiae, fatigue, thrombocytopenia	B12 deficiency
Deranged LFTs, jaundice, splenomegaly, bruising, thrombocytopenia	Chronic liver disease
Fever, fatigue, breathless, PCP on cultures, thrombocytopenia	Co-trimoxazole induced thrombocytopenia
Fever, diarrhoea, deranged LFTs, CMV positive, thrombocytopenia	Ganciclovir-induced thrombocytopenia
Isolated thrombocytopenia, easy bruising, gum bleeding, increased megakaryocytes on bone marrow biopsy	Immune thrombocytopenia (ITP)
Chest infection, penicillin, thrombocytopenia	Drug-induced ITP
Venous and arterial thrombi, thrombocytopenia, heparin, anti-PF4 antibodies	Heparin-induced thrombocytopenia (HIT)
Fondaparinux, argatroban	Treatment for HIT
Recent blood transfusion, bruising, thrombocytopenia, HPA-1a antibodies	Posttransfusion purpura (PTP)
Neonate, bruising, intracranial bleed, thrombocytopenia, HPA-1a antibodies	Neonatal alloimmune thrombocytopenia (NAIT)
Fragments, thrombocytopenia, anaemia	Microangiopathic haemolytic anaemia (MAHA)
MAHA, thrombocytopenia, fever, confusion, acute kidney injury	Thrombocytopenia thrombotic purpura (TTP)
ADAMTS13 deficiency/inhibition	Pathology of TTP
Thrombocytopenia, acute kidney injury, E. coli O157:H7	Haemolytic uraemic syndrome (HUS)
Left upper quadrant pain, early satiety, thrombocytopenia	Splenomegaly causing platelet sequestration
Factor II	Prothrombin
Factor VII, IX and X	Extrinsic pathway factors
Factor XII, XI, IX, VIII and X	Intrinsic pathway factors
Factor Xa, factor Va and factor II	Common pathway factor
Cleaves prothrombin (FII) to thrombin (FIIa)	Prothrombinase complex
Converts fibrinogen tofFibrin; further activates factors V, VIII and XI; activates FXIII	Thrombin functions
Vital component of coagulation; activates factors	Calcium
Factors II, VII, IX and X	Vitamin K-dependent factors
Inhibits vitamin K epoxide reductase	Warfarin
Prevents tissue factor-medicated initiation of coagulation	Tissue factor pathway inhibitor (TFPI)
Destroys activated cofactors Va and VIIIa	Protein C
Required cofactor for protein C	Protein S
Binds thrombin; activates protein C	Thrombomodulin
Potent inhibitor of thrombin, factor IXa, factor Xa and factor XIIa	Antithrombin (AT)
Potentiated by heparin	Antithrombin

Continued

Key findings	Diagnoses
Converts plasminogen to plasmin; activates fibrinolysis	Tissue plasminogen activator (tPA)
Degrades fibrin networks	Plasmin
Thrombin-activated fibrinolysis inhibitor, plasminogen activator inhibitor, α_2-antiplasmin	Antifibrinolytic factors
Reflects extrinsic pathway	Prothrombin time (PT)
Reflects intrinsic pathway	Activated partial thromboplastin time (APTT)
Degradation products of fibrin	D-dimers
Newborn baby; easy bruising; umbilical stump bleeding	Vitamin K deficiency
Deranged LFTs, bleeding, prolonged PT and APTT	Cirrhotic liver disease
Sepsis, deranged coagulation, thrombocytopenia	Disseminated intravascular coagulation (DIC)
Reduced von Willebrand factor activity	Von Willebrand disease
X-linked recessive, factor VIII deficiency, joint bleeds	Haemophilia A
X-linked, factor IX deficiency, joint bleeds	Haemophilia B
Venous stasis, endothelial injury, hypercoagulability	Virchow's triad
Acute calf erythema, swelling, tenderness, recent immobility, superficial vein dilation	Deep vein thrombosis
Validated risk score to estimate probability of DVT	Well's score
Pleuritic chest pain, dyspnoea, haemoptysis, tachycardia	Pulmonary embolism
Recurrent venous or arterial thrombosis; recurrent miscarriage; lupus anticoagulant; anticardiolipin antibodies	Antiphospholipid syndrome (APLS)
High haemoglobin, abdominal pain, deranged LFTs	Splanchnic vein thrombosis secondary to MPN
Haemolysis, thrombocytopenia, abdominal pain	Splanchnic vein thrombosis secondary to PNH
Measured prothrombin time (PT), used to monitor warfarin	International normalized ratio (INR)
Acute intracranial bleed; high INR; known to be on warfarin	Prothrombin complex concentrate (PCC)
Potentiates antithrombin; inactivates factors IIa and Xa	Heparin
Inhibits factor Xa, monitor anti-Xa levels	Low-molecular-weight heparin (LMWH)
Reverses dabigatran	Idarucizumab
Reverses apixaban and rivaroxaban	Andexanet alfa
Dabigatran	Direct thrombin inhibitor
Apixaban, edoxaban, rivaroxaban	Direct Xa inhibitor
Use of fibrinolytics; massive PE, ST-elevation myocardial infarct, acute ischaemic stroke	Thrombolysis
Therapeutic use of blood product	Transfusion
Focus on patient, reduce need for transfusion	Patient blood management
Screening questionnaire, travel history	Donor health check
Hepatitis B, C, E; HIV; HTLV; syphilis	Donor infection screening
Reduces risk of variant Creutzfeldt-Jakob disease (vCJD), CMV and graft versus host disease (GVHD)	Leucodepletion
Check patient for red cell antibodies	Forward grouping
Check patient red cell antigen	Reverse grouping
Stored at room temperature, shelf-life 5–7 days, constant agitation	Platelet transfusion

Key findings	Diagnoses
Corrects coagulopathy; stored frozen	Fresh frozen plasma (FFP)
Contains factors VIII and XIII, vWF and fibrinogen; treats hypofibrinogenaemia	Cryoprecipitate
Contains factors II, VII, IX and X; reverses warfarin	Prothrombin complex concentrate (PCC)
Haemolysis, fever, back pain, dark urine, hypotension, recent incompatible blood transfusion	Haemolytic transfusion reaction
Newborn baby, jaundice, phototherapy, haemolysis	Haemolytic disease of the foetus and newborn (HDFN)
Anaemia, jaundice, fever, haemoglobinuria, transfusion in previous 7–10 days	Delayed haemolytic transfusion reaction
Fever, normal heart rate and BP, during transfusion	Febrile non-haemolytic reaction
Wheeze, dyspnoea, lip/tongue swelling, recent transfusion	Severe allergic reaction to red cell transfusion
Platelet transfusion, itching, urticaria, normal BP and heart rate	Mild allergic reaction
Severe dyspnoea, frothy pink sputum, transfusion within last 2 hours, hypotension, fever	Transfusion-related lung injury (TRALI)
Acute onset dyspnoea, tachypnoea, desaturation, elevated JVP, recent transfusion within 6 hours, hypertension	Transfusion-associated circulatory overload (TACO)
Fever, tachycardia, hypotension, recent platelet transfusion	Bacterial contamination
Jaundice, pancytopenia, renal failure, diarrhoea, deranged LFTs, history of Hodgkin lymphoma	Transfusion-associated GVHD
Large volume transfusion, dilutional coagulopathy, hypocalcaemia, hypothermia	Major haemorrhage complications
First-line defence against pathogens; nonspecific	Innate immune system
Recognizes and provides protection against any pathogen; specific	Adaptive immune system
Specific molecules found on pathogens, recognized by innate immune system	Pathogen-associated immunostimulants
Small molecular units recognized on pathogens by adaptive immune systems	Antigens
Dynamic collection of organisms living in and on our body	Microbiome
Loss of gut homeostasis resulting in change of microbiome composition	Dysbiosis
Introduction of faecal matter from donor to intestinal tract of recipient	Faecal microbiota transplantation (FMT)
Antibiotics, watery diarrhoea, nausea, abdominal pain	*Clostridium difficile* infection
Phagocytes, natural killer cells, degranulating cells and dendritic cells	Cells of the innate system
Macrophages and neutrophils	Types of phagocytes
Acute sepsis, fever, high C-reactive protein	Raised neutrophils
Recent chemotherapy, fever, hypotension, tachycardia	Neutropenic sepsis
Receptors for complement and Fc portion IgG; cytokine receptors, MHC and B7 molecules	Expressed on macrophages
Cytokines, complement	Activate macrophages
Identify and target virally modified or cancerous cells	Natural killer cells

Continued

Key findings	Diagnoses
Chest tightness, face/tongue swelling, dizziness, breathlessness, raised tryptase	Anaphylaxis
IL-1, IL-6, IFN-γ and TNF	Cytokines released in acute phase response
Fever, cough, hypotension, tachycardia	High C-reactive protein
Bone pain, acute renal impairment, hypercalcaemia	High erythrocyte sedimentation rate in myeloma
Classical, alternative and lectin	Pathways which activate complement
Common terminal pathway	Membrane attack complex (MAC)
Triggered by antibodies	Classical pathway activation
C1 activates C2 and C4, which in turn activate C3	Classical pathway
Triggered by autoactivated C3	Alternative pathway Activation
C3 broken down to C3b -> binds factor B -> cleaved to Ba and Bb -> binds C3 convertase	Alternative pathway
Activated by ficolins and collectins	Lectin pathway activation
Mannan-binding lectin (MBL) binds proteases -> generates C3 convertase	Lectin pathway
C3 convertase cleaves C5 to C5a and C5b -> activates C6-C9 -> form membrane attack complex	Effectors of complement
Able to kill *Neisseria* bacteria	Membrane attack complex
Membrane cofactor protein, decay accelerating factor (CD55), C1 inhibitor, CD59, factor I	Complement pathway inhibitors
Anaemia, DAT negative, abdominal vein thrombosis, loss of CD55 and CD59 expression	Paroxysmal nocturnal haemoglobinuria (PNH)
Recurrent lip and face swelling, breathlessness, hypotension, C1 inhibitor deficiency	Hereditary angioedema
Anaemia, jaundice, DAT negative, factor I deficiency	Atypical haemolytic uraemic syndrome (aHUS)
Long-lasting immunity to pathogens	Adaptive immune system
Pathogen-mediated activation of adaptive immune system by innate immune system	Pathogen-associated immunostimulants
B-cell receptors, T-cell receptors, MHC molecules, immunoglobulin	Members of immunoglobulin superfamily
Part of the antigen bound by immunoglobulin superfamily molecules	Epitope
Process and present antigens	Antigen-presenting cells (APCs)
T cell receptor and CD3	Components of T-cell surface antigen receptor
Heterodimer of α- and β-chains	T-cell receptor structure
All nucleated cells express this	Major histocompatibility complex (MHC)
HLA-A, -B and -C	MHC class I
HLA-DR, -DP and -DQ	MHC class II
Present antigens to CD8$^+$ cytotoxic T cells	MHC class I molecules
Present antigens to CD4$^+$ T cells	MHC class II molecules
Th1, Th2, Th17 and T-regulatory cells	Express CD4
Cytotoxic T lymphocytes and T regs	Express CD8
Stabilize TCR-MHC interaction and promote T-cell signalling	CD4 and CD8 functions
Recurrent infections, fatigue, malaise, Kaposi sarcoma, low CD4 counts	HIV infection

Key findings	Diagnoses
Process that increases affinity of an immunoglobulin antibody for its antigen	Somatic hypermutation
Single B cell produces different classes of immunoglobulin	Class switching
Antibody production	Humoral immunity
Create lymphocytes and early development	Primary lymphoid organs (thymus and bone marrow)
Maintain lymphocytes and initiate immune response	Secondary lymphoid organs (spleen and lymph nodes)
Clonal selection of B cells that respond only to foreign antigen; ignore certain peptides	Tolerance
kappa (κ) or lambda (λ)	Types of light chains
IgM, IgG, IgA, IgE and IgD	Types of heavy chains
Hypervariable regions on light and heavy chains of immunoglobulin	Antigen-binding site
Allows movement and greater interaction with epitopes	Hinge region
Passive drainage system which returns interstitial ('lymphatic') fluid to circulation	Lymphatic system
Initiate adaptive immune response; filter lymphatic fluid	Lymph nodes
Lymphoid tissue found in gastrointestinal, respiratory and urogenital tracts	Mucosal-associated lymphoid tissue
Organized submucosal lymphoid follicles throughout large and small intestine	Peyer patches
T-lymphocytes, macrophages and natural killer cells	Components of cell-mediated immunity
Eliminate intracellular pathogens, tumour cells and foreign grafts	Functions of cell-mediated immunity
T-cell development and maturation with receptors that recognize foreign antigen	Thymus function
$\alpha\beta$-TCRs and $\gamma\delta$-TCR	Different types of TCR
Determine epitopes to be targeted by immune system	T-helper cell function
Recognize antigen with MHC class I molecules	Cytotoxic T lymphocytes
Activate T cells in nonspecific function	Superantigen
Fever, diffuse macular rash, tampon use, *Staphylococcus aureus*, superantigen response	Toxic shock syndrome
Negative selection; remove most self-reactive lymphocytes	Central tolerance
Nonspecific response following tissue injury	Inflammation
Rubor, calor, dolor and tumour	Signs of inflammation
Triggered by insult, short duration, innate and adaptive immune activation	Acute inflammation
Vasodilation, increased vascular permeability, entry of neutrophils	Vascular changes during inflammation
Neutrophils adhere to vessel wall -> pass between endothelial cells -> follow chemokines	Chemotaxis
Adherence of neutrophils to vessel wall	Margination
Neutrophils move between endothelial cells	Diapedesis
Fever, skin trauma, pus, erythema	Pyogenic bacterial infection
IL-6, IL-8, IL-1, TNF-α, IFN-γ	Cytokines involved in inflammation

Continued

Key findings	Diagnoses
Attract neutrophils, induce prostacyclin production, mediate acute phase response	Cytokine functions
Activated by factor XII, increases vascular permeability	Bradykinin
Activates complement, forms fibrin degradation products to increase vascular permeability	Plasmin
Infection, inflammation, cigarettes, stress, exercise, myeloproliferative neoplasms	Neutrophilia
Prolonged acute inflammation	Chronic inflammation
Joint swelling, fatigue, malaise, erythema	Rheumatoid arthritis
Low haemoglobin, normal MCV, inflammatory disorder	Anaemia of chronic disease
Fever, night sweats, haemoptysis, weight loss, granulomas	*Mycobacterium tuberculosis*
Antigen shift, virus expresses different immunological targets	*Influenza*
Fever, malaise, dermatomal rash, previous chicken pox	Latent varicella zoster virus
Don't require intracellular environment to replicate; examples include *Staphylococcus aureus*, *Haemophilus influenzae*, *Pseudomonas aeruginosa*	Extracellular bacteria
Require intracellular environment; cell-mediated immunity targets them; example includes *Mycobacterium tuberculosis*	Intracellular bacteria
Escape phagocytes; resistance to humoral defence; cytokine secretion; interfere with antigen presentation	Bacterial strategies to escape immune response
Intracellular infection; complex life cycles	Protozoa
Escape cytoplasm following phagocytosis	*Trypanosoma cruzi*
Prevent complement action	*Leishmania* spp.
Malaise, fever, headache, vomiting, diarrhoea, recent travel to Africa	*Plasmodium falciparum* infection
Fever, abdominal symptoms, weight loss, raised eosinophils	Parasite infection
Excessive, inappropriate inflammatory response to antigen	Hypersensitivity
Types I, II and III	Antibody-mediated hypersensitivity reactions
Type IV	Cell-mediated hypersensitivity reaction
Exposure to irritant, 'wheal and flare', bronchospasm, angioedema, IgE-mediated	Type I hypersensitivity reaction
Immune dysfunction from lack of exposure to antigens and microbes	Hygiene hypothesis
Multiple allergies, family history, high IgE	Atopy
Chronic inflammatory disorder of airways; reversible airflow obstruction; dry cough, wheeze	Asthma
Nasal congestion; watery nasal discharge; sneezing after exposure to allergen (grass/flower/pollen)	Allergic rhinitis
Superficial skin inflammation; contact with nickel; rash in flexural creases; itching, dry skin	Allergic eczema
Hypotension, wheeze, stridor, facial oedema, rapid onset	Anaphylaxis
Produce antibodies specific for cell surface antigens	Type II hypersensitivity reaction
Molecular mimicry; streptococcal antigens; mitral valve damage	Rheumatic fever
IgG antibodies against TSH receptor; palpitations; fevers; weight loss; exophthalmos	Graves disease

Key findings	Diagnoses
Antibodies react to soluble antigens; formation of immune complexes	Type III hypersensitivity reaction
Fever, rash and polyarthalgias; antithymocyte globulin	Serum sickness
Child with recent sore throat; hypertension; haematuria; proteinuria; acute renal failure	Post–streptococcal glomerulonephritis
Arthralgia, discoid rash, fever, malaise, glomerulonephritis, anti-dsDNA	Systemic lupus erythematosus (SLE)
Delayed reaction after antigen exposure; CD4+ T-cell mediated	Type IV hypersensitivity reaction
Erythematous purpuric rash, swelling, bullae, recently wore gloves	Contact dermatitis
Intradermal injection, local swelling and redness	Tuberculin type
Fever, hypercalcaemia, breathless, granulomas, raised ACE	Sarcoidosis
Severe skin and mucosal necrosis; hypovolaemic shock	Stevens-Johnson syndrome
Body exhibits immunological reactivity to itself	Autoimmunity
Polyuria, polydipsia, weight loss, raised sugars	Type I diabetes mellitus
Middle-aged female, weight gain, puffy face, bradycardia, cold intolerance, anti-TPO	Hashimoto thyroiditis
Swollen small joints of hands feet, symmetrical, anti-CCP	Rheumatoid arthritis
Predisposed to opportunistic infections	Immune deficiency
Inherited defects of immune system	Primary immunodeficiency
Malignancy, malnutrition, steroids, radiation, HIV	Causes of secondary immunodeficiency
Immunoglobulins, complement quantification, autoimmune antibodies	Immunological investigations
Temporary immunity; transfer of exogenous antibody from one person to another	Passive immunization
Maternal IgG crosses placenta; IgA in breast milk	Passive immunity in foetus/neonate
Contact with antigens; infection or vaccination	Active immunization
Induces specific immunity to particular pathogen	Vaccination
Vaccine with weakened organism	Live attenuated vaccination
Grafts moved from one part of the body to another	Autologous graft
Grafts between genetically identical individuals	Syngeneic grafts
Grafts between individuals of same species	Allogeneic grafts
Grafts between different species	Xenogeneic grafts
Hyperacute, acute and chronic	Types of graft rejection
Conditioning therapy, infusion of donor's haematopoietic stem cells	Allogeneic haematopoietic stem cell transplant
Transplant removes residual malignant cells	Graft versus leukaemia effect
Donor T cells recognize host cells and tissues as foreign	Graft versus host disease
Steroids, antimetabolites, T-cell signalling inhibitors	Immunosuppressive drugs
Abdominal pain, PR bleeding, weight loss, mouth ulcers, TPMT measurement	Azathioprine for IBD
Act on phagocytes, inhibitor mediators of inflammation	Glucocorticoid steroids
Steroid use, puffy face, rounder abdomen, bruising	Cushing syndrome secondary to glucocorticoids
Hypotension, tachycardia, hyperkalaemia, hyponatraemia	Addisonian crisis

Continued

Key findings	Diagnoses
Large complex molecules which block specific parts of immune system	Biologics
Programmed cell death 1 (PD-1) target, lymphoma, melanoma	Immune checkpoint inhibitors
Genetic modification of T cells to express antigen-binding domain from B-cell receptor	Chimeric antigen receptor (CAR) – T cells
T-lymphocytes from tumour tissue	Tumour-infiltrating lymphocytes
Targets CD3 and tumour antigen	Bispecific T-cell engager antibodies (BiTEs)
Recent CAR-T, hypotension, fever, peripheral oedema, tachycardia, high IL-6	Cytokine release syndrome

MLA Single Best Answer (SBA) Questions

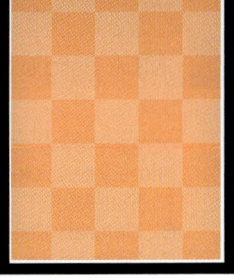

Chapter 1 Principles of haematology

1. Which of the following is a progenitor cell of lymphoid lineage?
   A. BFY-E
   B. CFU-Meg
   C. CFU-GEMM
   D. CFU-Eos
   E. Pre-B cell

2. Which of the following is a mature cell of the myeloid lineage origin?
   A. Natural killer (NK) cell
   B. T lymphocyte
   C. Platelet
   D. CFU-Eos
   E. CFU-Meg

3. Which of the following statements most accurately describes the spleen?
   A. The major site of haematopoiesis in adults
   B. The main site of blood filtration
   C. The major organ responsible for detoxification of digested molecules
   D. An organ accounting for ~5% of body weight
   E. The organ responsible for the majority of erythropoietin synthesis

4. Which of the following diseases is not associated with splenomegaly?
   A. Falciparum malaria
   B. Primary myelofibrosis
   C. Thalassaemia major
   D. Portal vein thrombosis
   E. Pernicious anaemia

5. Which of the following is a common cause for generalized lymphadenopathy?
   A. Mumps virus infection
   B. Lyme disease (borreliosis)
   C. Left ventricular failure
   D. Polycythaemia rubra vera
   E. Sickle cell anaemia

6. Regarding the management of asplenic patients, which of the following interventions is of lowest priority?
   A. Pneumococcal vaccination
   B. Annual influenzae vaccinations

   C. *Haemophilus influenzae* vaccination
   D. Testing for cytomegalovirus and Epstein-Barr virus status
   E. Prophylactic daily antibiotics

7. Which of the following growth factors stimulate CFU-Meg and megakaryocytes?
   A. Interleukin 1
   B. Erythropoietin
   C. Granulocyte-colony stimulating factor
   D. Thrombopoietin
   E. Interleukin 6

8. Which of the following would be appropriate in the clinical management of a severely neutropenic 18-year-old?
   A. Erythropoietin
   B. Thrombopoietin
   C. Interferon
   D. Granulocyte-colony stimulating factor
   E. Pegylated interferon

9. A 35-year-old patient with end-stage renal failure (awaiting renal transplant) complains to his nephrologist of breathlessness and palpitations on exertion. He is noted to be very pale. His lung function is normal. The nephrologist feels a regular subcutaneous infection of a synthetic growth factor would be appropriate. Which of the following is appropriate?
   A. Thrombopoietin
   B. Erythropoietin
   C. Granulocyte-colony stimulating factor
   D. Levemir
   E. Fragmin

10. Which cell typically resides in lymph nodes, secretes immunoglobulins and has a diameter of 6-9 μm, nongranular basophilic cytoplasm and a relatively large nucleus:cytoplasm ratio?
    A. Erythrocyte
    B. T cell
    C. Basophil
    D. Memory B cells
    E. Macrophage

11. Which of the following is derived from the BFU-E progenitor cell and responds to a growth factor

primarily synthesized in the kidney? Gas transport is its primary physiological role.

A. Platelets
B. Natural Killer cell
C. Erythrocyte
D. Monocyte
E. Macrophage

12. Which of the following is important for the destruction of multicellular parasitic organisms? The majority of this resides in tissues rather than the bloodstream.

A. Immunoglobulins
B. Interleukins
C. Macrophage
D. Natural killer cells
E. Eosinophils

Chapter 2 Red blood cells and haemoglobin

1. Regarding red cell structure, which of the following options describes the structure most accurately?

A. High-variable 3D structure
B. A biconcave discoid
C. Irregular polygonal
D. Nearly spherical
E. Elliptical (stretched ovoid)

2. The GP received a report about a peripheral blood film of a new patient who had routine health check bloods. The patient, a 35-year-old man, comes in for a consultation. In his past medical history, he reports that he takes daily antibiotics and needs to be registered for annual vaccines with the new GP. He reports this has been the case for the past 15 years, since he was in a bad motorcycle accident and had major abdominal surgery due to internal bleeding. What is the most likely finding on his peripheral blood film?

A. Howell-Jolly bodies
B. Heinz bodies
C. Pappenheimer bodies
D. Spherocytes
E. Immature lymphocytes

3. Regarding physiological iron levels, which of the following statements is the most accurate?

A. All iron intake accumulates over the lifespan of a person, since there is no mechanism for iron to leave the body
B. The primary regulation mechanism for iron excretion is via variable blood loss, since 1 mL blood contains 0.5 mg iron
C. Hepcidin, via downregulation of the iron exporter, represents the main regulation mechanism, affecting iron absorption

D. Most absorbed iron is removed from the body by faecal elimination
E. Iron elimination is mediated by albumin binding, then hepatic conjugation to glucuronide and finally biliary secretion

4. A 3-year-old patient is having elective complex hand surgery under regional anaesthesia. Using anatomical landmarks, the anaesthetist infiltrates a large volume of prilocaine; ultimately, the operation proceeds under general anaesthesia, as adequate numbness to the operating zone cannot be achieved. Shortly after the induction, the patient becomes deep cyanosed blue and the pulse oximetry oxygen saturations fall to 85% despite an inspired oxygen of 100%. Surprisingly, her heart rate, blood pressure and end-tidal CO_2 are unaffected. Which of the following is most likely to be the cause of the cyanosis?

A. An elevated proportion of haemoglobin with oxidized (ferric) iron
B. Hypoxia secondary to endotracheal tube being inserted into the right main bronchus
C. Hypoxia secondary to pulmonary embolism
D. Hypoxia secondary to tension pneumothorax
E. Hypoxia secondary to pulmonary aspiration

5. Which of the following sequences correctly describes part of haem metabolism?

A. Separation into protoporphyrin and iron components, protoporphyrin conjugation to bilirubin
B. Protoporphyrin conversion to bilirubin, bilirubin conjugation to acetyl groups
C. Conjugated bilirubin is secreted (in bile) into the gastrointestinal (GI) lumen, conversion to urobilinogen
D. Urobilinogen reabsorption from the GI lumen, intravascular metabolism (in hepatocytes) to urobilinogen for renal excretion

6. In which of the following scenarios would the patient be most likely to suffer from inadequate erythropoietin production?

A. Iron deficiency anaemia
B. End-stage renal failure awaiting transplant
C. Chronic haemolytic anaemia
D. Athlete following 2 months training at altitude
E. Patient with metastatic renal cell carcinoma

7. Regarding the oxygen dissociation curve, which of the following options is accurate?

A. A left shift in the curve describes a decrease in the affinity of haemoglobin (Hb) for oxygen
B. The presence of elevated levels of methaemoglobin shifts the curve towards the right

C. Under conditions of high pCO_2, low pH and high (2,3-DPG), the dissociation curve shifts to the left

D. A right shift means that a particular % of Hb oxygen saturation, for example, 50%, will occur at a high pO_2 value

E. Foetal Hb has a dissociation curve positioned to the right of that of adult Hb

8. Which of the following diseases is the least likely to carry a risk of iron overload?
   A. Thalassaemia
   B. Sickle cell anaemia
   C. B12 deficiency
   D. Haemochromatosis
   E. Prolonged oral iron ingestion

9. A patient with Child-Pugh C liver disease is admitted to the intensive care unit following a large variceal bleed. You receive a call from the haematology laboratory about the findings of the red cell morphology on the blood film, which was automatically requested given the patient is significantly anaemic. What finding is most likely to be found on the blood film?
   A. Acanthocytes
   B. Heinz bodies
   C. Band cells
   D. Anisocytosis
   E. Rouleaux

10. The medical junior doctor calls the Haematology team concerned about the blood film results of a patient. The patient, a 60-year-old lady, has been admitted with right temple and jaw pain, as well as some vision disturbance in the right eye. She is currently admitted to the acute medical unit, receiving IV methylprednisolone and awaiting Rheumatology review. The junior doctor is worried that the reported finding is found to be malignancy; which is the most likely comment on the blood film?
    A. Target cells
    B. Poikilocytosis
    C. Red cell fragments
    D. Rouleaux
    E. Sickle cell

11. Why may a patient with mixed iron and B12 deficiency have an increased red cell distribution (RDW) parameter reported on a blood film?
    A. Assay error
    B. Right shift
    C. Anisocytosis
    D. Haemolysis
    E. Dehydration

12. A Greek patient who vigilantly excludes broad beans from his diet experiences an acute fall in his Hb while hospitalized. He had an episode of diabetic ketoacidosis, precipitated by the pyelonephritis for which he was admitted and received cotrimoxazole. Bite cells and Heinz bodies are noted on his blood. Which of the following is the most likely trigger for this phenomenon?
    A. Anaphylactic reaction
    B. Diabetic ketoacidosis
    C. Pyelonephritis
    D. Cotrimoxazole
    E. B, C and D in combination

Chapter 3 Red blood cell disorders

1. In pyruvate kinase deficiency, what is the best statement to describe the biochemical disturbance in red blood cells?
   A. Increases susceptibility to oxidative stress due to inadequate availability of glutathione
   B. Increased structural fragility due to insufficient adenosine triphosphate (ATP) generation due to failure of glycolysis
   C. Abnormal precipitation of oxidized, denatured haemoglobin intracellularly
   D. Abnormal tetramerization of sceptrin dimers resulting in abnormal structure and reduced integrity
   E. Loss of normal membranal expression of phosphatidylinositol glycan protein A (PIG-A) leading to complement-mediated lysis

2. In clinical features associated with G6PD deficiency, which of the following is true?
   A. Chronic background haemolysis results in a mild but permanent normocytic anaemia
   B. Haemolysis is primarily extravascular; the spleen and reticuloendothelial system remove red cells prematurely
   C. In the African subtype, sufferers must avoid eating fava beans as they provoke haemolysis
   D. Insufficient glutathione regeneration occurs due to failure of the pentose phosphate pathway
   E. If this diagnosis is suspected, a sample drawn during active haemolysis is of greatest diagnostic use

3. Which diagnosis best accounts for the following findings? A 6-month-old baby with Portuguese parents presents with failure to thrive and is found to have Hb 35 g/L, MCV 62 fL; and electrophoresis showed HbF to be predominant and HbA to be absent.

A. Beta-thalassaemia minor (trait)
B. Alpha-thalassaemia major (no alpha globin chain)
C. Haemoglobin H disease (1 alpha chain)
D. Beta-thalassaemia major (2 abnormal beta genes)
E. Sickle cell anaemia (2 sickle variant beta genes)

4. Which of the following is more likely to be associated with iron than vitamin B12 deficiency?
   A. Peripheral paraesthesia and numbness
   B. Subacute combined degeneration of the cord
   C. Angular stomatitis and glossitis
   D. Megaloblastic anaemia
   E. Diffuse hair loss and koilonychia

5. Which of the following statements best describes a megaloblastic anaemia?
   A. A reduced haemoglobin (Hb), accompanied by a raised mean cell volume (MCV) and mean cell haemoglobin (MCH)
   B. A raised MCV, low Hb and megaloblasts visible on blood film
   C. A normal MCV, raised Hb and red cell count, erythropoietin (EPO) elevated
   D. Low Hb, raised MCV, megaloblasts seen on bone marrow examination
   E. A reduced Hb and MCV, basophilic stippling of red cells

6. Which of the following sets of investigation results are consistent with iron deficiency?
   A. Haemoglobin (Hb) 85 g/L, mean cell volume (MCV) 50 fL, total iron binding capacity (TIBC) 70 μmol, ferritin 280 μmol, transferrin 2.8 g/L
   B. Hb 75, MCV 110 fL, bone marrow iron stores increased, TIBC 80 μmol, transferrin 3.0 g/L, ferritin 350 μmol
   C. Hb 100 g/L, MCV 115 fL, TIBC 55 μmol, transferrin 2.9 g/L, red cell folate: low
   D. Hb 90 g/L, MCV 69 fL, TIBC 95 μmol, transferrin 5.5 g/L, ferritin 5 μmol.
   E. Hb 140 g/L, MCV 82 fL, TIBC 50 μmol, transferrin 3g/L, ferritin 300 μmol, red cell folate: normal

7. A 22-year-old patient complains of fatigue. On investigation she has a macrocytic, megaloblastic anaemia, Hb of 95 g/L and both low serum folate and low red cell folate. She is adamant she cannot be iron or folate deficient since as a vegan she eats so many dark green leafy vegetables. Which of the following options represents the best treatment strategy?
   A. B12 intramuscular injection, oral folate supplements
   B. Iron supplementations for at least 4 months
   C. Oral B12 supplementation
   D. Oral folate supplementation
   E. Two units of red cell transfusion

8. A patient is receiving a blood transfusion for severe anaemia of chronic disease. He becomes anxious, febrile and hypotensive. The transfusion is stopped, and he is transferred to the intensive care unit where he later receives temporary renal replacement therapy for anuric acute kidney injury and cryoprecipitate for disseminated intravascular coagulation (DIC). What is the underlying mechanism causing his deterioration?
   A. DIC
   B. Drug-induced haemolytic anaemia
   C. G6PD deficiency
   D. Alloimmune haemolysis
   E. Cold autoimmune haemolytic anaemia (AIHA)

9. A 25-year-old lady with hypothyroidism, type 1 diabetes and coeliac disease complains to her GP about cold intolerance. She states her fingers and toes become extremely painful and purple in colour when she is working in the garden. As she has just come from walking in the cold weather to the surgery without mittens on, the GP is able to see her hands. They also note she has mild jaundice. An FBC reveals Hb 95 g/L. She is referred to the Haematology team and commenced on treatment effectively in managing her symptoms. What is the most likely treatment she was commenced on?
   A. Antibiotics
   B. Nifedipine
   C. Iloprost
   D. Steroids
   E. Rituximab

10. A patient with severe burns develops disseminated intravascular coagulation (DIC). The blood film report highlights schistocytes. He becomes increasingly anaemic and the suspicion is that the cause is due to fibrin deposition in the microvasculature. What is the primary diagnosis?
    A. Hereditary spherocytosis
    B. Microangiopathic haemolytic anaemia (MAHA)
    C. Alloimmune haemolysis
    D. Drug-induced haemolytic anaemia
    E. Major external haemorrhage

11. A 27-year-old patient is started on cefalexin for streptococcal ear infection. She develops breathlessness and syncope and presents to the emergency department. She denies any other past medical or family history, on initial bloods she is found to have a new anaemia with Hb 90 g/L. What is the most likely diagnosis?
    A. Pyruvate kinase (PK) deficiency
    B. Paroxysmal nocturnal haemoglobinuria

C. G6PD deficiency

D. Drug-induced haemolytic anaemia

E. Disseminated intravascular coagulation

12. An 8-year-old Senegalese girl is brought in from school by the school nurse complaining of extreme pain in her back. She is crying with the pain. Examination is unremarkable; however, the pain does not respond to paracetamol or ibuprofen. The A&D doctor is hesitant to prescribe opiates at first; however, the school nurse reports that the girl has an important blood disorder diagnosis that needs consideration. What is the likely diagnosis?

A. Anaphylactic reaction

B. Functional disorder

C. Trauma

D. Sepsis

E. Painful infarctive crisis on a background of sickle cell anaemia

13. A 25-year-old man is in recovery following general anaesthetic for elective anterior cruciate ligament reconstruction. The nurse is extremely concerned because he is coming breathless and complaining of chest pain and has SpO_2 of 91%. A chest X-ray shows diffuse bilateral shadowing. On further review he admits that he has a diagnosis of sickle cell anaemia but did not want to mention it because it has been well controlled on medications and he wanted to get the surgery quickly. What is happening?

A. Acute chest syndrome

B. Severe anaemia

C. Sepsis

D. Splenic sequestration crisis

E. Aplastic crisis

14. You are the senior house officer called to see a 25-year-old man with sickle cell in theatre recovery, who you are suspecting acute chest syndrome. What is the next most appropriate step?

A. Sending off FBC, renal profile, CRP bloods with a venous blood gas

B. Trying to wean off oxygen aiming for lower oxygen targets

C. Commencing antibiotics and incentive spirometry

D. Prioritizing a commuted topography pulmonary angiogram (CTPA)

E. Sending off bloods and conducting an arterial blood gas, commencing analgesia and antibiotics

15. An 18-year-old female with known sickle cell anaemia attends to the emergency department with her mother. She has suffered from diarrhoea and vomiting for the past 48 hours, which her mother reports other family members have also been having. On examination, she is peripherally cool (capillary refill time 5 s), tachycardic (HR 140 bpm), tachypnoeic (RR 30 bpm), hypotensive (systolic blood pressure 60) and drowsy with a GCS of 13. What is happening?

A. Patient is having an aplastic crisis

B. Patient is tired from low nutrition these past 48 hours

C. Patient is in septic shock and need urgent resuscitation

D. Patient is drowsy from opiate use

E. Patient has viral gastroenteritis

16. A 1-year-old girl is brought into hospital with severe abdominal pain. On examination she has massive splenomegaly and the haematology laboratory calls to inform you that her Hb is 35 and they have seen some sickle-shaped red blood cells on the peripheral blood film. What is the likely treatment course she received?

A. Transfused, resuscitated and then when stable proceeded for splenectomy

B. Simple top up transfusion and discharged with safety-netting advise

C. Transferred to paediatric intensive care unit

D. Antibiotics and fluid resuscitation

E. Referred for urgent bone marrow transplant

17. A 14-year-old boy is brought into the emergency department looking unwell. He appears pale, is tachycardic and complaining of palpitations and a sore throat and feeling feverish. His mother reports his sister has been off sick from school as well with a runny nose and red rash on her cheek, almost appearing like a slap mark. You note widespread bruising and bleeding from his gums and inner nostrils. On review of his hospital notes, you see he is known to the Paediatric Haematology team for sickle cell disease. What do you expect to see on his FBC result?

A. Low Hb, low MCV and raised white cell count

B. Low Hb, normal white cell count and raised platelets

C. Normal Hb, low white cells and low platelets

D. Normal Hb, raised white cells and low platelets

E. Low Hb, low white cells count and low platelets

18. A 70-year-old man is asked to attend to the emergency department by his GP due to concern of abnormal results on a recent blood test. On review, he appears pale and short of breath when walking into the examination room. He reports feeling very tired over the past few weeks and has noticed his stool has been black in colour with a rather offensive smell in the past 2 days. On his FBC you find Hb 90, MCV 70 fL with

normal white cell and platelet count. What is the next most appropriate step?

A. Send home with oral iron supplementation
B. Transfuse two units of RBC and then discharge with requests for urgent outpatient endoscopy and colonoscopy on 2 week-wait cancer pathway
C. Check vital signs (BP, HR, SpO_2, temperature) and conduct a thorough physical examination including a PR exam
D. Give intravenous iron supplementation
E. Refer to the colorectal surgeons

Chapter 4   White blood cells

1. Which of the myeloid lineage leucocytes is the macrophage precursor?
   A. Lymphocyte
   B. Neutrophil
   C. Basophil
   D. Monocyte
   E. Eosinophil

2. Which of the following conditions is the most likely to be associated with lymphopenia?
   A. Ancylostoma (hookworm) infection
   B. Human immunodeficiency virus (HIV) infection
   C. Epstein-Barr virus (EBV) infection
   D. Acute lymphoblastic leukaemia (ALL)
   E. Toxoplasmosis

3. Which of the following neutrophil precursors is most likely to be present in the peripheral blood in 'left shift'?
   A. Band cell
   B. Metamyelocyte
   C. Promyelocyte
   D. Myelocyte
   E. Myeloblast

4. A 35-year-old female patient with rheumatoid arthritis and significant hepatosplenomegaly due to amyloidosis is being treated for septic shock on ITU with vancomycin for suspected methicillin-resistant *Staphylococcus aureus* infection of a recent total hip replacement. Her latest full blood count indicates that she is profoundly neutropenic, which was not on her admission bloods. Which of the factors revealed by the history is most likely to be responsible for her neutropenia?
   A. Recent surgery
   B. Vancomycin treatment
   C. Hypersplenism
   D. Rheumatoid arthritis
   E. Severe infection

Chapter 5   Haematological malignancies

1. Which of the following factors is not typically associated with 'apparent' erythrocytosis?
   A. Chronic obstructive pulmonary disease
   B. Thiazide diuretics
   C. Obesity
   D. Dapagliflozin
   E. Alcohol abuse

2. Which of the following statements most accurately describes the myelodysplastic syndromes?
   A. A clonal proliferation of abnormal plasma cells in blood and bone marrow
   B. Accumulation of abnormal lymphoid cells in nodal and extranodal tissues
   C. Replacement of normal marrow with dysplastic haematopoietic precursors
   D. Neoplastic proliferation of a myeloid precursor resulting in hypercellular marrow
   E. Accumulation of abnormal neoplastic white cells in the bone marrow

3. A 65-year-old man presents to A&E with 3-day history of headaches, blurred vision, breathlessness and productive cough of pink frothy sputum. Clinical findings are:
   Blood pressure 140/90 mmHg
   Heart rate 110 bpm sinus rhythm
   Temperature 37.1°C
   Saturations 88% on room air
   Investigations:
   Hb 50g/L
   White cell count 130×10^9/L
   Platelets 25×10^9/L
   Chest X-ray: bilateral infiltrates
   Which of the following is the most likely diagnosis?
   A. Acute pulmonary oedema
   B. Sepsis
   C. Hyperviscosity syndrome
   D. Pulmonary haemorrhage
   E. Atypical fungal infection

4. A 6-year-old boy with trisomy 21 presents with fever and recurrent infections. His mother states that he has been extremely tired recently and becoming breathless on exertion. On examination he is pale and has numerous bruises with palpable hepatosplenomegaly. Investigations are as follows:
   Hb 85 g/L
   White cell count 25×10^9/L
   Platelets 35×10^9/L
   Bone marrow biopsy: hypercellular with large numbers of lymphoblast cells seen

Cytogenetics: *MLL* gene rearrangement
What is the most likely diagnosis?
A. Nonaccidental injury
B. Acute lymphoblastic leukaemia
C. Chronic myeloid leukaemia
D. Primary myelofibrosis
E. Non-Hodgkin lymphoma

5. A 39-year-old man is undergoing preop assessment for knee surgery. On his routine blood tests, he has the following results:
Hb 110 g/L
White cell count 150 × 10^9/L
Neutrophils 90 × 10^9/L
Basophils 20 × 10^9/L
Platelets 90 × 10^9/L
Cytogenetics: *BCR-ABL* gene
What is the most likely diagnosis?
A. Acute myeloid leukaemia
B. Polycythaemia vera
C. Primary myelofibrosis
D. Chronic myeloid leukaemia
E. Chronic lymphocytic leukaemia

6. A 75-year-old female presents acutely with back pain and lower limb neurological symptoms. She reports recurrent chest infections, weight loss, polydipsia and polyuria. On examination she is pale and has widespread petechiae. Findings are as follows:
Hb 95 g/L
White cell count 1.9 × 10^9/L
Corrected calcium 3.5 mM
Erythrocyte sedimentation rate: raised
Film: rouleaux present
Serum electrophoresis: prominent monoclonal immunoglobulin present
Urine dip: protein +++
MRI spine: multiple vertebral body collapse fractures with lytic lesions
Bone marrow: 30% clonal plasma cells
What is the most likely diagnosis?
A. Monoclonal gammopathy of uncertain significance (MGUS)
B. Acute myeloid leukaemia
C. Chronic myeloid leukaemia
D. Multiple myeloma
E. Solitary plasmacytoma

7. A 25-year-old man presents with night sweats, fevers and weight loss of 15 kg over 6 months. On examination he has widespread, painless, nontender lymphadenopathy and moderate splenomegaly. Lymphoma is suspected and a superficial lymph node

is biopsied. Which of the historical features below would provide the best chance of discriminating between Hodgkin lymphoma (HL) and non-Hodgkin lymphoma (NHL) while waiting for the biopsy result?
A. Past Ebstein-Barr virus (EBV) infection
B. Complaint of fever, weight loss and night sweats
C. Known immunodeficiency
D. A complaint of severe itching
E. The patient's age

8. An 80-year-old man presents with an incidental leucocytosis on routine blood tests with his GP. Clinical history include night sweats but nothing else. Examination reveals generalized painless lymphadenopathy. Blood results are as follows:
Hb 120 g/L
White cell count 60 × 10^9/L
Lymphocytes 45 × 10^9/L
Platelets 100 × 10^9/L
Blood film: lymphocytosis with numerous smear cells seen
Which of the following is the most likely diagnosis?
A. Infective mononucleosis
B. Acute lymphoblastic leukaemia
C. Chronic lymphocytic leukaemia
D. Hodgkin lymphoma
E. COVID infection

9. A patient complains of nausea, vomiting, muscle cramps and widespread severe joint pains. He is 24 hours post commencement of R-CHOP chemotherapy for a high-grade non-Hodgkin lymphoma and the haematologist supervising his treatment informs you he had a particularly high tumour burden. His electrocardiogram (ECG) shows tall, peaked T waves and flattening of the P waves. Which of the biochemical findings correspond to the likely diagnosis?
A. K$^+$ 3.5 mM, Ca^{++} 1.9 mM, uric acid 800 µmol/L (normal range 180–420 µmol/L)
B. K$^+$ 7.2 mM, Ca^{++} 1.2 mM, uric acid 1500 µmol/L
C. K$^+$ 5.0 mM, Ca^{++} 3.5 mM, uric acid 220 µmol/L
D. K$^+$ 6.5 mM, Ca^{++} 1.9 mM, uric acid 250 µmol/L
E. K$^+$ 4.5 mM, Ca^{++} 2.7 mM, uric acid 1500 µmol/L

10. A 35-year-old patient with known acute myeloid leukaemia who has recently completed chemotherapy presents with a fever. He is acutely confused and sweating profusely. Clinical findings are as follows:
Blood pressure 65/20 mmHg
Heart rate 140 bpm sinus rhythm
Respiratory rate 30/min
Temperature 38.6°C
Blood gas:

pH 7.15
pO$_2$ 8.0 kPa
pCO$_2$ 2.5 kPa
Lactate 6.5 mM
Investigations:
Hb 75 g/L
White cell count 0.5 × 10^9/L
Neutrophils 0.0 × 10^9/L
Platelets 23 × 10^9/L
Uric acid 300 µmol/L
Of the following actions, which is the first priority in managing this patient?
A. Perform urgent red blood cell transfusion
B. Administer granulocyte colony stimulating factor (G-CSF) and discuss with haematology
C. Administer intravenous (IV) crystalloid and broad-spectrum antibiotics
D. Arrange urgent plasmapheresis
E. Administer allopurinol and rasburicase

Chapter 6 Haemostasis

1. Which of the following statements most accurately describes the sequence of events in primary haemostasis?
   A. Vasoconstriction, adhesion, aggregation, release reaction, fibrin deposition
   B. Vasoconstriction, transient tethering, release reaction, adhesion, aggregation
   C. Transient tethering, release reaction, vasoconstriction, adhesion, aggregation
   D. Adhesion, release reaction, transient tethering, aggregation, vasoconstriction
   E. Release reaction, transient tethering, vasoconstriction, adhesion, aggregation

2. Which of the following statements most accurately describes a stage in the extrinsic pathway?
   A. FXa unites with FVa and calcium ions to form prothrombinase
   B. Exposed subendothelial tissue factor binds to circulating FVII
   C. FXII is activated by the surface membrane of an activated platelet
   D. FVIIIa and FIXa unite with calcium ions to form 'tenase'
   E. FXIII is activated by thrombin to covalently cross-link fibrin polymers

3. Which of the following statements most accurately summarizes the common pathway?
   A. Products derived from intrinsic and extrinsic pathways integrate via the common pathway which culminates in the generation of thrombin

B. It is activated by exposure to procoagulants such as subendothelial tissue factor
C. Vasoconstriction, transient tethering, release reaction, adhesion, aggregation
D. It commences with activation of factor XII by an activated platelet and ultimately generated factor X
E. Tissue plasminogen activator binds to fibrin-bound plasminogen, forming plasmin which degrades fibrin

4. Which of the following does not act as an anticoagulant and limit the coagulation cascade?
   A. Protein C
   B. Protein S
   C. Plasmin
   D. Calcium
   E. Thrombomodulin

5. Which of the following coagulation assay results correctly correlates with the underlying disease?
   A. Normal PT, prolonged APTT, normal fibrinogen = vitamin K deficiency
   B. Normal PT, normal APTT, normal fibrinogen = factor XII deficiency
   C. Prolonged PT, normal APTT, normal fibrinogen = factor V deficiency
   D. Prolonged PT, prolonged APTT, reduced fibrinogen = liver disease
   E. Prolonged PT, prolonged APTT, normal fibrinogen = factor XI deficiency

6. A 15-year-old patient with easy bruising presents to his GP. He reports that his mother bruises easily and is largely asymptomatic, but has had bleeding complications following surgery as well as frequent nosebleeds. Which of the following gives the most likely diagnosis?
   A. Protein S deficiency
   B. Protein C deficiency
   C. Antithrombin deficiency
   D. Factor V Leiden
   E. Von Willebrand disease (vWD)

7. A 70-year-old man presents to his GP with widespread bruising. His platelet count has fallen to 10 × 10^9/L. All other investigations are normal. He had recently had a medication review where several new drugs were started. Which of the following is the most likely cause?
   A. Candesartan
   B. Paracetamol
   C. Codeine
   D. Quinine
   E. Adcal

8. A 45-year-old black female arrives in A&E with right hemiplegia, aphasia and low-grade fever (37.9°C). On examination by the haematology registrar, she is jaundiced with widespread bruising and petechiae. Surprisingly her neurological symptoms have resolved. Blood film reported includes features in keeping with microangiopathic haemolysis. She is correctly diagnosed and recovers with supportive treatment as well as plasma exchange. Which of the following accounts for this clinical presentation?
   A. Haemolytic uraemic syndrome (HUS)
   B. Disseminated intravascular coagulation (DIC)
   C. Transient ischaemic attack (TIA)
   D. Thrombotic thrombocytopenia purpura (TTP)
   E. Immune thrombocytopenic purpura (ITP)

9. An 85-year-old lady is found by her daughter lying on the floor. She had tripped 2 hours earlier but was unable to get herself back up. Her left leg is externally rotated and foreshortened. She has numerous extensive subcutaneous haematomas and is pale. She is taking warfarin for atrial Fibrillation. Admission bloods are as follows:

Hb	90 g/L
Platelets	425 × 10⁹/L
White cell count	13.0 × 10⁹/L
International normalized ratio (INR)	6.0
Activated partial thromboplastin time (APTT)	36 seconds
Fibrinogen	6.5 g/dL

   The orthopaedic team will not operate until her coagulation has been corrected and plan to take her to theatre in 2 hours. Which of the following options would be the best treatment to normalize her coagulation within this timeframe?
   A. Fresh frozen plasma
   B. Intravenous vitamin K
   C. Prothrombin complex concentrate (PCC)
   D. Recombinant factor VIIa
   E. Cryoprecipitate

10. Which of the following is not an inherited thrombophilia?
   A. Factor V Leiden
   B. Protein C deficiency
   C. Antithrombin deficiency
   D. Antiphospholipid syndrome (APLS)
   E. Prothrombin G20210A

11. Which of the following is considered a risk factor in the Well's score for deep vein thrombosis (DVT)?
   A. Age >65 years
   B. Smoker
   C. Previous cancer
   D. Major surgery in the last 12 weeks
   E. Recent long-haul flight >4 hours

Chapter 7 Blood transfusion

1. In relation to blood donation, which of the following statements is correct?
   A. Volunteers must be at least 16 years of age
   B. Women cannot donate more frequently than every 12 weeks
   C. Male donors must have a predonation Hb of 135 g/L
   D. All donations consist of whole blood
   E. Malaria infection will result in permanent exclusion from donating blood

2. Which of the following descriptions most accurately explains the mechanism underlying ABO incompatibility reaction?
   A. IgG binds to A or B antigens causing delayed intravascular haemolysis
   B. IgM binds to red cell H antigen causing extravascular haemolysis
   C. IgM and complement-mediated acute intravascular haemolysis
   D. IgG binds to the red cell H antigen causing acute intravascular haemolysis
   E. IgM and cell-mediated delayed extravascular haemolysis

3. A 75-year-old man is receiving his third unit of red cells following a total hip replacement. He complains of breathlessness and chest pain. His heart rate is 110 beats per minute, blood pressure is 155/95 mmHg, respiratory rate 35 breaths per minute and oxygen saturations 88% on room air. What is the first priority in managing this acute transfusion reaction?
   A. Help him to sit up and administer 20 mg of intravenous (IV) frusemide
   B. Stop the transfusion and clinically assess the patient
   C. Administer intramuscular adrenaline and elevate his legs
   D. Provide reassurance and administer intravenous paracetamol
   E. Take blood cultures and administer urgent intravenous antibiotics

4. In relation to haemolytic disease of the foetus and newborn (HDFN), which of the following statements is incorrect?
   A. If a rhesus (Rh) D −ve woman becomes pregnant with an RhD +ve foetus, she will become sensitized during pregnancy
   B. The risk of developing anti-D is highest during the first pregnancy
   C. The degree of immune haemolysis and subsequent anaemia is variable
   D. HDFN can also be caused by other red cell antibodies
   E. All RhD −ve women should receive anti-D prophylaxis between 28 and 30 weeks of pregnancy

5. Which of these scenarios is NOT a contraindication for electronic issue of blood?
   A. Positive antibody screen
   B. Historical presence of red cell alloantibodies
   C. ABO-incompatible bone marrow transplant
   D. Recent major surgery
   E. ABO-incompatible solid organ transplant within last 3 months

6. Which of the following blood products is stored at 2-5°C in a saline, adenine, glucose and mannitol solution with a shelf life of 35 days?
   A. Platelets
   B. Clotting factor concentrates
   C. Red cells
   D. Fresh frozen plasma (FFP)
   E. Immunoglobulin

7. Which one of the following blood products is stored at room temperature (22±2°C) with constant agitation?
   A. Platelets
   B. Clotting factor concentrates
   C. Red cells
   D. Fresh frozen plasma (FFP)
   E. Immunoglobulin

8. Which of the following are appropriate for platelet transfusion support?
   A. Patient with platelet count 35×10^9/L awaiting life-saving laparotomy
   B. Patient with platelet count 110×10^9/L and ongoing haemorrhage
   C. Patient with platelet count 45×10^9/L and acute liver failure with no active bleeding
   D. Patient with platelet count 15×10^9/L during induction chemotherapy with no active bleeding
   E. Patient with platelet count 50×10^9/L and a resolved gastrointestinal bleed

9. Which of the following combination scenarios regarding decision-making for transfusion of blood products, plasma derivatives and recombinant factors is incorrect?
   A. Red cell transfusion = A 32-year-old female following obstetric haemorrhage of 1.6 L with haemoglobin (Hb) 78 g/L and platelet 115×10^9/L
   B. Cryoprecipitate = A 35-year-old man following major surgery for large tumour complicated by major haemorrhage. Clotting shows prothrombin time (PT) 28 seconds, activated partial thromboplastin time (APTT) 52 seconds and fibrinogen 1.5 g/dL
   C. Platelet = A 64-year-old man with HIV admitted to intensive care unit with septic shock and has platelet 15×10^9/L
   D. Fresh frozen plasma = A 75-year-old man admitted to intensive care unit following major gastrointestinal haemorrhage. Bloods show PT 30 seconds, APTT 60 seconds and fibrinogen 1.6 g/dL
   E. Anti-D = A 34-year-old woman who is RhD −ve and 28/40 pregnant with second baby who is RhD +ve

10. Which of the following is a delayed and usually fatal transfusion reaction defined by lymphocyte implantation in the transfusion recipient?
    A. Posttransfusion purpura
    B. IgM-mediated haemolytic reaction
    C. Transfusion-associated graft-versus-host disease (GVHD)
    D. Chronic hepatitis C infection
    E. Transfusion-related lung injury

11. A 6-year-old girl is brought in by ambulance following a road traffic accident. She has a ruptured spleen and is haemorrhaging. She is drowsy, pale, clammy and peripherally cool. Type O −ve blood is prepared and transfusion about to commence when the parents arrive and adamantly refuse to let it go ahead since they are Jehovah's witnesses. Despite clear and frank explanation of the life-threatening consequences of withholding transfusion, the parents will not consent and produce an advanced directive signed by the child. What is the legally and ethically appropriate course of action?
    A. Abandon transfusion, attempt to maintain blood pressure with intravenous crystalloid
    B. Attempt to source cell salvager for recovery of blood during the laparotomy
    C. Seek a court order and proceed with transfusion in best interests in the interim

D. Continue to attempt to persuade the parents to give their consent, recruiting additional colleagues

E. Accept that the decision to refuse transfusion was made by the child herself and respect her wishes

12. Which of the following is least likely to be associated with massive transfusion?
A. Hypothermia
B. Hyperkalaemia
C. Hypercalcaemia
D. Dilutional coagulopathy
E. Transfusion-associated circulatory overload

13. As the night on-call doctor, you are called to attend to a medical emergency call on the gastroenterology ward. A 53-year-old lady, who is an inpatient, is having haematemesis when you arrive. She looks tired and pale and is complaining of epigastric pain as she continues to vomit frank blood with clots. The nursing staff are doing a set of vital observations at the same time: HR is 120 bpm, SpO$_2$ 92% on room air, BP 90/55 mmHg. The nurses deny any antihypertensive medications being given to the patient in the last 24 hours. A venous blood gas was done before you arrived and values are as following: pH 7.28, lactate 4.0, Hb 55. What is the next most appropriate step?
A. Prescribe anti-emetics and ask for cross-match blood transfusion of 2 units of red blood cells (RBC) from the blood bank laboratory
B. Ask the nurses to give 1 L of intravenous fluids while you wait for your senior registrar to review the patient
C. You are worried about the high lactate and abdominal pain, book and urgent abdomen and pelvis CT and ask surgeons to review the patient
D. Put out a major haemorrhage protocol, ensure patient has two large bore cannulas (× 1 in each arm), send off an FBC, renal profile, coagulation screen and group and screen, and give intravenous fluids (IVF) until the urgent blood products arrive.
E. Call the on-call upper-gastrointestinal bleed (UGIB) consultant

Chapter 9 The innate immune system

1. Concerning the innate immune system, which one of the following statements is correct?
A. It is a specific response to a particular antigen
B. Response improves on repeated exposure
C. It is composed of phagocytes and complement
D. It is good at combating intracellular pathogens
E. It takes a long time to develop

2. Which of the following cell types of the innate immune system does not perform phagocytosis?
A. Neutrophil
B. Basophil
C. Eosinophil
D. Macrophage
E. Monocyte

3. A 56-year-old man presents with high fever associated with sweats and persistent diarrhoea. He has recently completed a course of chemotherapy for bowel cancer. Which of the following is the likely diagnosis?
A. Viral gastroenteritis
B. Chemotherapy-induced toxicity
C. *Clostridium difficile* infection
D. Parasitic infection
E. Neutropenic sepsis

4. A general practitioner starts an 80-year-old lady on a course of ciprofloxacin for severe urinary tract infection. A few days later, she develops watery diarrhoea and abdominal pain. Which answer best describes the likely cause for these symptoms?
A. Anaphylaxis caused by an allergy to ciprofloxacin
B. Progression of the urinary tract infection to sepsis
C. Gastric ulceration caused by antibiotic
D. Flare-up of inflammatory bowel disease
E. Disruption of the patient's normal gut flora by ciprofloxacin, allowing colonization by pathogenic organisms

5. Which of the following is true of macrophages?
A. They have a shorter lifespan than neutrophils
B. They move and phagocytose quickly compared to neutrophils
C. They express high levels of MHC class I molecules
D. They can act as antigen-presenting cells
E. They are effective at killing intracellular pathogens such as *Mycobacterium*

6. Which of the following is true of natural killer cells?
A. They develop from myeloid progenitor cells
B. They require T-cell help to kill pathogens
C. They are induced to attack cells that do not express class I MHC molecules
D. They are clonally restricted
E. They have memory and are specific in their action

7. A 25-year-old woman with a history of nut allergy is taken to A+E after eating a dessert that contains peanuts. She has an audible wheeze, swollen lips and visible hives. Which cell of the innate immune system is likely to be responsible for this reaction?
   A. Neutrophil
   B. Macrophage
   C. T cell
   D. Mast cell
   E. Eosinophil

8. Protein and fat catabolism seen in infection is directly mediated by what?
   A. Acute phase proteins
   B. Bacterial antigens
   C. Immunoglobulins
   D. Cytokines
   E. Complement proteins

9. The membrane attack complex (MAC) mediates its action on pathogens by which one of the following mechanisms?
   A. Phagocytosis
   B. Opsonization
   C. Osmotic lysis
   D. Apoptosis
   E. Degranulation

10. A 79-year-old man presents with temporal tenderness and jaw claudication. You suspect giant cell arteritis (GCA). Which acute phase response would most support your suspicion?
    A. Raised white cell count
    B. Raised fibrinogen
    C. Raised C-reactive protein (CRP)
    D. Raised erythrocyte sedimentation rate (ESR)
    E. Raised complement levels

11. A 23-year-old woman with history of multiple allergies presents with facial swelling, stridor and abdominal pain. Physical examination reveals markedly swollen extremities. Medication review reveals she has been recently started on an ACE inhibitor. A deficiency of which of the following complement inhibitors would support your suspected diagnosis?
    A. Factor I
    B. CD59
    C. C4b-binding protein
    D. C1 inhibitor
    E. Decay accelerating factor

12. A 78-year-old man is brought to A+E with 3-day history of persistent cough, confusion and fever. He is tachypnoeic and hypoxic with normal blood pressure.

Which of the following is not part of immediate management in suspected sepsis?
A. Give high-flow oxygen
B. Take blood cultures and consider other sources
C. Give oral antibiotics
D. Measure serum lactate and other blood tests (full blood count, C-reactive protein, blood gases)
E. Give a fluid challenge

Chapter 10 The adaptive immune system

1. Which one of the following statements about major histocompatibility complex (MHC) is true?
   A. MHC chass II molecules present endogenous antigens
   B. The haplotype is found on chromosome 6
   C. CD4 positive cells bind MHC class I molecules
   D. MHC class I molecules are only present on antigen-presenting cells
   E. MHC class I molecules present peptides that are usually longer than MHC class II

2. What is the name of the process whereby a B cell can produce different types of immunoglobulin with the same specificity?
   A. Junctional diversity
   B. Somatic hypermutation
   C. Affinity maturation
   D. Positive selection
   E. Class switching

3. Which one of the following is not a member of the immunoglobulin superfamily?
   A. T-cell receptor
   B. CD4
   C. Major histocompatibility complex
   D. Immunoglobulin E (IgE)
   E. Toll-like receptor-4 (TLR-4)

4. Regarding B-cell activation, which one of the following statements is correct?
   A. B cells are activated in the follicles of primary lymphoid organs
   B. The expression of bcl-2 results in apoptosis
   C. Somatic hypermutation of immunoglobulin genes occurs in germinal centres
   D. B cells are activated following the presentation of antigen by neutrophils
   E. B cells can be activated and produce antibodies without help from T cells

5. Which antibody is important in the antiparasitic response?
   A. Immunoglobulin G (IgG)
   B. IgD
   C. IgM
   D. IgE
   E. IgA

6. Which of the following statements about T cells is correct?
   A. T cells are major histocompatibility complex (MHC)-restricted while developing in bone marrow
   B. Th1 cells are involved in response to intracellular pathogens more than Th2 cells
   C. Cytotoxic T cells express CD4
   D. Apoptosis is induced in T cells that bind to self-MHC
   E. Positive selection occurs in developing T cells that have high affinity for self-antigens

7. Which of the following statements is correct in relation to B and T lymphocytes?
   A. T helper cells induce B cells to become fully active and begin releasing antibodies
   B. B and T lymphocytes originate from myeloid stem cells
   C. Basophils contain vast amount of endoplasmic reticulin in order to secrete large quantities of immunoglobulin
   D. CD4 is a cell marker associated with cytotoxic T cells
   E. Memory B cells recognize antigen in conjunction with class I major histocompatibility complex

8. Concerning cell surface molecules, which of the following statements is not correct?
   A. Antigens are substances recognized by specific receptors of the adaptive immune system
   B. Collectins are pattern recognition molecules found in solution
   C. MHC class II molecules present antigens from intracellular pathogens
   D. Toll-like receptors are family of related molecules found on mammalian cell surfaces; they activate innate immune system after exposure to pathogen
   E. T-cell surface antigen receptor is made up of TCR and CD3

9. One winter, a 44-year-old surgeon develops fever, muscle pain, sore throat and vomiting. She self-diagnoses influenza and realizes she has not had the flu vaccine. She gradually improves after 4 days in bed. Which of the following is correct?
   A. The reason she had flu this year was because she had never encountered the flu virus previously
   B. She cleared the virus by secreting large quantities of antibodies against it

C. Natural killer and CD8+ cytotoxic T cells are responsible for clearing the flu virus
D. Her symptoms are caused by secretion of transforming growth factor-β (TGF-β)
E. Neutrophils and T helper (Th) 17 T cells are required to kill the flu virus

10. A 25-year-old woman is found unconscious and is taken to A+E. She is pale and sweaty, with a diffuse macular rash. Blood pressure is 75/38 with heart rate 138. After initial resuscitation she is diagnosed with toxic shock syndrome (TSS). Which of the following causes this syndrome?
    A. *Streptococcus pneumoniae*
    B. *Clostridium enterotoxin*
    C. Cholera toxin
    D. *Staphylococcal enterotoxin*
    E. *Escherichia coli*

Chapter 11 The functioning immune system

1. Which of the following mediators do not increase vascular permeability?
   A. C3a
   B. C5a
   C. Leukotrienes
   D. Prostaglandins
   E. Histamine

2. Which of the following statements relating to inflammation in disease is not correct?
   A. Persistent antigens cause continued activation and accumulation of macrophages and T cells
   B. Macrophages develop into epithelioid cells which then form a granuloma
   C. IFN-γ is required for granuloma formation and maintenance
   D. Fibroblasts migrate to granuloma resulting in increased collagen synthesis
   E. *Mycobacterium tuberculosis* induces persistent delayed-type hypersensitivity response resulting in granuloma formation

3. Which of the following is the reason that autoimmune disease results in chronic inflammation?
   A. Genetic predisposition
   B. Persistence of antigen
   C. Granuloma formation
   D. Prolonged increase in tumour necrosis factor-α (TNF-α)
   E. Inadequate immune response

4. Which of the following statements concerning the immune system in action is incorrect?
   A. Mast cells release histamine in response to immunoglobulin E stimulation
   B. Phagocytes destroy most extracellular bacteria
   C. Major histocompatibility complex (MHC) class I molecules present viral peptides to CD8+ T cells
   D. TNF-α is the cytokine secreted by virally infected cells to communicate with other cells
   E. IFN-γ is required for the transformation of macrophages into epithelioid cells as part of granuloma formation

5. A 56-year-old male presents with a 3-week history of dry cough and weight loss after visiting family in India. He is treated for suspected tuberculosis infection. Which of the following statements best describes how the immune system manages *M. tuberculosis* infection in the lungs?
   A. T helper 2 (Th2) cells release IL-4 activating B cells
   B. Neutrophils can phagocytose the pathogen directly
   C. Delayed type hypersensitivity response; the pathogen is surrounded by granulation tissue
   D. Antibodies can neutralize the pathogen directly as well as act as an opsonin against infected cells
   E. CD4+ T cells are able to destroy infected cells

6. A 38-year-old female healthcare worker goes to her GP for her annual flu vaccine. Which of the following correctly describes how her immune system would respond if she later encounters the seasonal flu virus?
   A. Antibodies can neutralize the pathogen directly as well as act as an opsonin against infected cells
   B. Interferon-gamma (IFN-γ) acts on neighbouring cells by inhibiting transcription and translation of pathogen
   C. Neutrophils phagocytose the pathogen directly
   D. CD4+ T cells are able to destroy infected cells
   E. Macrophages fuse to form multinucleate giant cells around the pathogen creating a granuloma

7. Which one of the following components of the immune system can prevent bacterial pathogens present on a mucosal surface from entering the body?
   A. Lysozyme
   B. C3b
   C. Neutrophils
   D. Dendritic cells
   E. Secretory immunoglobulin A (sIgA)

8. Which white blood cell count differential result would you expect to see in a parasitic worm infection?
   A. Raised neutrophils
   B. Raised eosinophils
   C. Raised lymphocytes
   D. Raised basophils
   E. Reduced neutrophils

9. Which of the following is the hepatitis B virus (HBV) serology result that implies the patient has previously cleared the virus without vaccination?

A.	HBsAg +	anti-HBc +	Anti-HBs +
B.	HBsAg –	Anti-HBc –	Anti-HBs –
C.	HBsAg +	Anti-HBc –	Anti-HBs –
D.	HBsAg –	Anti-HBc +	Anti-HBs +
E.	HBsAg –	Anti-HBc –	Anti-HBs +

10. A 24-year-old medical student presents to his GP with a 2-week history of headaches and a swinging fever following his elective in Columbia. He has no other medical conditions and has not taken any recent medication. Which of the following statements is true for the likely causative organism?
    A. The pathogen tends to cause extracellular infections
    B. The pathogen has a complex lifecycle which presents the immune system with a variety of challenges
    C. The pathogen causes significant damage selectively to CD4+ T cells, thus reducing the effectiveness of the adaptive immune system
    D. Infections with this pathogen are normally self-limiting
    E. The pathogen is pyogenic

Chapter 12 Immune dysfunction

1. What type of immune dysfunction is characterized by IgE-mediated degranulation of mast cells?
   A. Nickle hypersensitivity
   B. ABO incompatibility
   C. Allergic rhinitis
   D. Farmer's lung
   E. Rheumatoid arthritis

2. In relation to type I hypersensitivity reactions, which of the following statements is incorrect?
   A. Reactions are typically immediate, within minutes, of exposure to a target antigen
   B. IgE antibodies against target antigen need to be present
   C. Reexposure to sensitized antigens results in mast cell and basophil degranulation
   D. Atopy is a genetic predisposition to produce IgE in response to common, naturally occurring allergens
   E. Allergy testing can be done using blood test to measure tryptase levels

3. A child presents to his GP with a 2-month history of breathlessness, wheeze and dry cough following exercise. Their parent notes symptoms are worse at night. Which of the following statements in relation to this condition is incorrect?
   A. This is a chronic inflammatory disorder of the airways
   B. Common allergens include pollen, house-dust mites and airborne proteins from domestic animals
   C. Histological findings typically including infiltration by B cells and basophils
   D. Diagnosis is confirmed by reversible obstruction of ≥15% measured by peak expiratory flow
   E. Avoidance of triggers is part of management with short-acting β2-adrenoreceptor agonist

4. Which of the following conditions is caused by deposition of antibody-antigen complexes in tissues?
   A. Eczema
   B. Farmer's lung
   C. Asthma
   D. Haemolytic disease of the newborn
   E. Nickel hypersensitivity

5. A patient admitted under the haematology transplant team receives antithymocyte globulin. A few days later they become unwell with fever and rash. Which of the following statements in relation to this complication is incorrect?
   A. This reaction results from the formation of immune complexes between human and nonhuman proteins
   B. It is characterized by the triad of fever, rash and arthritis
   C. Symptoms typically occur 6-12 days after exposure
   D. This reaction resolves within a few days after discontinuation of the relevant culprit
   E. Antihistamines may be considered as well as glucocorticoids to treat this reaction

6. Type IV hypersensitivity is mainly mediated by which cells?
   A. Neutrophils
   B. Plasma cells
   C. CD8+ T cells
   D. Mast cells
   E. T helper cells

7. A 21-year-old man is brought to A&E suffering from breathing problems that he developed after eating a sandwich. He has an audible stridor, warm to touch and has facial oedema. Which of the following is the most appropriate next step in his management?
   A. Intravenous fluid challenge
   B. IV chlorphenamine

C. IV hydrocortisone
D. Intramuscular adrenaline (0.5 mL of 1:1000)
E. C1 inhibitor IV

8. A 23-year-old patient presents to their GP with a 3-week history of intermittent diarrhoea and fatigue. The patient appears pale and is found to have anti-tissue transglutaminase antibodies. Which is the likely diagnosis?
   A. Rheumatoid arthritis
   B. Type I diabetes
   C. Crohn disease
   D. Pernicious anaemia
   E. Coeliac disease

9. A 38-year-old lady presents to her GP with long-standing history of worsening pain and stiffness in the first and second metacarpophalangeal joints (MCPJs) of both her hands. An X-ray shows loss of joint space, bony erosions and subluxation of the affected joints. What serum antibodies would confirm the likely diagnosis?
   A. Anti–double-stranded DNA antibodies
   B. Anti-cyclic citrullinated peptide antibodies
   C. Anti-Ro antibodies
   D. Anti-nuclear antibodies
   E. IgE anti-IgA antibodies

10. What type of virus is the human immunodeficiency virus (HIV)?
    A. A double-stranded DNA virus
    B. A single-stranded DNA virus
    C. A single-stranded RNA retrovirus
    D. A double-stranded DNA retrovirus
    E. A single-stranded RNA virus

11. Which of the following HIV +ve patients would be classified as suffering from AIDS?
    A. A patient with CD4 count of 250 cells/μL
    B. A patient with a malignant melanoma
    C. A patient with a neutrophil count of 2 × 10⁹/L
    D. A patient with oesophageal candidiasis
    E. A patient with M. tuberculosis infection

12. Which of the following statements in relation to specific tests for immune dysfunction is incorrect?
    A. Measurement of IgG, IgA and IgM helps to measure the level of immunoglobulin
    B. A rise in C-reactive protein (CRP) can help to differentiate between acute appendicitis and constipation in acute abdominal pain
    C. Skin prick test involves an intradermal injection of purified protein derivative (PPD)

D. Enzyme-linked immunosorbent assay (ELISA) uses labelled antibodies to bind to and detect antigens or antigen-antibody complexes

E. Patch test is used to confirm nickel hypersensitivity

Chapter 13 Medical intervention

1. In relation to immunization, which of the following statements is incorrect?
   A. Passive immunization is a temporary immunity resulting from the transfer of exogenous antibody from one person to another
   B. Active immunization results from contact with antigens
   C. Vaccination is a form of active immunization that induces specific immunity to a particular pathogen
   D. Hepatitis B postexposure prophylaxis is a form of active immunity
   E. An ideal vaccine should be safe, immunogenic and heat stable

2. A 28-year-old man presents to A&E with an open tibial fracture following road traffic collision. There is dirt and debris in the wound. Since he cannot recall if he has had a full course of tetanus vaccinations, you opt to give him antitetanus immunoglobulin. Which of the following best describes how this treatment works?
   A. Clonal expansion of reactive B cells
   B. Vaccination booster
   C. Passive immunity
   D. Active immunity
   E. Initial sensitization

3. Concerning transplant rejection, which of the following is correct?
   A. Hyperacute rejection is caused by T cells
   B. Acute cellular rejection is primarily mediated by natural killer cells
   C. Chronic rejection responds well to long-term steroids
   D. Hyperacute rejection is prevented by human leucocyte antigen-matching the organ donor and recipient
   E. Acute cellular responses take days to develop

4. Regarding haematopoietic stem cell transplantation (HSCT), which of the following statements is correct?
   A. HSCT transplants are only used for the treatment of malignant haematological conditions
   B. Allogeneic HSCT uses the patient's own HSCs to replace the haematopoietic system
   C. Source of HSCs can be either the bone marrow, peripheral blood or umbilical cord

D. The graft-versus-leukaemia effect is typically seen in autologous HSCT with the removal of residual malignant cells

E. Graft-versus-host disease is a self-limiting complication of HSCT

5. A patient on regular corticosteroid therapy is followed up by their GP. Which of the following would be unlikely to be caused by the corticosteroids?
   A. Abnormal liver function tests
   B. Raised blood pressure
   C. Poor glucose tolerance
   D. Poor wound healing
   E. Repeated infections

6. An 89-year-old lady presents to her GP with knee pain related to her osteoarthritis. She also suffers from hypertension and has no known allergies. She does not suffer from asthma. You prescribe oral naproxen. Which of the following side effects of nonsteroidal antiinflammatory drugs (NSAIDs) would most concern you?
   A. Tinnitus
   B. Headache
   C. Bronchospasm
   D. Gastritis
   E. Rash

7. A 54-year-old woman is brought to A&E by ambulance. She is confused, generally unresponsive and pale. Initial observations show she is hypotensive, tachycardic but apyrexial. Blood tests show she is hyperkalaemic and hyponatraemic. Inflammatory markers are normal. You find a card in her bag which says she is on long-term steroids. What would your immediate management be?
   A. Administer oxygen, blood cultures, intravenous (IV) antibiotics, fluid challenge, bloods for full blood count, electrolytes; measure urine output (sepsis 6)
   B. IV hydrocortisone and IV fluids
   C. Oral antibiotics
   D. Oral prednisolone
   E. IM adrenaline

8. Which of the following statements in relation to immunological interventions is incorrect?
   A. Oral prednisolone is most likely to cause weight gain, hypertension and osteoporosis if used long term
   B. Methotrexate inhibits dihydrofolate reductase, therefore blocking the conversion of dihydrofolate to tetrahydrofolate and subsequent nucleotide synthesis
   C. Thiopurine methyltransferase (TPMT) activity should be checked prior to starting azathioprine

D. Tacrolimus causes immunosuppression by inhibiting calcineurin

E. Rituximab is a monoclonal antibody that targets tumour necrosis factor-α (TNF-α)

9. In relation to cancer immunotherapy, which of the following statements is incorrect?
   A. Immune-checkpoint inhibitors use antibodies targeting programmed cell death 1 (PD-1) and therefore enable tumour cell apoptosis
   B. Chimeric antigen receptor (CAR)-T cells are genetically modified to express antigen-binding domain with CD3 TCR
   C. IL-10 is used to promote T-cell activation and expansion for developing tumour-infiltrating lymphocytes (TILs)
   D. Bispecific T-cell engager antibodies (BiTEs) have been used in relapsed/refractory acute lymphoblastic leukaemia
   E. Cytokine release syndrome (CRS) is a life-threatening complication of CAR-T cell therapy and is managed with tocilizumab (anti-IL6 receptor)

MLA SBA Answers

Chapter 1 Principles of haematology

1. E. Option E is the only listed example of a lymphoid lineage progenitor. Pre-B cells are derived from a common lymphoid progenitor and ultimately develop into mature B cells. All other options describe myeloid projectors.
2. C. Options A, B and C are mature cells, but only option C is a mature cell of myeloid lineage origin. NK cells and T lymphocytes are of lymphoid origin. Options D and E are myeloid lineage, but they are progenitor cells not mature cells.
3. B. Option B is the only listed option describing one of the spleen's physiological roles; destruction of senescent erythrocytes and filtration of particulate matter from the bloodstream, initiation of immune response to blood-borne antigens, foetal haematopoiesis and a storage reservoir for platelets are the main physiological roles of this spleen.
4. E. Option E does not cause splenomegaly; this disorder results from impaired erythropoiesis secondary to B12 deficiency due to a failure of intrinsic factor-mediated gastrointestinal (GI) absorption. Options A–D are all causes associated with massive splenomegaly.
5. B. Only Lyme disease is commonly associated with generalized lymphadenopathy. Mumps causes local enlargement of the parotid glands. Options D and E are not associated with generalized lymphadenopathy and option C may lead to right ventricular failure, which may result in hepatomegaly and splenomegaly but not generalized lymphadenopathy.
6. D. Options A, B, C and E are mandatory features of caring for asplenic patients. Option D would not offer any additional benefit to the patient and would be costly. Once these viruses establish latency, they cannot be eliminated.
7. D. Thrombopoietin stimulates both megakaryocytes differentiation from CFU-Meg and megakaryocyte spawning of platelets, therefore option D is the answer. See Table 1.2 for details of the other growth factors' primary roles.
8. D. Option E is most commonly used in the treatment of hepatitis C virus. Option C has applications in multiple sclerosis. The remaining options are growth factors. Option A would promote erythropoiesis in a patient with a failure of endogenous synthesis. Option B could potentially reduce the chance of needing a platelet transfusion. Option D is the correct answer and could raise a dangerously low neutrophil count.
9. B. Options A, B and C are all clinically used growth factors, but only option B is appropriate in this scenario. The patient's symptoms are secondary to a normochromic normocytic anaemia, arising from his renal failure to synthesize erythropoietin. Iatrogenic replacement is appropriate and is common place in patients with end-stage renal failure.
10. D. This is describing memory B cells only. None of the other options typically reside in the lymph nodes or have the sole function of secreting immunoglobulins.
11. C. The only blood cell that has the capacity to transport gases in bulk is the red blood cell (erythrocyte), which contains haemoglobin. These are capable of binding and releasing oxygen in appropriate pO_2 environments.
12. E. Eosinophils are the primary effector cells for attacking parasitic organisms, in particular helminths. When in the blood stream, they typically travel between bone marrow and sites of inflammation and infection.

Chapter 2 Red blood cells and haemoglobin

1. B. Erythrocytes have a uniform appearance. The 3D structure is that of a thick disc with central depressions on each face: a biconcave disc. This shape allows the red cell to enjoy a large surface area: volume ration for maximum gas exchange, which still has a narrower leading edge for entering small vasculature.
2. A. The spleen normally removes these nuclear inclusions (Howell-Jolly) bodies from the circulating blood cells. The scenario describes that the patient very likely had his spleen removed after traumatic rupture, and now has to remain on prophylactic antibiotics and seasonal vaccinations.
3. C. Option E describes the sequence of events undergone by bilirubin as part of haem (not iron) catabolism. Option D refers to unabsorbed iron. There is no specific iron excretion mechanism, however, small continual losses occur via desquamation and background blood loss (hence options A and B are not correct). Option C represents the major mechanism for limiting uptake of ingested iron, which is the only step in iron metabolism that can be significantly controlled. Hepcidin reduces surface expression of the iron exporter molecule at basal surfaces of enterocytes.

Therefore limiting absorbed iron's access to the portal circulation.

4. A. Methaemoglobinaemia, is the correct answer. The discerning clue is that the cyanosis fails to improve with increased inspired oxygen developing soon after a drug administration. The hint is that the region anaesthesia was performed without ultrasound or electrostimulation and failed to obtain an adequate block. It is quite likely that the prilocaine was injected intravascularly, and is known to be predisposing drug for methaemoglobinaemia. The patient is blue due methaemoglobin rather than increased deoxyHb (which most certainly would cause tachycardia and reduced end-tidal CO_2). The options are all examples of perioperative emergencies which would accompany with cardiovascular collapse.

5. C. Haem is degraded into its iron and protoporphyrin components > protoporphyrin is degraded to bilirubin, which travels to the liver bound to albumin. It is there conjugated to glucuronide (not acetylated) and secreted into the GI lumen. Here it is converted to urobilinogen, which is either reabsorbed and renally excreted or further converted to stercobilinogen and stercilin and excreted in the faeces.

6. B. Loss of functional renal mass in end-stage renal failure. Renal tissue synthesizes the bulk of erythropoietin. Options D and E are associated with raised erythropoietin levels; in the case of option E, the resulting polycythaemia can lead to dangerous hyperviscosity complications. Options A and C would probably have a chronically raised erythropoietin secondary to impaired peripheral oxygen delivery due to reduced haemoglobin.

7. D. The p50 value (the pO_2 at which haemoglobin is 50% saturated) is used to compare different haemoglobins or same haemoglobin under different conditions. A rightward shift moves the p50 to a higher corresponding pO_2 value.

8. C. B12 deficiency is not treated with red cell transfusion nor iron supplementation, hence it carries no risk of iron overload.

9. A. Acanthocytes are associated with liver disease. Red cells display an irregular outline, with spike-like structures.

10. D. The scenario describes a patient with giant cell temporal arteritis (GCA). Rouleaux is seen in any scenarios characterized by raised erythrocyte sedimentation rate (ESR) due to increased globulins. ESR is significantly raised in acute temporal arteritis.

11. C. Anisocytosis describes varying sizes of red blood cells. A patient with mixed iron and B12 deficiency may have a combination of microcytic and macrocytic red blood cells, therefore increasing the overall range or distribution of red cell size.

12. E. The patient has glucose-6-phosphate dehydrogenase (G6PD) deficiency. Diabetic ketoacidosis, acute infections and sulphonamides (sulphamethoxazole component of cotrimoxazole) are all known factors which can provoke this episode of intravascular haemolysis.

Chapter 3 Red blood cell disorders

1. B. Option B is the most accurate description. Lacking mitochondria, erythrocytes are dependent on glycolysis. Failure of glycolysis leads to severe restriction of ATP availability. Options A and C describe G6PD deficiency. Option D refers to hereditary spherocytosis or elliptocytosis. Option E describes paroxysmal nocturnal haemoglobinuria.

2. D. Patients are typically asymptomatic but experience bouts of haemolysis (making option A incorrect). The Mediterranean (not African) subtype of G6PD deficiency renders sufferers at risk of haemolysis when exposed to oxidate stress including fava beans. Haemolysis is primarily intravascular (option B is incorrect). Bite cells and Heinz bodies are characteristic features of the blood film during active haemolysis. However, if the blood sample is drawn during active haemolysis, reticulocytes can confound the assay and a false negative diagnosis can be made (therefore, option E is incorrect).

3. D. Option D is correct. The age of presentation is typical for beta-thalassaemia major where the individual has homozygous (two copies) for the beta-globin mutations. At the time that foetal Hb synthesis would be expected to decline, the failure of normal HbA synthesis becomes apparent. Electrophoresis has absent HbA and persistence of HbF. Option B cannot be correct as these individuals die in utero due to severity of the anaemia. With both options C and E, you would expect to see additional abnormal bands on electrophoresis indicated the HbH and HbS, respectively.

4. E. Option E is classically associated with iron deficiency, which will most likely be accompanied with reduced Hb, MCV and MCH. All options except option E are typical of severe B12 deficiency. Epithelial symptoms precede or accompany haematological symptoms, which themselves precede neurological symptoms.

5. D. Option D is specific for a megaloblastic anaemia. Option A describes macrocytic anaemia, but this could be megaloblastic or any other cause of macrocytosis.

Option B is incorrect. The megaloblasts are the abnormal precursors and reside in the bone marrow and are rarely seen in peripheral films. Option C describes secondary polycythaemia and option E describes lead poisoning.

6. D. Option D shows a microcytic anaemia, low ferritin and raised TIBC/transferrin; which is what you expect in iron deficiency anaemia. Option A is beta-thalassaemia major; a microcytosis more pronounced than the level of anaemia. Option B is acquired sideroblastic anaemia; note the increased bone marrow and ferritin. Option C represents B12 deficiency or folate deficiency (we would need B12 serum to differentiate). Option E is a normal blood result.

7. A. The low serum folate and red cell folate inform us that the patient has long-term folate deficiency. However, this may be functional, that is, due to folate remaining trapped and methylfolate due to inadequate B12 availability. From the available information, a B12 deficiency cannot be excluded. The safest and best option is to treat them both in combination. Treatment of the folate deficiency alone (option D) risks correcting the anaemia but allowing neurodegeneration secondary to an occult B12 deficiency to progress unchecked.

8. D. Although the patient went onto develop DIC, the primary diagnosis is of an acute transfusion reaction. Major ABO incompatibility causes alloimmune haemolysis with rapid IgM-mediated destruction of donor red cells, triggered by anti-A or anti-B antibodies.

9. E. The skin discoloration arises as a result of vascular sludging. The jaundice is caused by unconjugated hyperbilirubinaemia. The pain is due to a Raynaud phenomenon. The underlying diagnosis is cold autoimmune haemolytic anaemia (AIHA). She is already at risk with a history of autoimmune diseases. Option D is incorrect as this is more effective in warm AIHA. Anti-CD20 monoclonal antibody, rituximab is effective in idiopathic cold AIHA. Option C is red herring and may very well be discussed given this lady's Raynaud phenomenon, however, it is not the underlying causative diagnosis and you would likely seek guidance from the Rheumatology or Vascular teams prior to commencement.

10. B. There is a high risk of DIC in patients with severe burns. The haemolysis seen secondary to DIC is secondary to red cell destruction due to shearing and mechanical damage in capillaries and arterioles from collision with fibrin strands. This type of haemolysis is referred to as microangiopathic haemolysis (MAHA). It is a feature of thrombotic thrombocytopenia purpura, haemolytic uraemic syndrome and DIC.

11. D. Cephalosporins are one of the most common causes of drug-induced haemolytic anaemia. In the absence of any other information on clinical picture, bloods, past medical or family history, we do not have enough information to ascertain the other options as correct, therefore option D is the single best answer.

12. E. Severe pain may be a feature of a painful infarctive crisis even before any external evidence of tissue hypoxia is present. Acute painful crises are characteristic of sickle cell anaemia. Often examination is normal. A high requirement for analgesia is also a feature of recurrent painful crises in these patients.

13. A. General anaesthesia is a stressor that frequently provokes decompensation in individuals with poor physical fitness. Perioperative features such as dehydration, fasting and hypothermia under anaesthesia combined to make general anaesthesia a major risk factor for precipitating various types of sickle cell crises. This gentleman is experiencing acute chest syndrome, which is important to recognize early and manage.

14. E. While all the options would certainly be sensible and conducted at varying stages, the question specifically asks what is the NEXT most appropriate step. It is important therefore to consider the priority of each action. Option E summarizes the acute management that you might likely take as the senior house officer attending first to the patient. An arterial gas (not venous, hence option A is incorrect) would guide on the level of hypoxia or type of respiratory failure and help inspired oxygen. It is important to administer adequate analgesia to prevent hypoventilation due to pain. Administering oxygen is an integral part of management; you would not wean while the patient is clearly hypoxic. An FBC with HbSS percentage would be useful as this patient may certainly require exchange transfusion and his case would need urgent discussion with the haematologist (why option E is superior to option C). While it is sensible to consider a CTPA, it would not delay immediate management if the clinical suspicion is more in keeping with acute chest syndrome rather than a pulmonary embolism. Not covered in options of the question, but the intensive care team should also be made aware of this patient as they have the risk of rapid deterioration and may require mechanical ventilation.

15. C. Sickle cell anaemia significantly increases susceptibility to infection and results in catastrophic complications even from minor infections, as is the case with this patient. She is periarrest due to septic

shock arising from gastroenteritis, and she requires urgent fluid resuscitation and circulatory support if she is to survive.

16. A. Patient has sickle cell anaemia as suspected on the peripheral blood film and is severely anaemic. Splenic sequestration crises typically present in patients younger than 2 years of age. We need to urgently restore her circulating volume with blood and fluid. Once stable it would appropriate to proceed with splenectomy. Option E has not place in acute management of sickle crises. Option D does not address the issue of severe anaemia. Option C may very likely be the end destination of the patient however the treating team would certainly attempt to stabilize the patient first.

17. E. This patient has been exposed to parvovirus B19 (also called slapped cheek syndrome). This is usually benign and self-limiting, although it can provoke a transient pure red aplasia. However, in sickle cell anaemia patients, it can result in aplastic anaemia, which we suspect given his symptoms of thrombocytopenia (bruising and bleeding) and leucopoenia (fever and systemic illness). We would therefore expect a pancytopenic profile on his FBC as is the case in option E. He will need admission and intravenous antibiotics.

18. C. Option C is the correct answer as it is the next more appropriate action you would take as an emergency department doctor. This man presents with symptoms of anaemia (pallor, fatigue and shortness of breath) and the FBC suggests it is likely iron deficiency (microcytic anaemia). Unexplained iron deficiency anaemia in an older male should trigger concerns for undiagnosed GI malignancy. We may very well consider options A, B and D; however, it is important to note the change in his stools is likely describing melaena, which is a sign of active upper GI bleed. It is important to check that he is not actively having melaena and his systemic vital signs suggest decompensation. He will likely need admission and discussion with the Gastroenterology for urgent endoscopy.

Chapter 4 White blood cells

1. D. Only the monocyte is a macrophage precursor, even though neutrophils, basophils and eosinophils are also of myeloid lineage. Monocytes are derived from CFU-M, which is derived from CFU-GM, derived from CFU-GEMM. They circulate in the bloodstream and when they leave the circulation to enter the tissues, they undergo further differentiation and acquire additional features, when they are referred as macrophages.

2. B. Only HIV infection would cause lymphopenia. Ancylostoma (hookworm) infection would be expected to cause eosinophilia. EBV infection would likely cause mononucleosis and lymphocytosis. ALL and toxoplasmosis would cause a lymphocytosis.

3. A. The band cells are most likely to be seen in "left shift", where immature neutrophil precursors are released into peripheral blood from bone marrow. The more severe the factor that provoked premature release of neutrophil precursors, the earlier the developmental stage of the immature cells released. Band cells are precursors immediately prior to a mature neutrophil and are most likely to be seen first.

4. B. The most common cause of neutropenia is drugs. Therefore, vancomycin is the correct answer. Recent surgery would be most likely to cause a neutrophilia. Hypersplenism results in increased splenic sequestration of neutrophils, and so may cause neutropenia by reducing neutrophil lifespan in the circulation. Rheumatoid arthritis is an autoimmune disease; recall that neutropenia may arise by immune-mediated neutrophil destruction that can be idiopathic or associated with existing autoimmune disease. The only clue we have is that she did not present with neutropenia (if she had, we would consider Felty syndrome more). Severe infection would be most likely to cause a neutrophilia, but it would also possibly result in neutropenia due to extortionately high demand created by overwhelming bacterial infection.

Chapter 5 Haematological malignancies

1. A. Chronic obstructive pulmonary disease causes chronic hypoxia which will cause a secondary erythrocytosis (i.e., 'absolute' erythrocytosis). The other options reduce plasma volume resulting in a rise in the haemoglobin, hence 'apparent' erythrocytosis. The different types can be confirmed with specialist testing, such as nuclear medicine red cell mass scan, which measures the true volume of red cells in the patient.

2. C. Cytopenias result from invasion of normal marrow by the dysplastic haematopoietic precursors. Clonal proliferation of abnormal plasma cells in blood and bone marrow describes multiple myeloma. Accumulation of abnormal lymphoid cells in nodal and extranodal tissues defines lymphoma. Neoplastic proliferation of a myeloid precursor resulting in hypercellular marrow defines myeloproliferative disorders. Accumulation of abnormal neoplastic white cells in bone marrow defines the leukaemias.

3. C. This scenario is typical of hyperviscosity syndrome secondary to excessively high levels of abnormal white cells. This is considered a medical emergency as the 'sludging' of these white cells affects tissue perfusion resulting in hypoxia. Sepsis is a potential option but the patient is afebrile in this case. Furthermore, pulmonary oedema would not be typically associated with neurological symptoms. In pulmonary haemorrhage, patients typically have haemoptysis while in atypical fungal infection; this is again associated with recurrent fevers as well as other constitutional symptoms such as weight loss.

4. B. The clinical presentation and examination findings are nonspecific in terms of haematological malignancy, but acute lymphoblastic leukaemia (ALL) should be a top differential as it is the most common childhood cancer. The elevated white cell count and cytopenias suggest a leukaemia but bone marrow biopsy is consistent with a lymphoid leukaemia. The *MLL* gene rearrangement is common in ALL. Chronic myeloid leukaemia (CML) exhibits myeloid lineage cells with 9:22 as defining translocation; anaemia and thrombocytopenia are not typical features. Nonaccidental injury should always be considered when bruising is noted in a child but would not present with the investigations above. Primary myelofibrosis is neither a childhood diagnosis nor does it present with lymphoblasts. Non-Hodgkin lymphoma also does not show lymphoblasts.

5. D. The presence of *BCR-ABL* fusion gene (also known as the 'Philadelphia chromosome') is pathognomonic for CML. Typically, patients with this condition are well and are often asymptomatic. Polycythaemia vera is typically associated with JAK2 mutation and typically patients have a high haemoglobin level. Primary myelofibrosis is not associated with *BCR-ABL*. Acute myeloid leukaemia is typically associated with symptoms and with this white cell count, patients will display features of leucostasis (i.e., hyperviscosity syndrome). Chronic lymphocytic leukaemia (CLL) does not cause raised neutrophils or basophils.

6. D. The polydipsia and polyuria are secondary to hypercalcaemia and renal involvement. The presence of protein on urine dip represents tubular damage and the presence of Bence-Jones protein. The serum electrophoresis and the presence of clonal plasma cells in the bone marrow excludes a leukaemia and is consistent with multiple myeloma. Widespread system involvement excludes solitary plasmacytoma and MGUS.

7. E. The patient's age would provide the best chance of discriminating between Hodgkin and non-Hodgkin lymphoma while waiting for the biopsy result because almost all subtypes of NHL present at older age (median age 60 years). Alcohol-induced painful lymphadenopathy and cyclical fever are also features of HL and are not seen in NHL, but are extremely rare. Past EBV infection and known immunodeficiency are nondiscriminatory because they predispose to both HL and NHL. Likewise, fever, weight loss, night sweats and pruritus can be presenting features of either HL or NHL.

8. C. Chronic lymphocytic leukaemia typically presents in older patients (median age 70 years) and classical feature from blood film is the presence of smear cells. Neither infective mononucleosis nor COVID infection would cause the symptoms or clinical findings described above, especially as viral illness is typically associated with painful lymphadenopathy. Acute lymphoblastic leukaemia is typically a childhood cancer, and patients are often more unwell with associated anaemia and thrombocytopenia. Hodgkin lymphoma is not typically associated with leucocytosis.

9. B. This patient would be at high risk of tumour lysis syndrome given his high tumour burden. The biochemical abnormalities in this option would correspond with this acute complication secondary to his treatment. The joint pain arises from acute crystal deposition of uric acid and the hypocalcaemia, the other symptoms. The high potassium accounts for the ECG changes and would warrant emergency intravenous 10% calcium gluconate and potassium-lowering treatments.

10. C. This patient presents with septic shock secondary to neutropenic sepsis with type 1 respiratory failure and metabolic acidosis. Urgent resuscitation via an ABC approach with early input from critical care would be an appropriate action. He requires urgent large-bore IV access and vigorous hydration and immediate broad-spectrum antibiotics (ideally after blood cultures). Performing an urgent red blood cell transfusion and administering G-CSF are not appropriate. Allopurinol and rasburicase would be used in tumour lysis syndrome, which does not apply to this case. Plasmapheresis would only be used in patients presenting with hyperviscosity secondary to a high paraprotein level in multiple myeloma.

Chapter 6 Haemostasis

1. B. Vasoconstriction is the most immediate event. Transient tethering then promotes platelet release reaction which allows more stable adhesion to occur. Finally aggregation follows.

2. B. Only option B correctly describes the first step of the extrinsic pathway. The events in options A, C and D are accurate, but refer to stages of the intrinsic pathway. Option E describes a stage in fibrin formation which only occurs after the common pathway.

3. A. Only option A summarizes the common pathway. Statement B describes the extrinsic pathway while option C describes primary haemostasis. Option D describes the intrinsic pathway and finally option E describes fibrinolysis.

4. D. Calcium plays a critical role in the coagulation cascade as it is a component of the tissue factor-factor VIIa-calcium complex (i.e., the tenase complex) as well as the prothrombinase complex (factor Xa-factor Va-calcium). In addition, the vitamin K-dependent factors require calcium ions as cofactors for their activation. The rest of the options are known anticoagulants and prevent spontaneous activation of the coagulation cascade.

5. D. Liver disease is typically associated with marked coagulopathy as impaired synthetic function results in deficiencies of multiple clotting factors. Vitamin K deficiency typically causes prolonged PT and APTT as it impacts both the intrinsic and extrinsic pathways through factors II, VII, IX and X. Factor V is a common pathway deficiency, and therefore both PT and APTT will be prolonged. Factor XII deficiency will cause prolonged APTT as it is part of the extrinsic pathway, as well as factor XI deficiency.

6. E. Option E describes a bleeding disorder, vWD, which is typically associated with mucocutaneous bleeding and prolonged bleeding after trauma or surgery. There are three subtypes of vWD with types 2 and 3 being more severe. Options A–D describe hereditary thrombophilias which manifest with thromboses.

7. D. D is the most common culprit for drug-induced immune thrombocytopenic purpura, where platelets are destroyed by drug-dependent immune mechanism, reducing their survival in the circulation.

8. D. She presents with traditional pentad of symptoms suggestive of TTP. While all options (excluding C) would present with bruising, the jaundice suggests haemolysis which is not a feature of either option C or option E. HUS (option A) would not present with transient neurological symptoms and in an adult would usually be preceded by a GI infection. DIC (option B) would be associated with a critically unwell patient, and blood results would show prolonged PT and APTT with reduced fibrinogen. Option C would not cause jaundice and option E would not include haemolysis nor any fever or neurological findings.

9. C. Options A-C all reverse warfarin, but only option C would achieve this within the specified timeframe. Dosage of PCC is best discussed with the on-call haematologist. Option D would only be appropriate in an acute bleeding patient with haemophilia or in a major haemorrhage. Option E only contains factors VIII, XIII, vWF and fibrinogen and therefore is only useful if fibrinogen <1.5 g/dL.

10. D. This is a trick question! Option D is an acquired, not inherited, thrombophilia. APLS results from antibodies targeting phospholipid-dependent proteins resulting in arterial or venous thrombotic events. The other options are known inherited thrombophilias and should be tested for in individuals presenting at a young age with a thrombosis event and there are more than two family members affected with thrombosis under 40 years of age.

11. D. The Well's score is a validated risk stratification tool used to estimate the probability of a deep vein thrombosis (DVT). A point is scored for risk factors which does include major surgery within the last 12 weeks as well as prolonged lower limb immobility, active cancer and previous venous thromboembolism. Age and smoking are not included, as well as long-haul flight.

Chapter 7 Blood transfusion

1. C. Male donors must have predonation Hb 135g/L while female donors require predonation Hb 125g/L. Volunteers must be at least 17 years of age and women cannot donate more frequently than every 16 weeks. Donations can consist of whole blood or of a single component (e.g., platelets). In relation to malaria, you can donate if it has been more than 4 months since you visited an endemic country or 3 years since clearance of active infection.

2. C. IgM binds to A or B antigens causing complement-mediated intravascular haemolysis.

3. B. This is the safest option. Option A would be appropriate for transfusion-associated circulatory overload while option C is appropriate for suspected anaphylaxis. Option D is part of the management of nonhaemolytic febrile transfusion reaction. Option E is the treatment for septic shock from bacterially contaminated blood products.

4. B. The risk of sensitization is highest during subsequent pregnancies with an RhD +ve foetus in RhD –ve women. This can result in previously developed anti-D antibodies crossing the placenta leading to HDFN. All RhD –ve women should receive

anti-D prophylaxis at 28-30 weeks gestation. HDFN can also be seen with anti-c and anti-K antibodies.

5. D. Recent surgery is not a contraindication for electronic issue – the options will preclude patients from having electronically issued blood products and therefore they will require serologic cross-match.
6. C. Red cells are typically stored in these conditions in SAG-M solution.
7. A. Platelets need to be stored at room temperature with constant agitation to avoid aggregation. They have a shelf life of 5 days.
8. A. A platelet count below 50×10^9/L is a high risk for haemorrhage during major abdominal surgery, and therefore transfusion is required to reduce this.
9. B. Although the fibrinogen is reduced, it is not at a level that requires urgent intervention and in major haemorrhage, a target >1.5 g/dL is required. However, the deranged PT and APTT do need correction and this is with fresh frozen plasma.
10. C. The mechanism described in this question underlies this potentially fatal complication. Leucodepletion is routinely performed to minimize this risk and patients with impaired cell-mediated immunity are transfused with irradiated blood products for this same reason.
11. C. The correct legal, ethical and clinical course of action is option C. Option A will not stabilize the child and haemodilution may worsen the situation. Option B is not appropriate as the child is in hypovolaemic shock and will not survive waiting for a cell saver to be on site. Option D wastes time while option E is not acceptable as a child cannot refuse life-threatening treatment and an advanced directive is not valid in someone so young.
12. C. Hypocalcaemia, not hypercalcaemia, is a complication of major transfusion. It can exacerbate myocardial dysfunction in haemorrhagic shock and cause platelet dysfunction.
13. D. This is a difficult scenario, but one you may likely come across as new qualified doctors. It is important to recognize that this patient is actively having a major/massive bleed and is unwell with it (severely low Hb and low blood pressure). This should trigger the Major Haemorrhage protocol (familiarize yourself with the hospital policies on how to activate when you are on clinical placements). Patient will need good-quality access to transfuse blood products quickly for resuscitation and while the patient ideally needs blood (given via a blood warmer), IVF can help to sustain perfusion of the organs by supporting the blood pressure. The scenario describes haematemesis which is an upper GI bleed, and this does require involvement of the UGIB consultant (less so the surgeons, hence

option C is incorrect). However, in reality, your priority "next steps" would be to resuscitate and stabilize the patient.

Chapter 9 The innate immune system

1. C. The innate immune system is composed of phagocytes and complement. The other options are typical of the adaptive immune system.
2. B. The basophil is the only cell not to perform phagocytosis – it mainly functions through degranulation of leucotrienes which then attract eosinophils to the site of infection.
3. E. Chemotherapy-induced toxicity does not usually cause fevers while *Clostridium difficile* is typically seen in patients who have had prolonged courses of antibiotics while admitted into hospital. Viral and parasitic infections are possible but given the history of chemotherapy, this patient is at high risk of neutropenic sepsis and this should first be ruled out and managed accordingly.
4. E. Hospitalized patients are at higher risk of developing *Clostridium difficile* infection due to disruption of the patient's normal gut flora by recent antibiotics. Typical symptoms include abdominal distension, pain and watery diarrhoea. Key management is isolation and good hand washing techniques, as well as antibiotics.
5. D. Macrophages can act as antigen-presenting cells. They have a longer lifespan compared to neutrophils but move and phagocytose more slowly. They express high levels of MHC class II molecules and are unable to kill intracellular pathogens, requiring help from T cells.
6. C. Natural killer cells attack cells that do not express MHC class I molecules as this does not activate the inhibitory killer-cell immunoglobulin-like receptors (KIRs). This can make them effective at targeting certain viral infections (e.g., herpes).
7. D. Mast cells play an important role in the development of type I hypersensitivity reactions including anaphylaxis.
8. A. The acute phase proteins (APPs), including C-reactive protein, fibrinogen and haptoglobulin, catabolize muscle proteins and fat deposits as part of the systematic response to infection.
9. C. The membrane attack complex (MAC) attacks pathogens by inserting a hole in their cell membrane causing its death via osmotic lysis. Phagocytosis is mainly mediated by phagocyte cells (e.g., neutrophils and macrophages) while opsonization is the means of enhancing phagocytosis through coating of pathogens with C3b. Degranulation is a function of basophils and mast cells, while apoptosis is triggered by cytotoxic T and natural killer cells.

10. D. Raised ESR is a classical feature of giant cell arteritis and should raise suspicion for this condition when patients present with temporal headaches.
11. D. This patient has hereditary angioedema due to deficiency of the C1 inhibitor. C1 inhibitor typically inhibits C1 and therefore the subsequent activation of the classical complement pathway. Loss of this inhibitor leads to spontaneous activation of the early complement pathway resulting in life-threatening swellings.
12. C. This patient has sepsis and needs to be treated as part of the 'Sepsis 6' management plan which includes:
    (i) Giving high-flow oxygen
    (ii) Taking blood cultures as well as other sources
    (iii) Giving intravenous (not oral) antibiotics
    (iv) Giving a fluid challenge (e.g., 500 mL of 0.9% sodium chloride)
    (v) Measuring serum lactate and other blood tests
    (vi) Monitoring urine output

Chapter 10 The adaptive immune system

1. B. The haplotype is found on chromosome 6. MHC class I molecules present endogenous antigens, CD8 positive cells bind MHC class I, MHC class II are only present on antigen-presenting cells and there is no difference in peptide length that MHC class I and II present.
2. E. Somatic hypermutation and affinity maturation are different names for the same process that increases the affinity of an antibody for an antigen. Junctional diversity is the increased variability in antibodies due to the formation of junctions between various gene segments. Positive selection is the process in which T-cells are able to recognize self-MHC survive and those that cannot recognize self-MHC do not.
3. E. TLR-4 are not members of the immunoglobulin superfamily but are pattern-recognition molecules. The others all contain immunoglobulin domains and therefore are members of the immunoglobulin superfamily.
4. C. Somatic hypermutation occurs in the germinal centres. B cells are activated in the follicles of secondary lymphoid organs. Bcl-2 expression prevents apoptosis of the B cell, and B cells are activated by antigen presented by dendritic cells. Activated T helper cells enable B cells to activate and produce antibodies.
5. D. IgE.
6. B. Th1 cells express IL-2 and TNF-α which can target intracellular pathogens while Th2 cells target extracellular bacteria and parasites. MHC restriction occurs in the thymus. Cytotoxic T cells express CD8. T cells must bind self-MHC as part of their function. However, if they bind self-MHC with self-antigens, they undergo apoptosis (i.e., negative selection).
7. A. T-helper cells induce B cells to become fully active through cytokines. B and T lymphocytes originate from Lymphoid stem cells. Plasma cells contain vast amount of endoplasmic reticulin to secrete large quantities of immunoglobulin. CD8 is a marker associated with cytotoxic T cells and these cells recognize antigen in conjunction with class I MHC.
8. C. MHC class I molecules present antigens from intracellular pathogens while MHC class II recognize exogenous antigen that has been phagocytosed into intracellular vesicles.
9. C. Cytotoxic T cells and Th1 lymphocytes are crucial to eliminating the influenza virus. She may have encountered this virus before but the strain mutates annually. The flu symptoms are mainly due to interferon rather than TGF-β.
10. D. Staphylococcal enterotoxin causes cross-linking of the V-β domain of the TCR and MHC class II molecule on an antigen-presenting cell, resulting in enhanced activation of the adaptive immune system. The other options do not act as a superantigen.

Chapter 11 The functioning immune system

1. D. Prostaglandins do not increase vascular permeability but do cause vasodilation and pain response.
2. C. TNF-α is required for granuloma formation and maintenance, while IFN-γ is required for the transformation of macrophages into epithelioid cells. IFN-γ also stimulates the production of multinucleate giant cells.
3. B. Persistence of antigen is the main factor in the progression of inflammation from acute to chronic.
4. D. Interferon-α rather than TNF-α is the cytokine secreted by virally infected cells to communicate with other cells.
5. C. *M. tuberculosis* is an intracellular pathogen so phagocytes cannot easily engulf these bacteria and antibodies are unable to neutralize it. Th2 cells release IL-4 against extracellular pathogens and are involved in allergic responses. Primary tuberculosis infection in an immunocompetent patient is managed by granulation tissue forming caseous necrosis.
6. A. IFN-Y activates macrophages and natural killer cells – it does not affect viral transcription or translation. Neutrophils phagocytose bacteria not viruses. CD8+ T

cells destroy infected cells and granuloma formation is not associated with flu infection.

7. E. sIgA can bind bacteria and prevent them from binding to epithelial cells.

8. B. Mast cells and eosinophils interact with parasitic worms on mucosal surfaces and are responsible for the immune response to parasitic worms.

9. D. If the virus has been cleared, HBSAg would be -ve. Vaccinated immunity only produces anti-HBs as vaccinations are used against the surface antigen. If a person has cleared the virus, they would have antibodies against the core and surface antigens (i.e., anti-HBc and anti-HBs).

10. B. The pathogen is *Plasmodium* and this typically has a complex lifecycle which can make the immune response more challenging.

Chapter 12 Immune dysfunction

1. C. IgE-mediated degranulation of mast cells is the cause of type I hypersensitivity reactions. Nickel hypersensitivity and rheumatoid arthritis are type IV hypersensitivities and are cell-mediated. ABO incompatibility is type II hypersensitivity which is antibody-mediated but not IgE-mediated. Farmer's lung is a type III hypersensitivity reaction.

2. E. Allergy testing can be performed using a skin prick test where a small amount of the suspected allergen is inoculated into the skin – a positive reaction will result in an itchy red lesion within 15–20 minutes. Tryptase is typically a marker of mast cell activation and is typically measured following a suspected anaphylactic reaction.

3. C. Histological findings within the airway walls in asthma patients include infiltration by eosinophils, neutrophils and lymphocytes. This is a chronic inflammatory disorder and is characterized by reversible airflow obstruction. Management includes avoiding triggers, short-acting β2-adrenoreceptor agonist and steroids.

4. B. This is a hypersensitivity pneumonitis (a type III hypersensitivity reaction). Eczema and asthma are due to IgE-mediated mast cell degranulation (a type I hypersensitivity reaction). Nickel hypersensitivity is cell-mediated (type IV) and haemolytic disease of the newborn is antibody-mediated, with red blood cell destruction secondary to complement activation and antibody-dependent cell-mediated cytotoxicity (type II hypersensitivity).

5. D. Serum sickness is a type III hypersensitivity reaction resulting from formation of immune complexes between human and nonhuman proteins. It typically occurs within 6–12 days of exposure and is characterized by triad of fever, rash and arthritis. Symptoms can last several weeks, not days, and can be managed with antihistamines, NSAIDs and glucocorticoids.

6. D. These cells secrete cytokines on contact with the antigen resulting in the attraction and activation of macrophages. This process takes 24–72 hours to peak hence the name delayed-type hypersensitivity.

7. D. This is the immediate treatment required in anaphylactic reaction. Options A, B and C can be used but later. C1 inhibitor is used in hereditary angioedema.

8. E. The antitissue transglutaminase test is very sensitive and specific for coeliac disease.

9. B. Given the clinical history and radiographic findings, the most likely diagnosis is rheumatoid arthritis. Anti-CCP antibodies are typically present in this condition as well as IgM anti-IgG antibodies (rheumatoid factor).

10. C. HIV possesses reverse transcriptase which allows it to manufacture double-stranded DNA, which is incorporated into host cells' genetic material.

11. D. This is an AIDS-defining infection. AIDS can also be diagnosed with CD4 count of less than 200 cells/μL. The other conditions do not indicate the patient has progressed to AIDS.

12. C. Tuberculin skin test is used to measure previous exposure to *Mycobacterium tuberculosis* or the bacilli Calmette-Guerin (BCG) vaccine. Previous exposure to either results in a firm, red lesion at the site of injection 48–72 hours later. It is caused by the infiltration of macrophages and T cells. Skin prick test is used to diagnose IgE-mediated response to allergens (i.e., type I hypersensitivity reactions).

Chapter 13 Medical intervention

1. D. Hepatitis B postexposure prophylaxis is a form of passive, not active immunity. This is through the injection of immunoglobulins to that specific antigen taken from blood donors who are immune to the pathogen.

2. C. The immunoglobulin administered does not directly stimulate the immune system and therefore is not active immunity. No immunological memory is created, therefore once the immunoglobulin is excreted no immunity will be conferred.

3. E. Hyperacute rejection is rapid because antibodies have been induced prior to transplantation, for example, by blood transfusion. It is prevented by cross-matching the donor cells and recipient serum. Chronic rejection is not well understood and, if it occurs, cannot be treated. Acute cellular rejection is mediated by T cells (i.e., a type IV hypersensitivity reaction).

4. C. Haematopoietic stem cell transplant (HSCT) can be used for both malignant and nonmalignant conditions, a good example for the latter being multiple sclerosis. Autologous HSCT uses the patient's own HSCs while allogeneic HSCT uses a donor. As a result, graft-versus-leukaemia effect is typically observed in allogeneic HSCT recipients, where the donor lymphocytes target any residual malignant cells. Graft-versus-host disease (GVHD) is not self-limiting and can be both acute and chronic.

5. A. Raised blood pressure is seen due to the mineralocorticoid activity of the steroids. The glucocorticoid action of steroids means they act as an antiinsulin and promote gluconeogenesis, affecting glucose tolerance. Wound healing is attenuated by systemic steroids and immunosuppressive action of them also predisposes patients to infections.

6. D. While all the side effects listed are concerning, the major adverse effect to monitor for is gastric ulceration in elderly patients.

7. B. This patient is in an Addisonian crisis, likely due to the sudden interruption of interruption of long-term high-dose systemic steroids. Management is to correct hypotension and restart steroid therapy (i.e., IV hydrocortisone).

8. E. Rituximab is a monoclonal antibody targeting the CD20 surface marker on B cells and is typically used to treat lymphoma. Infliximab is an anti–TNF-α antibody used in various rheumatological conditions (including rheumatoid arthritis, psoriatic arthritis and ankylosing spondylitis), as well as adalimumab. These antibodies are also used in GI inflammatory conditions including Crohn disease.

9. C. IL-2, not IL-10, is co-cultured with T cells, causing their activation and expansion. These result in the development of tumour-infiltrating lymphocytes (TILs). TIL therapy has been used to treat a variety of solid cancers, including head and neck cancers as well as melanomas.

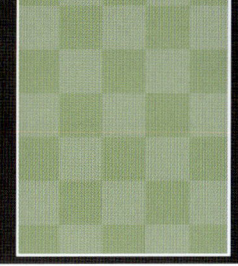

Case 1

A 48-year-old Greek patient is admitted with a legionella lower respiratory tract infection (LRTI). He is noted to be pale several days after admission. His blood count is as follows:

Hb 65g/L
White cell count 13×10^9/L
Platelets 350×10^9/L
Blood film is shown below:

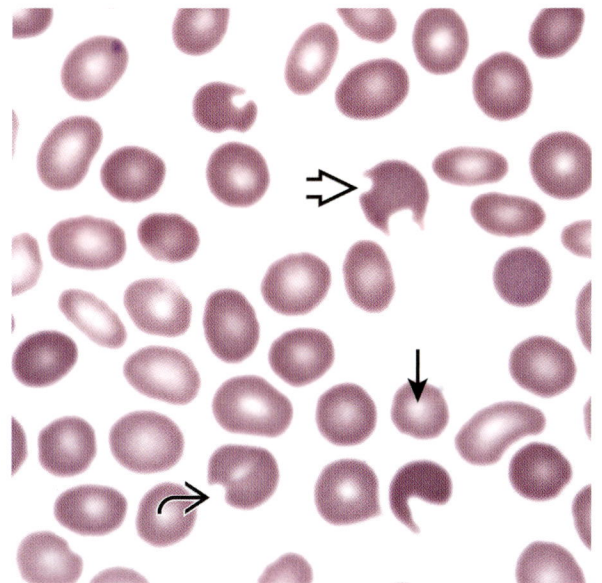

Figure Case 1 Marked anaemia with bite cells noted (black arrow). (From Foucar K. *Diagnostic Pathology: Blood and Bone Marrow*. 3rd ed. Philadelphia, PA: Elsevier Health Sciences; 2023).

a. What is the most likely diagnosis?
b. Based on your diagnosis, what other investigations would you request?
c. Please list the typical triggers for this complication.
d. How would you manage this patient?

Answers:

a. G6PD Deficiency
   – The ethnicity of the patient as well as the blood film features are typical for this condition.

b. As with any patient presenting with haemolysis, the following markers should be sent:
   – Full blood count: typically, Hb is reduced and white cells may be raised
   – Reticulocyte count: typically raised in acute haemolysis
   – Lactate dehydrogenase: raised
   – Haptoglobin: reduced
   – Unconjugated bilirubin: usually raised with normal liver enzymes
   – Direct Coombs test: typically negative in G6PD deficiency but will be positive in autoimmune haemolytic anaemia

c. Potential triggers for G6PD deficiency are listed below:
   – Infections
   – Acidosis
   – Broad (fava) beans
   – Mothballs
   – Medications (aspirin, dapsone, primaquine, sulphonamides)

d. Management of G6PD deficiency is mainly focused on symptom control. Ideally potential triggers should be reviewed or corrected. If haemodynamically stable, patients can be cautiously transfused, especially if their Hb is less than 70 g/L. All patients should be started on folic acid supplementation.

Case 2

An 84-year-old man presents to his GP with a 3-month history of worsening cognitive impairment. His family also report that he is struggling to walk and has had recurrent falls at home. He has also lost weight and has become increasingly depressed. Past medical history includes hypertension and type 2 diabetes for which he takes amlodipine and metformin, respectively. He is a nonsmoker but does drink 20 units per week. Clinical examination reveals impaired vibration sense and proprioception in his lower limbs as well as loss of light touch sensation. Blood results are as follows:

Hb 95 g/L
MCV 120 fL (normal range 80–100 fL)
White cell count 3.1×10^9/L
Neutrophil 1.3×10^9/L
Platelets 110×10^9/L

a. What are your differentials for the above presentation?
b. What is the most likely diagnosis and how would you confirm this?

c. What are the different causes for this condition?

d. The patient is initially started on treatment but then returns to his GP a few weeks later with worsening neurological symptoms – what do you think might have happened?

Answers:

a. This patient has a high MCV with low haemoglobin suggestive of a macrocytic anaemia – typical differentials include:
   – B12 deficiency
   – Folate deficiency
   – Haemolysis
   – Myelodysplastic syndrome
   – Alcohol excess

b. Based on his neurocognitive symptoms combined with macrocytic anaemia, this is typical for B12 deficiency. To confirm this, the following investigations should be sent:
   – Vitamin B12 levels (usually reduced)
   – Methylmalonic acid (MMA; typically increased)
   – Blood film: this will show 'megaloblastic' changes including macrocytic red cells, 'oval macrocytes', hypersegmented neutrophils

c. Vitamin B12 deficiency can be due to either dietary or nondietary conditions:
   – Dietary: vegan diet (most B12 is obtained from animal-derived food products); food cobalamin malabsorption; intestinal malabsorption; small bowel diverticulae
   – Nondietary: alcohol excess; pernicious anaemia; metformin use

d. The patient has been started on B12 replacement alone meaning all tetrahydrofolate becomes trapped as a nonfunctional compound. This compound cannot participate in usual reactions resulting in folate deficiency. As a result, patients can develop symptoms of folate deficiency including neuropsychiatric complications. Therefore, it is important that B12 and Folate are coadministered together in patients with suspected deficiency.

Case 3

1. A 25-year-old woman presents with jaundice and right upper quadrant pain to her GP. She reports that she has had recurrent episodes of jaundice since childhood, but this is the most severe episode. She did note these episodes typically followed a viral illness. She is not taking any regular medication or any over-the-counter supplements. The woman has two siblings, one of whom had surgery when they were young, but she is unclear what this was. She is a nonsmoker and does not drink excess alcohol. Examination reveals icteric

sclera and she is tender in the right upper quadrant on deep palpation. She also has palpable splenomegaly. Investigations are as follows:

Hb 100 g/L
MCV 95 fL
White cell count 11 × 10⁹/L
Platelets 100 × 10⁹/L
Bilirubin 47 μmol/L (normal range <21 μmol/L)
Blood film:

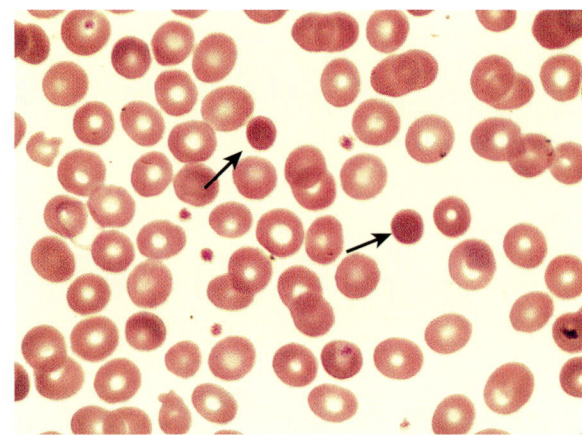

Figure Case 3 Black arrow shows numerous spherocytes on this blood film. (From *Crash Course: Haematology & Immunology*. 5th ed. 2019.).

a. What is the most likely diagnosis?
b. What type of complication has this patient developed from this condition?
c. What is the most appropriate next step in diagnosis?
d. Which cytoskeletal defect results in this condition?
e. What would be the management for this patient?

Answers

a. Hereditary spherocytosis
   – The patient is presenting with a history of likely recurrent haemolysis and based on her blood results as well as the film features, this is typical for this condition.

b. Pigment gallstones
   – Patients with chronic haemolysis can develop pigment gallstones as a result of excess bilirubin levels.

c. The following investigations are required to confirm her diagnosis as well as her acute complication:
   – Haemolysis markers on blood tests including reticulocyte count, lactate dehydrogenase (LDH), haptoglobin and direct coombs test (this is typically negative).

- Osmotic fragility: this is typically increased in this condition.
- Eosin-5-maleimide (EMA) binding is typically reduced in this condition and is the gold standard investigation.
- Ultrasound abdomen to investigate potential gallstones and also confirm if any associated splenomegaly which is typically associated with this condition.

d. Patients with hereditary spherocytosis typically have a defect in spectrin, one of the key cytoskeletal proteins, resulting in membrane abnormality.

e. Management for this patient would be as follows:
- Supportive management for acute haemolysis – this will include managing triggers (usually infection) and commencing folic acid supplements.
- Referral to the gastroenterology surgeons to consider cholecystectomy for pigment gallstones.
- In severe cases of hereditary spherocytosis, some patients have a splenectomy (which is potentially what happened to this patient's sibling).

Case 4

1. A 21-year-old man presents with severe leg pain which he has developed over the last few days – score is 9/10. He has tried his usual analgesia at home with no effect. The man mentions that he did have a recent viral upper respiratory tract infection which may have triggered this. He does have an ongoing dry cough but denies any haemoptysis or breathlessness. Clinical examination reveals BP 110/75 mmHg, heart rate 110 bpm sinus rhythm, temperature 37.6°C and saturations 95% on room air. Initial investigations are as follows:

Hb 75 g/L
MCV 67 fL
White cell count 15×10^9/L
Platelets 450×10^9/L
Blood film as shown below:

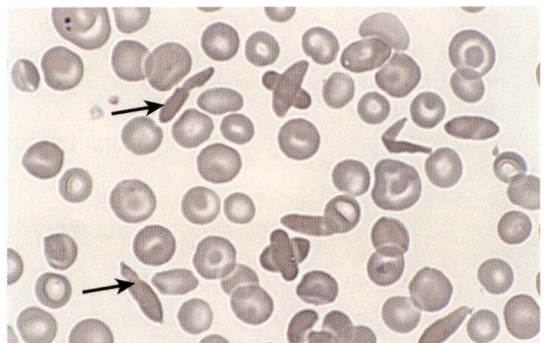

Figure 1 Case 4 Numerous sickle cells (black arrow) are present on this blood film. (From *Microscopic Haematology: A Practical Guide for the Laboratory*. 3rd ed. 2011.).

a. What is the most likely diagnosis?
b. What are the most appropriate next steps in managing this patient?
c. A few days later, the patient develops worsening breathlessness with productive cough. He is only managing to talk in short sentences and reports chest pain. Clinical examination reveals temperature 37.8°C, heart rate 110 bpm sinus, BP 100/70 mmHg, respiratory rate 28/min and saturations 85% on room air. There is bilateral crepitations on auscultation and mobile chest X-ray is as below.

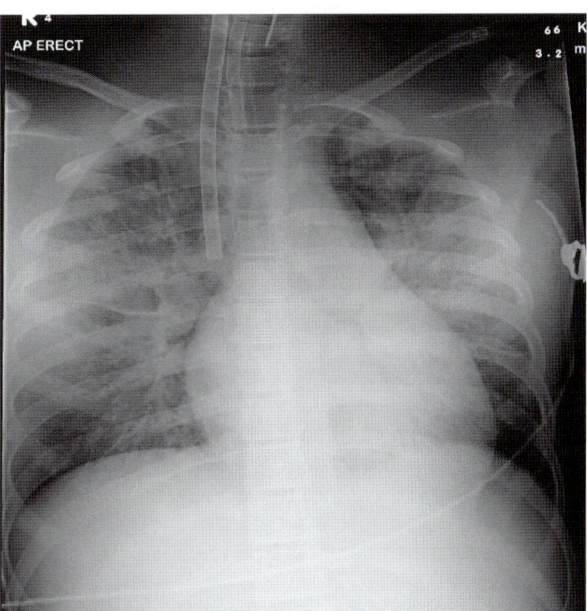

Figure 2 Case 4 Chest X-ray showing bilateral infiltrates. (From Systemic diseases and the lung. 2005.). (From YPRRV. 2005s).

What type of complication has this patient developed?
d. What is the definitive management for this complication?
e. The patient is later stabilized and discharged on new medication as this is his fourth admission to hospital. What treatment would he have started for his underlying condition?

Answers:

a. Sickle cell disease with vasoocclusive crisis (VOC)
- The marked anaemia with presence of numerous sickle cells on blood film is typical for sickle cell disease. The clinical history is in keeping with vasoocclusive crisis.
b. Patients presenting with VOC on background of sickle cell disease require urgent admission to hospital for

management of their pain and reducing any triggers. Management therefore should be as follows:

- Oxygenation to aim saturations >95% on room air
- Hydration with intravenous fluids
- Pain control – this is either orally or can be administered via patient-controlled analgesia (PCA) which is typically subcutaneous
- Antibiotics if any suspected infection
- Thromboprophylaxis for venous thromboembolism – the presence of sickle cells can make blood flow more viscous so the risk of thromboembolic complications is high
- Incentive spirometry is encouraged to ensure adequate oxygenation and reduce the risk of developing a chest crisis
- Transfusion is typically discussed with the Haematologist managing these patients

c. Acute chest crisis
  - This is a haematological emergency and requires urgent intervention. Patients with sickle cell disease can develop this complication as a result of infection or vasoocclusion within the pulmonary vasculature. Patients with this complication can become acutely unwell very quickly and early critical care input is recommended.

d. Exchange blood transfusion
  - This can be performed manually or automated and is where the patient's blood is removed and replaced with donor blood, thus reducing the amount of sickled cells in their bloodstream. The overall aim is to reduce the amount of HbS to <30%.

e. Hydroxycarbamide
  - This medication is usually prescribed for all sickle cell patients who have recurrent vasoocclusive or chest crises. Hydroxycarbamide helps to reduce the frequency of these complications by increasing the amount of HbF, and therefore causes a relative reduction in the amount of HbS.

Case 5

1. A 78-year-old man presents to his GP with a 6-month history of worsening fatigue, sweats and itching. For the latter, he notes it is worse following a shower. On further questioning, he admits his appetite has been reduced and he has found it difficult to finish his meals. Past medical history includes ischaemic heart disease, chronic obstructive pulmonary disease and hypertension. His medications include aspirin, bendroflumethiazide and salbutamol inhalers. On clinical examination, he has a plethoric face. Abdomen is mildly distended with palpable splenomegaly. Blood results are as below:

Hb 175 g/L
Hct 0.58
White cell count 14 × 10⁹/L
Platelets 650 × 10⁹/L
Ferritin 35 ng/mL

a. What is the most likely diagnosis?
b. Which genetic mutation is pathognomonic for this condition?
c. List other causes of raised haemoglobin/haematocrit levels.
d. What are the potential complications associated with this condition?

Answers:

a. Polycythaemia rubra vera (PRV)
  - The clinical history is typical of myeloproliferative disorders, with PRV being associated with aquagenic pruritus in particular. The raised haemoglobin and haematocrit levels support this diagnosis and usually patients will also have raised white cell and platelet counts.

b. JAK2
  - The *JAK2* gene mutation is pathognomonic for this condition and is positive in >90% of patients presenting with PRV.

c. Erythrocytosis can be 'absolute' or 'apparent':
  - 'Absolute' erythrocytosis is defined with there being a truly raised red cell mass with normal plasma volume. Common causes including chronic hypoxia (e.g., chronic obstructive pulmonary disease; cyanotic heart disease; long-term smoker) as well as erythropoietin-secreting tumours (e.g., renal cell cancer; cerebellar haemangioma).
  - 'Apparent' erythrocytosis is defined with a normal red cell mass but reduced plasma volume. Causes include alcohol excess, dehydration, diuretics and SGLT-2 inhibitors.

d. Potential complications can be short- or long-term in association with PRV:
  - Short term (acute): hyperviscosity; venous thromboembolism; arterial thrombotic events (e.g., myocardial infarct; cerebrovascular event).
  - Long term: increased risk of developing secondary myelofibrosis or acute myeloid leukaemia.

Case 6

1. A 35-year-old woman presents to A&E acutely unwell with fevers and extensive bruising. She reports she has had recent nosebleeds and has been feeling more fatigued over the last few weeks. She has no significant medical history and is not taking any regular medication. Clinical examination demonstrates extensive bruising and purpura over her arms and legs. She has a palpable liver and spleen edge. Blood results are as follows:

Hb 65 g/L
White cell count 2.5×10^9/L
Neutrophil 0.4×10^9/L
Platelets 23×10^9/L
INR 6.5 (normal range <1.5)
APTT 45 seconds (normal range 20–35)
Fibrinogen 0.9 g/dL (normal range 1.5–4.0)

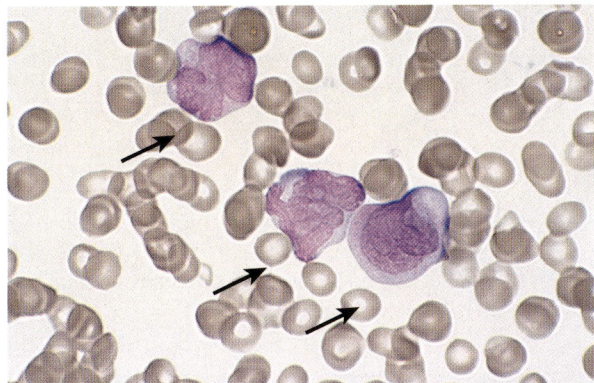

Figure Case 6 Blood film showing promyelocytic blasts. (From *Microscopic Haematology: A Practical Guide for the Laboratory*. 3rd ed. 2011.).

a. What is the most likely diagnosis?
b. What immediate management is required for this patient?
c. Urgent cytogenetic analysis reveals PML-RARA translocation (t[15;17]) – what haematological condition is this typically associated with?
d. What definitive treatment is given for this condition?

Answers:

a. Acute leukaemia with disseminated intravascular coagulation (DIC)
   - The clinical history of fever and bruising together with the low blood counts and presence of immature cells on the blood film are typical features in those presenting with acute leukaemia. The abnormal clotting factors are in keeping with DIC with global coagulopathy.
b. Chemotherapy and correction of coagulopathy
   - Treatment is a two-pronged approach with urgent chemotherapy aimed to reduce the acute leukaemia as well as correction of the coagulopathy. The latter includes vitamin K (for INR), fresh frozen plasma (for APTT) and cryoprecipitate (for fibrinogen).
c. Acute promyelocytic leukaemia (APML)
   - APML is typically associated with this translocation and usually patients do present with an associated DIC.
d. All-trans retinoic acid (ATRA)
   - ATRA is a vitamin A derivative and specifically targets the PML-RARA abnormality. By doing so, this enables immature promyelocytes to mature into healthy white blood cells.

Case 7

1. A 45-year-old man presents to A&E with breathlessness and headaches, associated with facial swelling. He reports over the last 6 months he has had cyclical fevers associated with pruritus and has lost 15 kg weight. Clinical examination shows temperature 37.5°C, heart rate 100 bpm sinus, respiratory rate 25/min, saturations 90% on room air. He has distended veins along his anterior chest wall and notable facial oedema. Investigations are shown below:

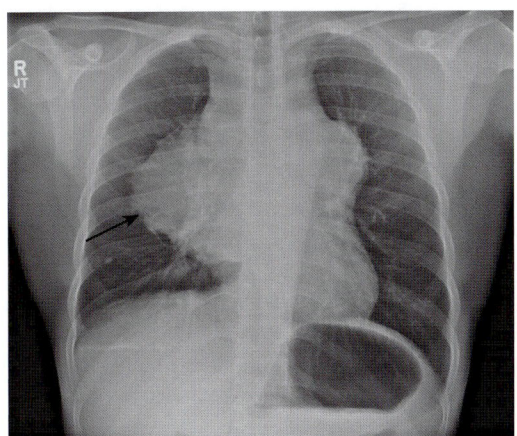

Chest X-ray demonstrates large mediastinal mass (black arrow) (From *Kumar and Clark's Clinical Medicine*. 10th ed. 2021.).

a. What is the most likely diagnosis?
b. What immediate management is required for this patient?

c. The patient has an urgent biopsy of the mediastinal mass – histology notes the presence of Reed-Stenberg cells. Which haematological condition are these typically associated with?

d. The patient is started on chemotherapy. However, 2 days later he reports worsening joint pains as well as abdominal cramps and is confused. Blood results are as follows:

Hb 110 g/L
White cell count 3.0×10^9/L
Platelets 120×10^9/L
K^+ 6.0 mM
Creatinine 150 µmol/L
Ca^{++} 1.9 mM
Uric acid 1500 µmol/L (normal range 180–420 µmol/L)

What complication has this patient developed?

e. How would you manage this complication?

Answers:

a. Given the presence of 'B' symptoms, it is likely this patient has lymphoma with associated superior vena cava obstruction (SVCO) given his clinical features.

b. SVC obstruction is a medical emergency and requires urgent intervention. Management can be medical and surgical. The former includes using corticosteroids while the latter includes stenting to relieve the pressure.

c. Hodgkin lymphoma
   – Reed-Sternberg cells typically have an 'owl's eye' appearance and are associated with Hodgkin lymphoma. These cells usually make up 1–2% of lymph node cellularity.

d. Tumour lysis syndrome
   – This complication arises from the breakdown of malignant cells and results in the excessive release of proteins and uric acid from tumour cells resulting in renal failure as well as electrolyte disturbance. The symptoms reported by this patient are due to hypocalcaemia causing muscle spasms and abdominal discomfort.

e. To prevent this complication, patients receive medication to reduce the production of uric acid. These include either allopurinol or rasburicase. Furthermore, patients should be aggressively hydrated and electrolyte abnormalities corrected.

Case 8

1. An 85-year-old woman presents to her GP with worsening back pain associated with lower leg weakness and bowel incontinence. She reports over the last few months, she has had recurrent infections as well as fatigue. Clinical examination reveals reduced power and sensation in the lower limbs with sensory level at T11. Blood results are as follows:

Hb 90 g/L
White cell count 5.5×10^9/L
Platelets 250×10^9/L
Creatinine 240 µmol/L
Ca^{++} 3.0 mM
Erythrocyte sedimentation rate raised

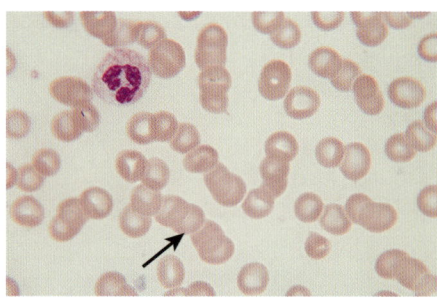

Blood film: red cell rouleaux (black arrow). (Goldman L, Ausiello D. *Cecil Medicine*. 23rd ed. Philadelphia, PA: Saunders; 2008. [Fig. 161–19]).

a. What is the most likely diagnosis?

b. What are the four clinical criteria typically associated with this condition?

c. The patient has an urgent MRI scan for her back pain which is shown below:

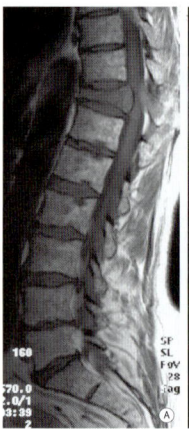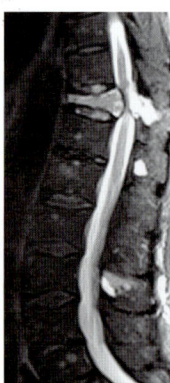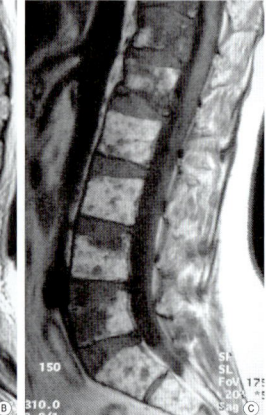

(From Grant LA. *Grainger & Allison's Diagnostic Radiology Essentials*. 2nd ed. Philadelphia, PA: Elsevier; 2019.).

What complication has this patient developed?

d. What is the management for the above complication?

Answers:

a. Multiple myeloma
   - The symptoms together with anaemia and renal impairment, as well as raised erythrocyte sedimentation rate and red cell rouleaux are features typically associated with this condition.
b. The 'CRAB' criteria are the most common clinical symptoms associated with multiple myeloma and are as listed below:
   - Calcium elevated above normal range
   - Renal impairment
   - Anaemia
   - Bony lesions
c. Spinal cord compression
   - The MRI images demonstrate vertebral collapse with spinal cord compression. This is a medical emergency and requires urgent intervention. Patients typically present with acute back pain associated with limb weakness and paraesthesia. Some patients can also develop bowel and bladder disturbance.
d. Management of spinal cord compression can be one of the following options:
   - Neurosurgical intervention
   - Radiotherapy to target lesion
   - Corticosteroids (usually patients are commenced on dexamethasone 16 mg daily)

Case 9

1. A 33-year-old woman presents to A&E with fever, confusion and headaches. She has no medical history and is not taking any regular medication. Clinical

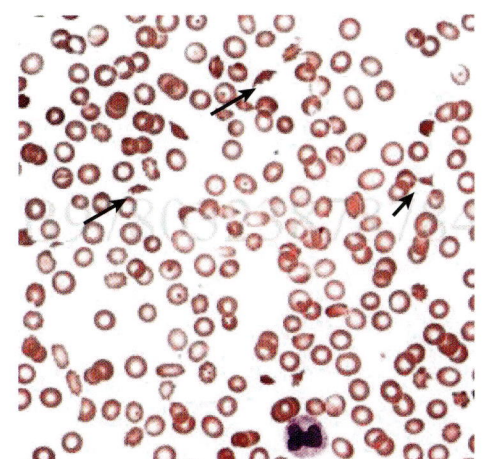

Blood film: numerous schistocytes (i.e., fragments) can be seen (black arrow). (From *Diagnostic Pathology: Blood and Bone Marrow*. 3rd ed. 2024)

examination did not reveal any significant findings with normal neurology. Investigations are as follows:

Hb 85 g/L
White cell count 11 × 10⁹/L
Platelets 11 × 10⁹/L
Lactate dehydrogenase 1100 IU/L
Creatinine 85 µmol/L

a. What is the most likely diagnosis?
b. What immediate management is required for this patient?
c. What novel treatments are available for this condition?
d. What other conditions are associated with microangiopathic haemolytic anaemia (MAHA)?

Answers:

a. The clinical symptoms together with the presence of schistocytes on the blood film are typical for thrombotic thrombocytopenic purpura (TTP). It should be noted that patients often have a marked thrombocytopenia with elevated lactate dehydrogenase as well as normal coagulation screen.
b. TTP is considered a haematological emergency which requires early recognition and intervention. Currently, any patient presenting with TTP is immediately transferred to a tertiary TTP centre for urgent plasma exchange. As a holding measure, patients have a large-bore cannula inserted and are infused with fresh frozen plasma (FFP) that contains ADAMTS13 which is typically reduced/absent in this condition.
c. Novel treatments include caplacizumab which is a nanobody that targets von Willebrand Factor (vWF) and its interaction with platelets. Other treatments include corticosteroids and rituximab.
d. MAHA can be seen in the following conditions:
   - Thrombotic thrombocytopenic purpura (TTP)
   - Haemolytic uraemic syndrome (HUS) – this is associated with renal impairment and is commonly due to E.coli infection
   - Disseminated intravascular coagulation (DIC)
   - Severe burns
   - Malignant hypertension
   - Systemic lupus erythematosus (SLE)
   - Drugs (ciclosporin, gemcitabine, mitomycin-c)
   - Mechanical heart valves

Case 10

1. A 29-year-old woman presents to her GP with facial rash (butterfly distribution) as well as arthralgia and malaise. She has no significant medical history and is

not taking any regular medication. Investigations are shown below:

Prothrombin time (PT) 14 seconds (normal range 13–15)

Activated partial thromboplastin time (APTT) 45 seconds (normal range 27–35) – no correction with mixing studies

Fibrinogen 3.5 g/dL (normal range 1.5–4.0)

a. What is the most likely diagnosis?
b. What is the cause for her prolonged APTT?
c. Does this patient have an increased risk of bleeding?
d. How would you manage this clotting abnormality?

Answers:

a. The clinical symptoms are typical for systemic lupus erythematosus (SLE).
b. The prolonged APTT is likely secondary to the presence of lupus anticoagulant (LA). This is an antibody directed against phospholipid-binding proteins resulting in phospholipid-dependent prolongation of phospholipid-dependent coagulation assays. To differentiate between the presence of an LA or clotting factor deficiency, mixing studies are performed in the laboratory. If the APTT corrects on mixing, this confirms a clotting factor deficiency but if it does not correct, this is more in keeping with the presence of a lupus anticoagulant.
c. The patient is not at increased risk of bleeding as there is no clotting factor deficiency, as confirmed by the mixing studies. The patient is actually at increased risk of thrombosis and therefore should be risk assessed for this should they be hospitalized or require any surgery.
d. The presence of a lupus anticoagulant is a laboratory artefact and is not clinically significant, so it does not require any intervention.

Glossary

Active immunity Resistance to an infection or disease that develops as a result of prior infection or vaccination.

Adaptive immunity An immune response that is slow to respond but produces lasting immunity and is adapted to produce the most effective eradication of the pathogen.

Adjuvant A substance that enhances the immune response to a vaccine.

Agglutination The process by which suspended bacteria, cells or particles clump together.

Allergen An antigenic substance that stimulates an immediate hypersensitivity reaction.

Antibody A protein produced by B lymphocytes in response to the presence of an antigen.

Antigen Molecules that are recognized specifically by receptors on cells of the adaptive immune system.

Antigen-presenting cells Cells capable of presenting antigenic material to cells of the adaptive immune system.

Antineutrophil cytoplasmic antibody (ANCA) A type of autoantibody directed against proteinase-3 (cANCA) or against myeloperoxidase (pANCA).

Apoptosis Programmed cell death.

Atopy Possessing a genetic predisposition to allergy.

Autoimmunity Occurs when the body's own defences are targeted against normal body components.

Cell-mediated immunity Immune response mediated by T lymphocytes, macrophages and natural killer (NK) cells to eliminate intracellular pathogens.

Chemotaxis The movement of cells in response to chemicals, often to a site of infection.

Collectins A family of pattern-recognition molecules, present in solution, that stimulate the innate immune system in response to a pathogen.

Complement A series of enzymatic reactions stimulated by the presence of a pathogen.

Cytokine Intercellular molecules used to transmit messages from one cell to another.

Degranulation The release of the preformed secretory granule contents by fusion with the plasma membrane.

Ecchymoses (bruises) Diffuse flat haemorrhages under the skin.

Erythropoietin A hormone, secreted by the kidney, that regulates erythropoiesis.

Essential thrombocythaemia A type of blood cancer that results from the uncontrolled proliferation of megakaryocytes causing high platelets.

Haematocrit The relative volume of erythrocytes in the blood.

Haematoma Distinct local swelling caused by loss of blood into a muscle or subcutaneous tissue.

Haemoglobinopathies Abnormalities of haemoglobin due to either abnormalities of the haemoglobin structure or from reduced synthesis of normal haemoglobin.

Haemolysis Accelerated destruction of the red blood cells reduces their lifespan and therefore results in anaemia.

Haemorrhage Loss of circulating blood.

Haptens Small molecules that need to be bound to a large carrier molecule in order to become immunogenic.

Human leucocyte antigen (HLA) The human form of major histocompatibility complex (MHC): cell surface proteins that present antigen.

Humoral immunity Immune response mediated by antibodies targeting extracellular antigens.

Hypersensitivity The inappropriate response of the immune system to an antigen.

Immunity A state of relative resistance to a disease.

Immunoglobulin (Ig) A protein substance secreted from plasma cells in response to infection.

Immunoglobulin domain An amino acid sequence, common to many proteins that are involved in pathogen recognition.

Inflammation Localized response to tissue damage characterized by redness, swelling, pain, oedema and increased white cell count.

Innate immune system Produces a nonspecific response to an infection or disease.

Interferon A cytokine that is targeted against viruses and intracellular bacteria.

Left shift Phenomenon where observed increased proportion of immature neutrophils (including early progenitors) within the peripheral blood.

Leucocytosis Increased total white cell count (i.e., $>11 \times 10^9$/L).

Leucopenia Total white cell count is less than 4×10^9/L.

Major histocompatibility complex (MHC) A cluster of genes encoding for cell surface receptors that present antigen on the surface of cells.

Monoclonal antibody Identical immunoglobulin that has been synthetically produced to target a specific antigen for therapeutic or diagnostic purposes.

Myelodysplasia Rare blood cancer due to a genetic mutation in the myeloid progenitors within the bone marrow. This causes inadequate production of blood cells.

Myeloproliferative neoplasms These are a group of cancers that result from the uncontrolled proliferation of one type of blood cell within the bone marrow.

Opsonin A substance that binds to a molecule to enhance its uptake by a phagocyte.

Packed cell volume (PCV) A measure of the proportion of blood occupied by red blood cells.

Passive immunity The passage of immunity from one individual to another.

Pathogen An organism that causes disease.

Pattern recognition molecules Are present either in solution or on the surface of cells and are capable of recognizing molecules characteristic of infection.

Petechiae Punctate haemorrhages <2 mm in diameter, usually clustered.

Polycythaemia vera A type of blood cancer which results from the uncontrolled proliferation of erythroid cells causing high haemoglobin.

Polymorphism Slight differences in the genetic material of individuals within a population.

Purpura Any condition with bleeding into the skin or mucous membrane.

Right shift Leucocytes persist longer than normal in the peripheral blood with 'hypermaturity'.

Sepsis Immune dysregulation caused by infection, potentially resulting in organ failure and death.

Thymus A mediastinal organ in which T cells develop.

Tolerance The ability of the immune system to ignore molecules that it has the capacity to attack.

Toll-like receptor A family of pattern recognition molecules on the cell surfaces that stimulate the innate immune system in response to a pathogen.

Urticaria Also called hives or nettle rash, characterized by an area of red inflammation and raised white bumps.

Vaccine A suspension of antigenic material injected to produce immunity against infection and disease.

Vertical transmission Transmission of an infection from mother to foetus.

Index

Note: Page numbers followed by *f* indicate figures, *t* indicate tables and *b* indicate boxes.

239